The Cytotoxics Handbook

Third Edition

Edited for
The Cytotoxics Services Working Group

by

Michael Allwood
BPharm, PhD, MRPharmS, Director, Pharmacy Academic Practice Unit,
School of Health and Community Studies, University of Derby, Derby

Andrew Stanley
BSc, MSc, MRPharmS, Director of Oncology Pharmacy,
St Chads Unit, City Hospital, Birmingham

and

Patricia Wright
BPharm, MPhil, MRPharmS, Chief Pharmacist,
West Middlesex University Hospital, Isleworth, Middlesex

RADCLIFFE MEDICAL PRESS
OXFORD AND NEW YORK

Radcliffe Medical Press Ltd
18 Marcham Road, Abingdon, Oxon OX14 1AA, UK

Radcliffe Medical Press, Inc.
141 Fifth Avenue, New York, NY 10010, USA

First edition 1990
Second edition 1993
Third edition 1997

British Library Cataloguing in Publication Data

A catalogue record for this book is available from the British Library.

ISBN 1 85775 141 8

Library of Congress Cataloging-in-Publication Data is available.

Typeset by Advance Typesetting Ltd, Oxon
Printed and bound by Redwood Books, Trowbridge, Wilts

Contents

The past 30 years have witnessed impressive changes in the drug treatment of cancer.

A better understanding of the nature of neoplastic disease has led to the development of cancer chemotherapeutic drugs, encompassing a wide spectrum of chemical compounds, which kill or impair susceptible tumour cells by blocking a drug-sensitive biochemical or metabolic pathway. The ability to use a number of agents in combination has improved clinical outcome in a variety of conditions and increasingly complex regimens continue to be developed.

However, cytotoxic therapy has its limitations: poor selectivity between neoplastic and normal cells, especially in the bone marrow and reproductive organs, can produce severe side-effects; many of the agents are carcinogens and mutagens and have been implicated in causing secondary neoplasms in patients being treated for cancer and most agents cause local damage to skin and mucous membranes due to their irritant, vesicant or allergenic action.

The obvious toxicity of these drugs has led to concern over their possible hazard to health care workers who prepare and administer the drugs and care for patients during treatment. In response to a number of reports indicating skin absorption and droplet inhalation of cytotoxics prepared in uncontrolled environments, guidelines for the safe handling of antineoplastic drugs have been drawn up by a number of countries. All make the same basic recommendations: controlled handling procedures; a high level of staff training and, where practicable, centralized reconstitution of IV cytotoxics in pharmacy departments with suitable controlled working areas.

The development of centralized pharmacy cytotoxic services in many countries has occurred in a non-uniform manner depending on local requirements, legislation, the availability of funding and existing service commitments. The diversity of services, both within some countries and between countries, is still significant although a huge amount of progress has been made in the last five years. Where services have been established, much time has been spent researching the literature for information on drug stability, designing documentation, establishing training programmes and ensuring that facilities comply with health and safety requirements. That services have been established is commendable considering the general lack of information on the safe handling and stability of IV cytotoxics and the divergent and conflicting views of much published work.

In response to the obvious need for more practical information on the procedures involved in setting up and running such units, a group comprising pharmacists and technicians in the UK met for informal, 'round table' discussions during the winter of 1987–88. All members had a substantial interest and expertise in cancer chemotherapy and the development of pharmacy-based hospital cytotoxic services and represented hospital pharmacy, pharmaceutical industry and academic interests. Early in the discussions, it was agreed that the Cytotoxic Services Working Group would produce, as quickly as possible, a manual on how to set up and operate pharmacy-based cytotoxic services, with specific detail on equipment, facilities, health and safety, documentation and training; and a compendium of cytotoxic drugs detailing their pharmaceutical properties, reconstitution details and stability in secondary packaging systems based on an informed review of the literature. This in-house edition was printed in late 1988.

An extensively updated and expanded, first complete edition was published in 1990. In this, the manual and compendium were combined into a single handbook designed primarily for use by pharmacists wishing to establish or update centralized cytotoxic services, but also aimed at other health care workers in this specialty.

The second edition, further updated, was geared towards a more international readership. Contributions from the US and Europe were included. Much superfluous and overlapping information was removed to aid information retrieval and all information pertaining to stability was added to individual drug monographs.

In this third edition the information given is representative of the current state-of-the-art cytotoxic reconstitution services and reflects international recommendations and the contributors' own experience. New material has been added and several chapters have been extensively revised.

The compendium of monographs on injectable cytotoxic drugs has, as in previous editions, been prepared for specific use by those hospital pharmacists and experienced pharmacy technicians who have responsibility for the provision of reconstituted and ready-to-administer cytotoxic drugs. Information on stability refers to preparation in controlled environments, where the sterility of the final product can be assured. The object of each monograph is to provide the basic information relevant to the preparation; stability during storage in the primary container; stability in secondary packaging systems; administration and disposal of the drug. Use of the monographs should obviate the need for extensive literature searching and interpretation of data. The author of each monograph is named and can be consulted on specific queries.

Interferon, interleukins and granulocyte-stimulating factors are now included in the handbook for completeness.

The section on investigational agents has been updated. However, readers are referred to the National Cancer Institute book of *Investigational Drugs* (available from The Pharmaceutical Resources Branch, NCI, Executive Plaza North, Suite 818, Bethesda, Maryland 20892, USA) and specialist oncology centres for further information.

Michael Allwood
Andrew Stanley
Patricia Wright
August 1996

Contributors

Michael Allwood
Director
Pharmacy Academic Practice Unit
University of Derby
Mickleover
Derby
DE3 5GX

Yaacov Cass
Regional Pharmaceutical Officer
Ministry of Health
PO Box 12052
Jerusalem
Israel
91120

Lynnette Ferguson
Director, Centre for Mutagen testing
Cancer Research Laboratory
Faculty of Medicine and Health Sciences
University of Auckland
Private Bag 92019
Auckland
New Zealand

Jeff Koundakjian
Pharmaceutical Services Manager
Clatterbridge Hospital
Bebington
Wirral
L63 4JY

Gerard Lee
Director of Quality Control
Pharmacy Practice Unit
70 Pembroke Place
Liverpool
L69 3GF

Tony Moore
Principal Pharmacist
Pharmacy Department
Royal Hallamshire Hospital
Glossop Road
Sheffield
S10 2JF

Richard Needle
Principal Pharmacist
Pharmacy Support Unit
Colchester General Hospital
Turner Road
Colchester
CO4 5JL

Margaret Nicolson
Senior Clinical Pharmacist
Pharmacy Department
Christie Hospital
Wilmslow Road
Manchester
M20 9BX

Jonathan Oakes
Principal Pharmacist
Pharmacy Department
Countess of Chester Hospital
Chester
CH2 1UL

Tim Root
Chief Pharmacist
Pharmacy Department
The Royal Marsden Hospital
Fulham Road
London
SW3 6JJ

Graham Sewell
Research and Technical Services Manager
Department of Pharmacy
Derriford Hospital
Plymouth
PL6 8DH

Robert Shaw
Director
Academic Pharmacy Practice Research Centre
The Queen's Building
University of East Anglia
Norwich
NR4 7TJ

Andrew Stanley
Director of Oncology Pharmacy
St Chads Unit
City Hospital
Dudley Road
Birmingham
B18 7QH

Helen Streeter
Staff Pharmacist
Pharmacy Department
University Hospital of Wales
Heath Park
Cardiff
CF4 4XW

Max Summerhayes
Principal Pharmacist
Pharmacy Department
Guy's Hospital
St Thomas Street
London
SE1 9RT

Jayne Wood
Clinical Pharmacy Services Manager
Pharmacy Department
Hope Hospital
Salford
M6 8HD

Patricia Wright
Chief Pharmacist
Pharmacy Department
West Middlesex University Hospital
Twickenham Road
Isleworth
Middlesex
TW7 6AF

PART ONE: Cytotoxic Services

Introduction to cytotoxic services

The introduction and use of new drugs over the past decade represents a major advance in the treatment of cancer. Because of the nature and presentation of these compounds, different techniques of reconstitution and administration have been developed. The reconstitution of cytotoxic chemotherapy in a safe and effective manner is an essential component in the treatment of patients suffering from cancer. The drugs must be prepared in a way that assures the quality of the product and also protects the operator and the working environment.

After a series of incidents in 1974, a working party under the chairmanship of Alistair Breckenridge examined all aspects of aseptic dispensing. The report from this working party (HC(76)9)[1] concludes that the addition of drugs to intravenous infusion fluid is an aseptic pharmaceutical procedure, which ideally should be carried out in appropriate environmental conditions under the direct control of a pharmacist.

IS THERE A NEED FOR A CYTOTOXIC RECONSTITUTION SERVICE?

There are a number of areas to be studied in order to justify to doctors, nurses, managers and pharmacy staff the introduction of such a service. Before proceeding, the following questions should be answered to establish need.

1 Range of current service and workload

▼ What is the workload?
  It will be necessary to establish:
    the type of preparations used
    the number of individual doses administered annually
    the stability of the preparations administered
    who the prescriber is
    who prepares the reconstitution and who administers the drug (is it the same person?)
    how long it takes to reconstitute the preparation
    if there is adequate time allowed for documentation
    the preferred method of administration.
▼ Competence issues
  Are doctors and nurses adequately trained to prepare cytotoxic drugs?
▼ Health and safety
  Are existing arrangements satisfactory and appropriate for patient safety and operator protection?

▼ Risk management
Is there a risk management approach to drug ordering, preparation and delivery?

▼ Cost
What is the current expenditure in terms of drugs, equipment, facilities and staff?
Are there sufficient amounts of nursing and medical time which could be better utilized providing direct patient care?
Can the value of some of the time saved be attached to the pharmacy budget?
Is drug wastage a significant financial issue (e.g. paediatrics)?
Will the provision of a pharmacy-led service reduce or increase expenditure?

▼ Quality issues
Are preparation areas suitable?
Are there checks for drug compatibility?
What is the administration time v. the prescribed time?
Are there interruptions in preparation or administration?
Are medication errors documented?
Are vial/ampoule contents stored and re-used?
Are administration methods appropriate?
Is duration of the injection appropriate?

2 Problems with the current service

▼ Identify existing problems and their importance.

3 Potential benefits of a reconstitution service

▼ Standardization of drug concentration and administration route and method.
▼ Consequent reduction in errors of administration.
▼ Drug administration at the correct time and rate.
▼ Improved monitoring and control of health and safety issues.
▼ Comprehensive documentation.
▼ Increased confidence in drug stability and sterility.

4 Potential disadvantages of a reconstitution service

▼ Capital expenditure.
▼ Communication of requirements to colleagues.
▼ Distribution and storage of drugs.
▼ Increase in staff.
▼ Out of hours service.
▼ Increase in expenditure if commercial services are employed.

5 Running a pilot scheme

A pilot scheme can give the opportunity to test proposed procedures, gain valuable feedback from staff and to collect 'local' data.

A reconstitution service is a major development and thorough planning and research should be completed before such a service is introduced. Additional resources may well be required, or existing resources may need to be redeployed.

An awareness of strategic plans is vital to ensure an appropriate balance of commitments to resources is achieved.

A multidisciplinary working party should be appointed. Clear objectives should be set, which are then backed up by information gathered in the pilot, which will evaluate whether the introduction of a reconstitution service is appropriate.

SETTING UP A WORKING PARTY

1 Membership

Membership of the working party should include:

Clinicians	Medical oncologists
	Clinical oncologists
	Haematologists
Nurses	Specialists
	Nurse managers
	Tutors
	Community/homecare
Pharmacy staff	Pharmacists (including a quality control pharmacist)
	Technicians
Management	General manager or representative
	Risk manager, or member of risk management team
Occupational health	Senior representative

2 Objectives

▼ To establish and co-ordinate a pilot study in accordance with previously agreed aims and objectives.
▼ To assess the capital and revenue implications of a service and allocate resources as appropriate.
▼ To decide what type and level of service is required.
▼ To monitor the performance of the service.
▼ To formulate policy and to provide advice on relevant issues.

WHAT TYPE OF SERVICE IS REQUIRED?

When deciding on the type of service to be provided, certain areas should be considered.

1 Workload

The volume of work, measured as individual patient doses per annum, and annual expenditure on cytotoxic chemotherapy are key considerations.

2 Range and presentation of doses

The range and pattern of cytotoxic prescribing needs to be determined. The key areas to consider are:

▼ range of cytotoxics used
▼ stability in solution of the drugs used
▼ methods of administration (e.g. bolus injections, infusions and continuous infusions)
▼ whether treatment regimens are established
▼ whether there is any standardization of doses.

3 Level of service

▼ Determine a level of service pharmacy can provide.
▼ Can a total service be provided during normal working hours, or does a 24 hour service need to be established?
▼ Will 'on-call' arrangements be required?

Skill level on wards will need to be addressed as there may be a loss of skills due to the reduction or disappearance of medical or nursing preparation.

4 Quality assurance and sterility assurance

Quality assurance procedures should be agreed, documented and adhered to. In order to achieve high levels of sterility assurance, procedures should include rigorous standards for equipment maintenance, operator training and environmental monitoring.

5 Facilities

Utilize existing facilities if available. If these are not available, convert facilities and purchase appropriate equipment.

6 Health and safety needs

Local and national guidelines must be adhered to (*see* Chapter 3, Health and safety).

7 Risk management

Modern risk management methods should be employed.

8 Funding

Resources should be identified.

▼ Can potential savings on medical and nursing time, or savings on drug expenditure be utilized?
▼ Is the hospital prepared to pay for increased safety, quality and proactive risk management?

9 Personnel

Are there staff available and what is their level of expertise? Are funds available for recruitment and training?

10 Logistics

Points for consideration are:

▼ the physical geography of the site
▼ how many sites are being serviced
▼ communication and transport systems
▼ consultants' prescribing habits
▼ recovery and re-use
▼ distribution
▼ weekends
▼ costing arrangements
▼ location of inpatients and outpatients in relation to pharmacy.

11 Clinical commitment

The level of clinical involvement by pharmacy can be enhanced by providing a service. However, the level of involvement with patient care should not detract from the efficiency of the service and will depend on the attitudes of local personnel and their managers.

SERVICE OPTIONS

A list of the possible service options with the advantages and disadvantages of each follows.

1 Pharmacy controlled centralized unit

Advantages	Disadvantages
Existing facilities.	Potential large capital cost.
High sterility/stability assurance.	Extended lines of communication between pharmacy/nurse/doctor.
Cost/efficiency savings on a high workload.	Problems of distribution to clinical areas and off-site locations.
Planned workload.	Slower reaction/lead times.
Suitably trained/skilled staff.	Out of hours service may not be provided.
High level of operator/product protection.	Potential long-term pharmacy staff exposure.
Easier supervision.	High level of long-term pharmacy commitment.
Standardization of presentation of doses.	Loss of expertise at ward level.
Comprehensive documentation.	

2 Pharmacy controlled satellite unit

Advantages

Workload centralized in designated hospital areas.

Short lines of communication.
Reduced distribution problems.
Increased interprofessional contact.
Ability to respond more quickly to requests.
Cost/efficiency savings on high workload.
High sterility/stability assurance.

Easier to provide an extended hours service.
Potential for access by non-pharmacy staff out of hours (working to strict pharmacy procedures).
High level of operator/product protection.

Disadvantages

Deployment of staff away from pharmacy, with potential for increased staff requirements and labour costs.
Increased stock holdings.
Potential for greater wastage.
Fragmentation of pharmacy service.
Negotiating space within another department.
May also be required to supply oral medication and adjuvant therapy.
Potential long-term pharmacy staff exposure.

3 Ward/clinic-based in an uncontrolled environment (nurse/doctor operated)

Advantages

Status quo

Disadvantages

Health and safety aspects/operator protection.
No product protection.
High level of wastage.
High stock holdings.
Limited pharmacy control.
No record of preparation process; therefore no recall traceability.
Possibility of untrained staff preparing doses.

4 Ward/clinic-based in a controlled environment (nurse/doctor operated)

Advantages	*Disadvantages*
Reduced pharmacy labour costs.	High nursing and medical staff turnover, leading to increased training requirements.
Rapid response, 24 hour service.	Less time for direct patient care.
Short lines of communication.	Decreased assurance of sterility/stability.
No distribution or delivery problems.	Higher level of wastage.
	Limited pharmacy control.
	No record of preparation process; therefore no recall traceability.
	Increased stock holdings.
	Difficult to maintain high standard of quality assurance.
	Pharmacy activity undertaken by non-pharmacy staff.
	Management responsibilities and level of control poorly defined.
	Formal accreditation/validation system would be required, which would lead to increased quality assurance costs.

5 Commercial service

Advantages	*Disadvantages*
No additional capital or staff costs (full off-site service).	Potential for increased revenue expenditure.
Provision of a full range of drugs in a ready-to-use form.	
Health and safety aspects of a local reconstitution eliminated.	Communication and supply logistics (if service is off-site).
Standardization of presentation of doses.	Further distribution of drugs from a central delivery point to the ward/clinic.
Planned workload.	
Comprehensive documentation.	
Minimal stock holdings.	
Reduced wastage.	
High sterility/stability assurance.	

SERVICE OPERATION

The following operational areas need to be considered in the cytotoxic reconstitution service. For further information see the chapters listed in brackets.

▼ Facilities and equipment (Chapter 2).
▼ Health and safety issues (Chapter 3).

▼ Documentation (Chapter 4).
▼ Training (Chapter 5).

Points to consider for the service operation of a cytotoxic reconstitution service are:

1 Receipt of requests

▼ Is the request direct from the prescriber or via the nurse? Consider documentation.
▼ Consider transmission of request (paper, computer prescribing, hospital information systemic mail (e-mail), telephone or FAX).

2 Processing the request

▼ Ensure that sufficient information is provided for checking doses, method of administration and computer input.
▼ Consider computerization but ensure regular backups or manual backup.

3 Documentation

▼ Design of worksheets and labels.
▼ Patient and drug records.
▼ Quality assurance procedures and records.
▼ Data for workload statistics.
▼ Financial and budgetary information.
▼ Personnel, training and maintenance records.
▼ Procedures for the creation and maintenance of documents.
▼ Procedures for documents must be numbered and indexed.
▼ Consider computerization.

4 Reconstitution

▼ Selection of equipment – isolator, laminar airflow cabinet (LFC) and cleanroom.
▼ Method of equipment use.
▼ Changing procedures.
▼ Transfer of preparation in and out of cleanroom, LFC or isolator.
▼ Checks during preparation.

5 Labelling and checking

▼ Inspection of product.
▼ Labelling.
▼ Final check.
▼ Release.

6 Distribution and storage

▼ Packaging, including protective outer wrap.
▼ Transport and role of porters, drivers, nurses and reconstitution unit staff.
▼ Unit storage.
▼ Ward storage.
▼ Recovery and re-use.

7 Cleaning

▼ Cleaning and disinfection of cleanroom, LFC or isolator.
▼ Spillage and decontamination.

8 Quality assurance

▼ Documentation e.g. worksheets, procedures.
▼ Validation of operators and environments.
▼ Monitoring of operators, environment, containers and product.
▼ Temperature control of storage facilities.
▼ End-product testing (chemical and sterility).

9 Training

▼ Induction.
▼ Broth tests.
▼ Use of equipment and computers.
▼ Testing of knowledge and technique.
▼ Continuous training and validation schedules.

10 Stock control

▼ Ordering, stock control and stock rotation.
▼ Receipt and storage.
▼ Expiry dates and batch number records.

11 Computers

▼ Cytotoxic prescribing and reconstitution programs.
▼ Interface with hospital/finance/pharmacy/prescribing systems.
▼ Validation.

REFERENCE

1 DHSS (1976) *Report of the working party on the addition of drugs to intravenous fluids, chaired by A Breckenridge.* DHSS Health Circular HC(76)9. HMSO, London.

FURTHER READING

The following are important international documents.

American Society of Hospital Pharmacists (1992) ASHP Technical Assistance Bulletin on Handling Cytotoxic and Hazardous Drugs. In *AHFS Drug Information.* ASHP, Bethesda, US, pp. 610–18.

Canadian Society of Hospital Pharmacists (1993) *CSHP Guidelines for the Handling and Disposal of Hazardous Pharmaceuticals.* CSHP, Ottawa, Canada.

Society of Hospital Pharmacists of Australia (1990) *SHPA Guidelines for the Safe Handling of Cytotoxic Drugs in Pharmacy Departments.* SHPA, Melbourne, Australia.

2

Facilities

INTRODUCTION

The risks associated with handling and administering cytotoxic drugs have resulted in the widespread use of safety cabinets for the preparation and dispensing of these products. Such cabinets must achieve a balance between operator and product protection in order to provide adequate levels of safety for both the patient and the staff preparing and administering the drug. There are two broad options for facilities and equipment that can be used for the preparation of sterile cytotoxic doses. These are:

▼ conventional cleanroom with a vertical laminar flow cabinet (VLFC)
▼ isolators in a suitable environment.

Vertical laminar flow cabinets with similar operating characteristics to Class II microbiological safety cabinets have limitations which have led to an increased use of isolators. Isolators have an advantage over cleanrooms in that they do not require an expensive air handling plant, nor do they need costly and time-consuming gowning procedures.

The selection of equipment and the working environment is dependent upon a number of factors:

▼ expected workload
▼ existing facilities and commitments
▼ resources available (capital/revenue, personnel etc.).

1 Vertical laminar flow cabinets

1.1 Standards

There are no nationally agreed standards in the UK for vertical laminar flow drug safety cabinets. The British Standard for Microbiological Safety Cabinets, BS 5726, 1992[1] makes reference to vertical laminar flow protection cabinets, but this standard is not readily applicable to hazardous drugs because:

▼ bacteria have a defined mass or bulk and are of known particle size, whereas cytotoxic contaminants are of variable size and may be in a solid, liquid or gaseous state
▼ for the materials handled in microbiological safety cabinets, operator protection is more critical than product protection.

The Australian Standard, AS 2567, 1982[2] has been written to apply only to cytotoxic cabinets. Some of the features of this standard are:

▼ all potentially contaminated zones are under negative pressure

▼ all filter seals which may come into contact with potentially hazardous material are under negative pressure with respect to the uncontaminated zones
▼ stainless steel construction
▼ incorporation of carbon exhaust filter.

In Germany a 'cytostatic work station' is defined in a document describing principles of operation and test procedures, GS-GES-04, published by the Professional Association of Health Service and Welfare Care[3] (GS DIN 12590). Filters are tested to DIN standard 24184 and are of 99.99% efficiency. These work stations are, in essence, compact laminar downflow cabinets with a front visor having two apertures for the worker to access the work zone. Whilst manufacturers vary the machine dimensions and number of filters used, the principles and tests in GS-GES-04 are common to all. In the US, the American Society of Hospital Pharmacists has produced guidelines on cytotoxic drug handling.[4] Laminar downflow safety cabinets that comply with US National Sanitation Foundation Standards[5] are described.

1.2 Operating principles

A vertical downflow of laminar-flow air, filtered through a HEPA filter (efficiency 99.997% in UK, 99.990% in Germany), passes over the work surface. The air then passes through vents at the front and back of the cabinet, and is recirculated. Depending on the manufacturer there may be one or more filters in the recirculation and exhaust air flows. Approximately 30% of the recirculated air is exhausted from the cabinet and, to compensate for this, air is drawn in through the front opening. This creates a negative pressure within the cabinet. The balance between the cabinet downflow and the air drawn in at the front of the cabinet produces an air curtain, which is the basis of the operator and product protection properties of the cabinet. The air exhausted from the cabinet may be recirculated into the room or ducted to the outside.

1.3 Cabinet details

Cytomat (Medical Air Technology Ltd)

Cabinet dimensions: ($w \times d \times h$ (mm)) $1200 \times 695 \times 2135$

Tray area: ($w \times d$ (mm)) 1075×450

Filters: The Cytomat is available in two formats. The fixed format has a downflow HEPA filter, 1100 mm × 500 mm × 150 mm and an exhaust HEPA filter, 1000 mm × 450 mm × 300 mm. The movable format has an additional in-line exhaust HEPA filter, 825 mm × 375 mm × 75 mm. Filters are sealed on both the upstream and downstream faces.

Design characteristics: The manufacturer states that this machine is built to AS 2567,[2] but it does not fully comply as the working chamber tank is not entirely of stainless steel construction. The air flow through the cabinet is generated by a fan in the terminal exhaust duct. Therefore the cabinet and exhaust system will be under negative pressure. The ducting is fitted with anti-blowback flaps. The filter case forms the walls of the air ducts; so air cannot bypass the filter. The exhaust duct can be fitted with either a carbon, or an HEPA, exhaust filter.

Figure 2.1 shows the airflow pattern for the total dumping (exhaust) and recirculating versions of this cabinet.

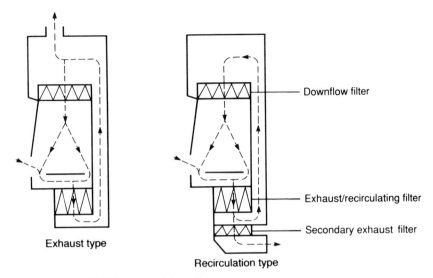

Figure 2.1: *MAT Cytomat airflow diagram*

Downflow filter

Exhaust/recirculating filter

Secondary exhaust filter

Exhaust type

Recirculation type

Cytogard (Gelman Hawkseley Ltd)

Cabinet dimensions: $(w \times d \times h \text{ (mm)})$

model CG 900 – $1180 \times 768 \times 2310$
model CG 120 – $1340 \times 770 \times 2310$
model CH 180 – $1950 \times 770 \times 2310$

Tray area: (CG 900) $(w \times d \text{ (mm)})$ 875×590

Filters: Filters are Gelman microseal 7531 series (dimensions not stated). One downflow HEPA filter and one exhaust HEPA filter is fitted, plus an activated carbon bed in the exhaust. The exhaust filter is sealed on the upstream face.

Design characteristics: This cabinet complies with AS 2567.[2] The cabinets are bulkier and taller than the Cytomat. They have no normal provision for exhaust ducting, but this can be done. Manometers are optional and do not allow measurement downstream of the main filter.

Figure 2.2 shows the airflow pattern for this type of cabinet.

1.4 General comments on VLFCs

A carbon exhaust filter is not a true filter but a gas adsorption cell that can be subject to channelling. It can release carbon particles into the room and it is not possible to test the adsorption capacity non-destructively. There seems little need for a carbon exhaust filter, particularly if the air exhaust is ducted to the outside.

Where cabinets are sited in aseptic suites, product protection is simplified because the cabinet itself is in an EC GMP Grade B environment.[6] If situated in a dispensary or on a ward, local air turbulence will be a more critical determining factor of operator and product protection than the cabinet's design. Since isolators are now commonly available, it is recommended that VLFCs are not sited in an unclassified environment. Isolators would be the cabinets of choice in such areas.

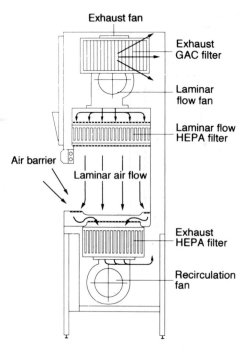

Figure 2.2: *Gelman, Cytogard airflow diagram*

UK, US, Australian and German cabinets are not strictly comparable and it is necessary to ensure that equipment complies with regulatory requirements in the country of use.

2 Isolators

2.1 Standards

Within the UK there is now a guidance document on isolators for pharmaceutical applications.[7] This refers to design principles and operational characteristics for negative pressure (type 2) isolators that can be used for handling cytotoxics. BS 5726[1] includes a reference to Class III containment, microbiological safety cabinets. The International Standards Organisation Committee ISO TC 209 is currently reviewing the standard for cleanrooms and clean air equipment to include isolators within a section on mini-environments.

2.2 Operating principles

Isolators are enclosed work stations supplied with filtered air which should meet EC GMP Class A[6] in the controlled work space. Operators use either glove ports, or a half-suit arrangement to access the working area. Materials are introduced through a transfer device. Isolators can be of a rigid or a flexible structure and their design can have a considerable impact upon their potential use and upon operating, monitoring and disinfection procedures.

Transfer devices include rigid boxes (filtered or unfiltered air supply), rapid transfer docking ports or another isolator which can be connected to the main working enclosure. Many different designs exist and are acceptable. The choice of device will depend upon the design of the isolator, the application for which it is to be used, and the external environment of the isolator.

2.3 Flexible film isolators

The dimensions and configurations of flexible isolators are variable as there are a large number of working, bank, transfer and sterilization chambers marketed. Companies will meet the design needs of the customer.

Design characteristics: Flexible film isolators have an enclosure made entirely of flexible PVC film supported on a chrome or stainless steel framework. Sizes can vary and two, three or four glove port models, half-suit or double half-suit designs are available. Inlet and outlet air is HEPA filtered (99.997% efficiency in UK models) and the air supply can be designed so that the working environment is under positive or negative pressure. The air supply is not necessarily laminar flow and normally provides the controlled work space with no fewer than 20 air changes per hour.

The half-suit system offers greater flexibility and all-round movement but appears at first to be claustrophobic. The suits are double layered and are fed with an air supply that both inflates and lifts the suit so that it does not press against the operator while providing a flow of air across the face and body. By their very nature, flexible isolators are more easily damaged and require care during use.

For cytotoxic reconstitution, isolators should be under negative pressure. Extra support frames are required for this and the relative pressures may cause ingress of contaminated air if the PVC canopy is pin-holed. Monitoring procedures must be capable, therefore, of detecting pin-hole leaks.

Flexible film isolators are available from a large number of cleanroom equipment manufacturers, to a wide range of specifications.

2.4 Rigid isolators

The walls of the cabinet are rigid with an enclosed workspace. The inlet air and outlet air supplies are HEPA filtered (99.997% efficiency in UK models) and the air can be turbulent or laminar flow. The front panel is typically clear plastic and may be fitted with up to four glove ports. Standard models available from UK manufacturers are listed below.

Amercare Limited:

A range of standard and bespoke negative pressure units is available including the following.

Compact isolator, code CIN 23PR: Consists of two modules; the transfer chamber and process isolator, which is fitted with three glove ports.

Cabinet dimensions: ($w \times d \times h$ (mm)) $1620 \times 600 \times 1950$

Workspace area: ($w \times d$ (mm)) 1200×600

Full compact isolator, code FCN 25PR: Consists of three modules; a type D transfer isolator, a process isolator and a type D transfer chamber. The transfer isolator is fitted with two glove ports and the process isolator is fitted with three.

Cabinet dimensions: ($w \times d \times h$ (mm)) $2420 \times 600 \times 1950$

Workspace area: ($w \times d$ (mm)) 1200×600

Compact throughflow isolator, code CTN 24PR: Consists of three modules; two type D transfer chambers and a process isolator, which is fitted with four glove ports.

Filters: Filters are cylindrical cartridge filters 244 mm in diameter × 305 mm in length.

Design characteristics: These isolators are rigid 4 mm thick stainless steel constructions. The inlet air supply is HEPA filtered (99.997% efficient). All enclosures are under negative pressure, air being drawn through the system into the controlled workspace through small bore distribution tubes, creating rapid turbulent flow. Air is either ducted to outside or units can be designed to recirculate air. Inner and outer door sets are fitted with timed interlocks and are pneumatically sealed.

Figure 2.3 shows the airflow pattern of a compact isolator with Class D transfer device.

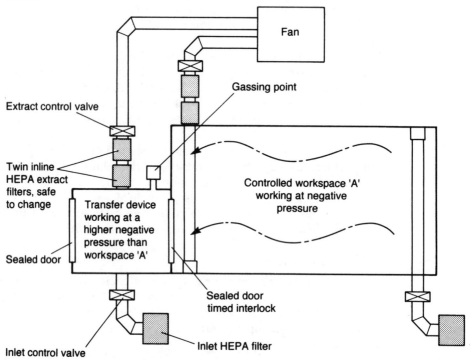

Figure 2.3: *Schematic diagram of Amercare compact isolator with Class E transfer device*

Envair UK Limited

Containair dispensing cabinet

Cabinet dimensions: (w × d × h (mm))
Two glove recirculating 2432 × 695 × 2430
Two glove ducted 2432 × 695 × 2280
Four glove recirculating 3030 × 695 × 2430
Four glove ducted 3030 × 695 × 2280.

Workspace area: (w × d (mm))
Two glove 1097 × 480
Four glove 1700 × 480.

Filters: Downflow HEPA (minipleat): Two glove – 1220 mm × 508 mm × 150 mm, four glove – 1828 mm × 508 mm × 150 mm
Main (primary exhaust) HEPA (minipleat): Two glove – 1130 mm × 456 mm × 66 mm, four glove – 860 mm × 456 mm × 124 mm (×2)
Secondary exhaust HEPA (minipleat): 590 mm × 420 mm × 66 mm
Hatch HEPAs: 460 mm × 320 mm × 66 mm
Prefilters: 600 mm × 180 mm × 25 mm.
The filters are sealed on the upstream and downstream faces.

Design characteristics: The Containair is a rigid, polyester-coated mild steel carcase with an electro-polished 316 stainless steel work surface. Two or four glove ports are fitted into the front viewing panel which is hydraulically assisted and may be lifted to allow the installation of large pieces of equipment. The cabinet is supplied with vertical laminar flow HEPA filtered air (99.997% efficient) and is fitted with dual exhaust HEPA filters. The air supply provides approximately 1000 air changes per hour in the two glove and 700 in the four glove unit.

Transfer devices constructed of polyester-coated stainless steel are fitted on the side panels of the cabinet and are independently flushed with HEPA filtered air, providing 4000 changes per hour.

Airflow patterns for controlled work zone and the transfer hatch of the Containair cabinet with a C2 type[7] transfer hatch are shown in Figure 2.4. A class D hatch is being developed.

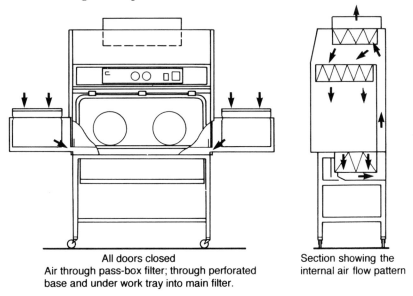

All doors closed	Section showing the
Air through pass-box filter; through perforated	internal air flow pattern
base and under work tray into main filter.	

Figure 2.4: *Envair Containair airflow diagram for CDC 'C', two glove isolator*

Medical Air Technology Limited (MAT)

Isomat 2

Cabinet dimensions: (*w* × *d* × *h* (mm)) Two glove 2400 × 630 × 2465, four glove 3200 × 630 × 2465.

Workspace area: (*w* × *d* (mm)) Two glove approximately 1200 × 600, four glove approximately 2000 × 600.

Filters: Downflow HEPA (minipleat) 1090 × 500 × 66
Exhaust HEPA (minipleat) 900 × 305 × 88.
The filters are sealed (gel-seal) on the upstream and downstream faces.

Design characteristics: The Isomat is a rigid powder-coated mild steel carcase with a stainless steel work chamber and work surface. The front viewing panel is hinged and may be opened to allow the installation of large pieces of equipment. The cabinet is available in recirculating or total exhaust versions, the recirculating version having a second exhaust HEPA filter in-line. The air supply to the controlled workspace provides 1800 air changes per hour.

The airflow to the controlled work zone and the transfer device is shown diagrammatically in Figure 2.5.

MDH Limited

Microflow isolators

The standard range of isolators that is available includes a two glove model with either one or two transfer chambers and a four glove model with two transfer chambers.

Cabinet dimensions: ($w \times d \times h$ (mm))
Two glove, single transfer chamber 1625 × 950 × 2065
Two glove, double transfer chamber 2050 × 950 × 2065
Four glove 2850 × 950 × 2065.

Workspace area: ($w \times d$ (mm)) Two glove 1100 × 550
Four glove 1900 × 550.

Filters: HEPA inlet and exhaust filters (99.997% efficient) fitted with a pre-filter sheet. Both filters are standard 305 mm² minipleat. Transfer hatches (lock chambers) are fitted with HEPA filters on inlet and exhaust.

Design characteristics: This is a computer controlled system where chamber working pressure is monitored and controlled. The chambers are of epoxy-coated mild steel. The work tray is stainless steel. Airflow is vertical laminar downflow. Airflow rate and chamber pressure are displayed digitally and high and low set pressure alarms are provided.

Filters are changed from within the isolator using a safe-change bagging technique. Power supplies can be fitted to the chamber. Sterilization and disinfection can be achieved with formaldehyde, Citanox® or by alcoholic surface treatment.

Bassaire Containments Limited

Bassaire high integrity isolator

Cabinet dimensions: ($w \times d \times h$ (mm))
Two glove 1600 × 775 × 200
Three glove 2000 × 775 × 2000
Four glove 2500 × 775 × 2000.

Workspace area: ($w \times d$ (mm))
Two glove 800 × 650
Three glove 1200 × 650
Four glove 1700 × 650.

Filters: Downflow HEPA: Two glove 525 mm × 457 mm × 66 mm
Three glove 915 mm × 457 mm × 66 mm
Four glove 1425 mm × 457 mm × 66 mm.

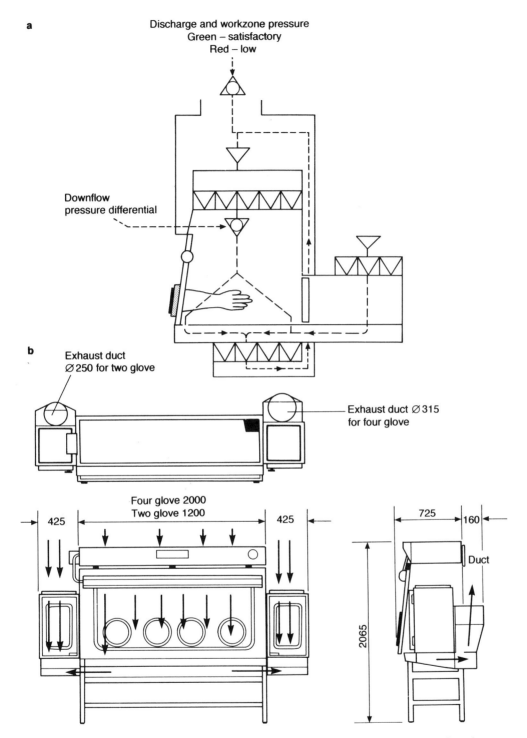

Figure 2.5: *MAT Isomat 2 airflow diagram (all dimensions are in mm, and are approximate)*

Design characteristics: The Bassaire isolator is a rigid cabinet constructed of 316 stainless steel and fitted with Class D hatches.[7] The front visor is bolted on and the hatches are fitted with vertical sliding doors. The cabinet is available in a recirculating or total exhaust version. The air supply to the controlled workspace provides between 1800–2000 air changes per hour.

A schematic diagram of the airflow to the controlled workspace and the transfer device of the total exhaust version is shown in Figure 2.6.

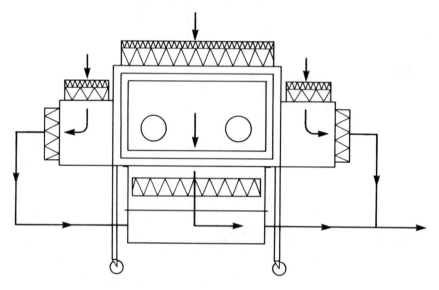

Figure 2.6: *Bassaire high integrity isolator airflow diagram*

2.5 General comments on isolators

Rigid isolators are relatively easy to clean and disinfect using hard-surface disinfectants. Since they may be used in an unclassified environment and will operate under negative pressure, high efficiency seals in all cabinets are essential.

In addition, units with non-laminar airflow may have dead spots within the EC GMP Grade A area.[6] Purging of contaminants from the cabinets is largely dependent on air turbulence created within the cabinet.

3 Sterilization and sanitation of internal surfaces

Gaseous sterilization is a practical means of sterilizing large, flexible-film isolators. The filtered output air is ducted to the outside above the roof of the building, or the exhaust air is passed through a suitable chemisorbant filter pack, which adds considerably to the cost.

It is possible to link two or more flexible isolators via the transfer ports. Components, containers and equipment can be surface-sterilized, by gaseous sterilization, in one isolator overnight then transferred the following day to the adjoining isolator prior to use.

Formaldehyde, peracetic acid and hydrogen peroxide vapour are the usual sterilants. Peracetic acid is most effective and easier to use but is the most toxic. Formaldehyde is absorbed by PVC and therefore time must be allowed for the gas to desorb from the canopy.

It is possible to validate sterilization cycles that use gaseous sterilants but there are many problems associated with this process and there is still little information on it in published literature.

Gaseous sterilization cannot be recommended for the surface sterilization of articles within isolators unless the user can fully validate the system with respect to gas desorption from packaging, closures, syringes, etc. There is also a risk of gas entry into drug or diluent containers if stress cracks are present or if the closure of individual containers is not guaranteed impervious to gas ingress.

Any sterilization process will be ineffective unless adequate cleaning has preceded it. Any spillages of nutrient solutions will provide ideal growth media for bacteria and also protect bacteria from the effects of sterilants.

In the UK COSHH regulations[8] require that a safe and effective means of gas desorption, removal and disposal must be included in any protocol for use of sterilization equipment.

Sanitization of small flexible film isolators by hard-surface disinfectants is not precluded but the effect of the alcoholic sprays on PVC film needs to be evaluated. Chlorhexidine-based alcoholic sprays should be used with caution, or not at all, as a film of chlorhexidine residue builds up on surfaces, potentially causing contamination of solutions.

For rigid isolators, surface sanitization with an alcoholic solution is the simplest and quickest option, but some manufacturers do not advocate the practice. However, direct questioning has revealed that the reservations expressed relate to long-term soaking in alcoholic solutions leading to crazing of some types of clear plastic. The routine use of alcohol solutions by swab or spray applications with subsequent rapid evaporation is not seen as problematic.

Sanitization is not a validated sterilization process and is not guaranteed to leave a surface free from viable microorganisms. Whilst alcohols are very effective against vegetative organisms they have no sporicidal activity.

4 Gauntlets and glove ports (*see also* Chapter 3)

All isolators, whether they be rigid, flexible film or half-suit isolators, are accessed via a glove port. These are glove/sleeve arrangements designed to maintain the aseptic environment within the isolator. Several types of gauntlets and glove/sleeve systems, made from various materials are available and careful selection will be necessary.

Gloves and gauntlets used with isolators should, as a minimum, comply with the limits for perforations specified in BS 4005: 1984, the British Standard for sterile latex gloves[9] or its equivalent International Standard. Because pin-holes are unavoidable, the integrity of the gloves and gauntlets should be tested frequently. Most manufacturers of isolators have available a simple, relatively inexpensive device for this purpose.

4.1 Gauntlets

These are one piece, full-arm-length gloves. They are available in a range of materials. Pin-holes do occur because manufacturers are not always aware of the need for stringent testing for perforations during manufacturing.

Gauntlets are usually changed on a weekly (or longer) basis due to the high cost, resulting in a potential risk of drug penetration and poor general hygiene, as a number of operators will use the same gloves. For these reasons, double-gloving is generally used. However, as gauntlets do not fit well, particularly under conditions of negative pressure, operator sensitivity will be reduced. They are normally thicker than surgeons' latex gloves, which may offset the risk of drug penetration to a degree. They are not normally available pre-sterilized.

4.2 Glove/sleeve systems

These are multi-component systems consisting generally of a replaceable sleeve piece, a connecting cuff piece and the glove. The sleeve should be mechanically strong enough to remain in position without deterioration for a number of weeks. It should not be too rigid to allow comfortable working and should be resistant to chemical attack. The cuff piece should allow an easy, safe, aseptic glove change-over.

A glove/sleeve system allows gloves of an appropriate specification, particularly with respect to perforations and pin-holes, to be used. It will, if correctly designed, allow the individual operator to fit and change gloves of correct size as frequently as required and enable the glove material to be altered without jeopardy to the isolator environment. Risk of drug penetration can be minimized in this way and general hygiene is improved as each operator can fit a fresh sterile pair of gloves each time the equipment is used.

5 Monitoring

Aseptic preparation facilities in hospitals enable the preparation of injections in controlled environments with greater assurance of sterility. The British Pharmacopoeia currently recommends that unpreserved injections, prepared aseptically from sterile ingredients, should have a 24 hour shelf-life. Furthermore, the product licences of lyophilized injections often restrict their shelf-lives to 24 hours after reconstitution. The overriding reason for the 24 hour shelf-life is the risk of microbial contamination of the product during preparation or reconstitution. However, in centralized cytotoxic dispensing facilities, where a licensed sterile product is used for the preparation of sterile medication and is prepared under conditions of good manufacturing/dispensing practice in suitably monitored and audited premises, then the shelf-life may be extended beyond 24 hours, provided the microbiological integrity of the process has been validated and the physicochemical stability of the product justifies it.

It is essential, therefore, that a monitoring programme is implemented to:

▼ confirm that aseptic dispensing facilities continuously meet performance requirements
▼ indicate and identify system breakdown before product sterility is affected.

Such a programme will include physical tests of the cabinets and isolators and the surrounding environment, in addition to active and passive microbial sampling of the controlled environment.

Units should determine their optimum programme for monitoring of facilities. The frequency of testing will be a function of the design of the facility and will be dependent on the workload and frequency of service use. Data obtained during commissioning studies will help in deciding the frequency of monitoring. Each unit should agree a programme of daily, weekly, monthly, quarterly and annual testing, which should be implemented and all results documented. Each of these programmes should be a combination of the following tests:

5.1 Physical tests

▼ pressure differentials

▼ alarm checks
▼ integrity tests
▼ airflow
▼ particle counts
▼ installation leak test
▼ operator protection test.

5.2 Microbiological tests

▼ settle plates
▼ surface swabs
▼ airborne viable counts
▼ finger dab plates.

For some tests, e.g. pressure differentials, daily data will be expected. Tests such as the installation leak test need only be undertaken annually.

Testing of VLFCs is similar to that for horizontal LFCs, but in addition to particle counts and filter challenge tests, operator protection factors should be measured regularly. Particle counts and filter challenge tests are equally applicable to isolators. Furthermore, there is a need to monitor for pin-holes and defects in gloves, and in the canopies of flexible isolators, so regular leak tests are also required. Suggested limits for the monitoring results are given in Table 2.1. These limits are based on those in the EC GMP guide,[6] in BS 5295[10] and on those in the Parenteral Society's technical monograph on environmental microbiological contamination in controlled environments.[11] Because of imprecision of the methods, expected low levels of contamination and the natural variability of the levels, the microbiological data require most careful analysis. It is recommended that the levels given in Table 2.1 are regarded as target levels. Exceeding target levels on isolated occasions may not require more action than examination of control systems. However, the frequency of exceeding the limit should be examined and should be low. If the frequency is high or shows an upward trend, then action should be taken.

6 Summary

Isolators offer significant advantages over cleanrooms for small-scale aseptic operations. They can be housed in a socially clean room and a minimum of gowning is required. Revenue and maintenance costs are substantially less than conventional cleanrooms. Rigid isolators are generally fairly compact and not designed for industrial-scale use. However, these cabinets are very suitable for small-scale operations and particularly for one-off aseptic dispensing operations, since sanitization is quick and easy and materials can be introduced very simply.

Flexible isolators address the problem of space but create other problems, such as the detection of pin-holes (particularly when under negative pressure), sanitization, and loading ready for use. Ideally they need to be loaded for a complete session of work and rapid, aseptic transfer of items that have been omitted is not easy.

The problems of turbulence, due to the immediate environment or the operator, limit the effectiveness of VLFCs as cytotoxic dispensing cabinets. Isolators offer an enclosed work area. Aseptic transfer into and out of isolators is more complicated than for VLFCs since there is no simple front aperture. In this respect the transfer hatches of the rigid isolators have an advantage over docking ports.

Table 2.1: *Environmental monitoring: centralized cytotoxic dispensing services – limits for physical testing and target microbiological levels*

	Controlled areas		Laminar flow	Isolators	
	Filling room	Change area		Work station	Transfer device
Pressure differentials[10]	>10 Pa between classified area and adjacent area of lower classification >15 Pa between classified and unclassified area				
Airborne particle counts[6,10] (particles M^{-3})					
>0.5 μ	3500	350 000	3500	3500	350 000
>5 μ	0	2000	0	0	2000
>10 μ	0	450	0	0	450
Airflow velocity/ exchange rate[1,7,10]	>20 air changes/hr		Horizontal: 0.45 ± 0.1 m/s Vertical: 0.30 ± 0.05 m/s	Vertical LF: 0.3 ± 0.05 m/s	
Installation leak test[10]			Max. conc. 0.001%	Max. conc. 0.001%	
Settle plates[11] (90 mm: 4 hr exposure)	5	20	1 per 2 plates	1 per 2 plates	5
Surface swabs[11] (55 mm plate)	5		2	2	
Airborne viable[6,11] counts (cfu. M^{-3})	10	100	<1	<1	5

Notes:

1 Where a number of classified areas are connected in cascade, the differential over-pressure need not exceed 30 Pa provided an over-pressure can be demonstrated between each classified area.[10]

2 Airborne particle counts will only be possible in transfer devices that allow access by monitoring equipment.

3 If settle plates are exposed for less than four hours, target levels should be adjusted accordingly.

4 The source documents for each of the limits are referenced. Where no reference is indicated, the limit is suggested best practice.

Isolators should be sited within a designated room which provides an appropriate external environment to the isolator.[7] When installing VLFCs and isolators with external ducting, there may be problems of filtration of the air supply to the cabinet and in balancing air pressures within the room in which the cabinet is sited. Adequate consideration should also be given to the discharge of the exhaust duct.

Gaseous sterilization should only be used on those cabinets fitted with external ducting or other appropriate means of removal of the toxic sterilant gas. Isolators that lend themselves to sanitization with hard-surface disinfectants and do not require fumigation with formaldehyde or peracetic acid are generally preferred by users and allow more flexibility.

For very large-scale operations and for batch manufacturing, a traditional cleanroom may be preferable because of the flexibility it allows, but the costs of operation will be higher and the increased risk potential should be recognized.

Choice of gloves and glove changing procedures are important practical considerations and these should be thoroughly investigated before purchasing decisions are made.

It should be possible to change gloves without loss of EC GMP Grade A[6] conditions within the isolator.

FACILITIES FOR NON-STERILE CYTOTOXIC DRUG MANIPULATION

Cytotoxic chemotherapy regimens often include oral cytotoxic preparations and health care personnel should be aware of the potential hazards when handling them. Care in the supply and administration of solid dosage forms is essential to ensure that staff and, when appropriate, patients and their carers, are given suitable advice on the safe handling of cytotoxic drugs.

Developments in paediatric oncology have resulted in more babies and young children receiving cytotoxic chemotherapy. The treatment regimens for these patients can result in doses being prescribed that cannot be administered in commercially available solid oral dosage forms. In addition, liquid oral preparations are often required for babies and children, and also for adult patients who are unable to swallow solid dosage forms.

The extemporaneous preparation of medicines containing cytotoxic drugs must be avoided whenever possible. In addition, any manipulation of dosage forms on wards which may cause release of a drug into the atmosphere should be discouraged.

Any dosage manipulation or extemporaneous preparation must be restricted to the pharmacy department.

The extemporaneous preparation of liquid oral or any other non-parenteral cytotoxic drug should be performed in such a way that the operator is protected from dust from capsules, tablets and powders, and from aerosols of liquids.

Facilities for non-sterile manipulation of cytotoxic preparations need to provide satisfactory levels of operator protection, but product protection is less critical since product sterility is no longer necessary.

The use of appropriate personal protective clothing is essential, and the preparation should be carried out in fume cupboards or containment enclosures.

1 Fume cupboards

Fume cupboards and exhaust hoods with a negative air inflow and a filtered or ducted exhaust airflow will provide suitable working environments. In the UK fume cupboards should comply with the British Standard for fume cupboards BS 7258, 1990.[12] This standard, in its various parts, covers safety and performance, design and installation and use and maintenance of laboratory fume cupboards. An ancillary document, BS DD191,[13] describes methods for testing such equipment. However, such installations are not always appropriate to hospital pharmacy departments, since they are bulky, of fixed construction, and require ducted exhaust airflow. Some smaller bench-top designs are now available that have a filtered air outlet but the size and bulk of these can still be a problem.

2 Enclosed work stations

Another option is the use of glove box containment cabinets. These are simplified, smaller designs of isolators with sealed glove ports. Inlet and outlet air supplies are HEPA filtered and they may also have activated carbon exhaust filters. Such cabinets are available from: Amercare Ltd and Miller-Howe. They can be free-standing or bench-top units. They are, however, bulky (typically ($w \times d \times h$ (mm)) $600 \times 600 \times 800$), expensive and not easily moved, and their class F^{10} environment is an unnecessary luxury for handling non-sterile cytotoxic manipulations.

3 Portable containment or extraction systems

Bench top, negative pressure extract systems which are portable or movable and allow flexibility, are preferred. They should have a filtered exhaust air supply and the velocity of the inlet airflow should give satisfactory operator protection. Systems are available that provide a localized contained work station or localized extraction at low cost.

It should be recognized that these systems are not designed to the same specification as clean air devices and may not provide total containment of any dust generated. The system should be evaluated and its suitability for its intended task confirmed.

Gelman Sciences

Safetech fume bubble FX1 (Figure 2.7)

Dimensions: ($w \times d \times h$ (mm)) $500 \times 600 \times 580$

Weight: 15 kg

Volume: 0.053 m³

Work surface area: 1500 cm²

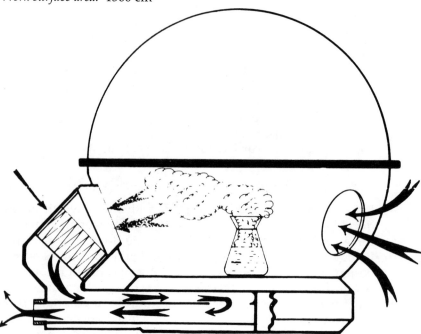

Figure 2.7: *Safetech fume bubble FX1 (Gelman Sciences)*

Filters: Exhaust filter cartridges are available as either HEPA, activated carbon, or in combination. Filter cartridges have a 5 µ pre-filter. The HEPA filter is 99.997% efficient.

Design characteristics: This safety cabinet is a spherical, clear, acrylic construction with two hand ports. Air is drawn through the hand ports and is exhausted via the filter. The minimum negative air velocity at the hand ports is 0.7 m/s.

Nederman Limited

Nederman 2000 extractor (Figure 2.8)

Dimensions: $(w \times d \times h \text{ (mm)})$ $385 \times 175 \times 272$

Weight: 10 kg

Filters: The filter comprises a particle filter and an activated carbon filter, size $(w \times d \times h \text{ (mm)})$ $288 \times 388 \times 285$. The particle filtration is 99.97% efficient.

Design characteristics: The extractor is a multi-component system. An aluminium, rectangular hood, which covers the work area, clips on to a polypropylene extraction arm; the extraction arm is clamped to the working surface and can be pivoted about its foot for manoeuvrability. It is connected, via a 2.5 M PVC flexible hose, to the fan which is attached to the exhaust filter. The fan fits directly on to the filter element and the total depth of the fan and filter is 555 mm.

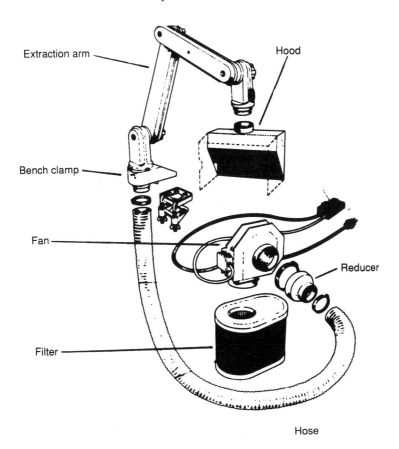

Figure 2.8: *Nederman 2000 extractor (Nederman Ltd)*

Industri Filter UK

Alsident system

Work surface area: Dome 350 mm diameter; canopy 150 × 200 mm

Filters: Available both as a two-stage filter, which comprises a pre-filter and a HEPA filter, and a three-stage filter, which has a carbon filter as well as a pre-filter and HEPA filter.

Design characteristics: A filter unit is connected by flexible tubing to an extraction tube. This comprises short lengths of 50 mm diameter, rigid, aluminium or polypropylene tubes connected together with polypropylene swivel joints. The extraction tube is clamped on to the work surface and terminates in a circular extraction dome or a rectangular extraction canopy.

DISPOSABLES

1 Introduction

Despite the range of items available for drug reconstitution, transport and disposal, the overriding aim when selecting disposables for use with cytotoxic drugs should be suitability, safety and simplicity. Devices listed in this chapter meet all three criteria, although choice of particular items will depend on the level of service provided. The cost of many of the devices may seem prohibitive but their use can be justified for health and safety reasons. No one particular manufacturer is recommended; the choice is left to each individual. Most hospital supplies departments stock a wide range of disposables.

2 Syringes and administration systems

It is recommended that syringes used for cytotoxic drugs be luer-lock and made of polypropylene, as the material is chemically inert.[14,15] Styrene syringes are specifically not recommended for cytotoxic drugs. Standards for syringes are given in BS 5081, Part 1 (1987)[16] and ISO 7886.[17]

Syringes are usually made in three parts – the barrel and piston of plastic materials and the plunger of rubber. Certain grades of rubber have been found to release water-soluble materials on prolonged contact with drug solutions.[18,19] Hence, chemical interactions between rubber extractives and the drugs are possible. If it is intended to store drugs in a particular brand of syringe for prolonged periods, it is advisable to check that there are no such interactions. Two-piece polypropylene luer-lock syringes are available, overcoming the possibility of an interaction between plunger and drug. In addition to ensuring that a drug is stable on storage, it is necessary to check that there is not an unacceptable degree of water loss from the syringe.[20]

Syringes must be fitted with blind-hub closures, not needles, when prepared in the pharmacy. The blind hubs should be luer-lock, must be a good fit and not permit leakage. They must be of a suitable size to be easy for medical and nursing staff to remove safely.

Instillations of cytotoxic drugs are better presented in syringes or containers with catheter tips. Some bladder syringes have luer-lock connections in addition to the usual catheter tip. However, the addition of a luer-lock fitting to a bladder irrigation container may be potentially hazardous as it could facilitate IV administration of the bladder irrigation solution. Recently a catheter-tip adapter with a luer-lock connection has been marketed in the UK enabling cytotoxic bladder instillations to be prepared in luer-lock syringes. Devices are made specifically for the instillation of fluids into the bladder. In certain countries, a fitting for converting a mini-bag into a bladder instillation device is available.

Information on disposables used in ambulatory pumps is provided in Chapter 5.

3 Needles and filtration systems

3.1 Needles and quills

When removing solutions from vials or ampoules, it is essential to use as wide a bore needle as possible to prevent undue pressure building up in the system. This is particularly important with viscous solutions such as etoposide. Specifications for needles are included in BS 5081, Part 1 (1987)[16] and ISO 7886.[17] The length of the needle used will depend on the nature of the procedure being carried out.

Butterfly needles, which consist of a winged needle attached to a length of tubing with a luer-lock connector at the end, can be useful for multiple additions or withdrawals from infusion bags or vials. They are available in standard needle sizes. However, newer devices with one-way valves and luer-lock connections are easier and safer to use than systems such as butterfly needles for multiple additions and withdrawals.

Quills are useful for drawing up solutions from ampoules, the rate of flow being greater than with a needle.

3.2 Filtration systems

Sterilizing filters are not recommended for use with solutions of cytotoxic drugs because of the risk of pressurizing the system (*see* section on Reconstitution devices and air vents, below). If a solution requires clarification, a filter with a pore size of not less than 5 µm can be used but with great caution. Filter straws are quills with a 5 or 10 µm filter attached. Filters are not recommended for use with etoposide as there is a potential chemical interaction with the material of which most filters are made.[21]

4 Reconstitution devices and air vents

The hazard of aerosol production during the preparation of cytotoxic drugs is well recognized. To prevent the risk of exposure to individuals carrying out cytotoxic drug reconstitution, substantial positive or negative deviations from atmospheric pressure within drug vials and syringes should be avoided.[14,15,22] The practice of using needles to 'vent' cytotoxic drug vials is not recommended because the risk of exposure is high. 'Venting' of cytotoxic drug vials can be carried out in one of several ways.

▼ Using a negative pressure procedure: The negative pressure procedure described by Wilson and Solimando[23] requires consistent, impeccable technique. Some operatives find it difficult to maintain and it may not always be possible with partially pressurized vials.

▼ Using a non-filtered air vent: Even though these equilibrate the pressure within the system they are not recommended because of the risk of escape of cytotoxic drug.

▼ Using a reconstitution device: A number of reconstitution devices are available, but not all are suitable for use with cytotoxic drugs. The devices usually have a short, fine plastic spike attached to a filter. Spikes can make large holes in rubber bungs, with the possibility of leakage of the solution from around the spike. In addition, there is a risk of producing a 'core' of rubber. Where devices with spikes are used for cytotoxic drug reconstitution they should be single use only and the spike should not constitute more than 50% of the surface area of the rubber bung of the vial. Reconstitution devices are useful for the repeated aspiration of measured volumes of diluent by syringe.

▼ Using a hydrophobic filter-needle unit: Several types are available incorporating a 0.2 μ hydrophobic filter supplied as a reconstitution device or a unit which can be used separately. The latter type can be difficult to use with smaller vials as both the filter unit and the needle of the reconstituting syringe need to be accommodated in the rubber bung of the vial. Hydrophobic filter-needle units are relatively expensive but it is prudent to balance cost with increased safety to the individual.

5 Incidental items

5.1 Cleaning equipment

All cleaning equipment should only be used in the designated cytotoxic reconstitution area. Any cloths, sponges or mop-heads can be used provided they are low-lint. Cloths, ideally, should be disposable. Where in-house sterilizing facilities are available it may be cheaper to buy unsterile cleaning equipment. If there are several areas to be cleaned, the use of colour coding may be applicable.

5.2 Trays

These can be used for many purposes, including collection of waste inside an isolator or VLFC, as a confined environment for cytotoxic drug reconstitution and for setting up each preparation prior to reconstitution. They come in a variety of materials and sizes. It is important that they can be easily cleaned or sterilized depending on their use.

5.3 Absorbent mats

These are used for lining work surfaces. Their use in VLFCs is not ideal because recirculation of air is hampered, but they may have a use in isolators. Their ease of disposal once contaminated is an advantage. Any absorbent material of suitable size can be used provided it can be sterilized for use within an aseptic area.

5.4 Tamper-evident seals

The injection ports of infusion bags and the tops of infusion bottles should ideally be sealed after addition of a drug or reconstitution. This prevents the further addition of drugs and indicates any loss of integrity during storage and transport. A variety of caps and seals are commercially available.

5.5 Packaging

All cytotoxic preparations should be packed in leak-proof containers after preparation. Polythene tubing which can be heat sealed to give an air/water tight seal and which can be cut to enclose any size or shape of container is recommended.

Grip-top bags should be avoided as the seal is easily broken. Opaque polythene can be used for drugs requiring light protection. Polythene of gauge 200–250 g is suitable for most purposes; however 500 g polythene may be required for outer-packaging of items being transported to off-site centres.

Heat sealers are available from a number of sources. The sealer selected must create an adequate seal and must be durable enough to endure repeated use. Domestic heat sealers are not suitable for the grades of plastic recommended.

REFERENCES

1 Anon. (1992) *Microbiological safety cabinets, BS 5726*. British Standards Institute, London.
2 Anon. (1982) *Cytotoxic drug safety cabinets, AS 2567*. Standards Association of Australia, Sydney.
3 GS-GES-04 (1988) *DIN standard 24184*. Professional Association of Health Service and Welfare Care.
4 Anon. (1990) *ASHP technical assistance bulletin on handling cytotoxic and hazardous drugs. Am. J. Hosp. Pharm.* **47**, 1033–49.
5 Anon. (1987) *National Sanitation Foundation Standard: Class II (laminar flow) Biohazard Cabinetry. Standard 49*. National Sanitation Foundation, Ann Arbor, MI.
6 European Commission (1992) *Good manufacturing practice for medicinal products, Vol. IV*. Brussels.
7 Lee MG, Midcalf B (1994) *Isolators for pharmaceutical applications*. HMSO, London.
8 Anon. (1988) *The control of substances hazardous to health regulations*. HMSO, London.
9 Anon. (1984) *Sterile latex surgeons' gloves, BS 4005*. British Standards Institute, London.
10 Anon. (1989) *Environmental cleanliness in enclosed spaces, Parts 1,2,3, BS 5295*. British Standards Institute, London.
11 Anon. (1989) *Environmental contamination control practice. Technical Monograph No. 2*. The Parenteral Society, Swindon, Wiltshire.
12 Anon. (1990) *Laboratory fume cupboards, Parts 1,2,3, BS 7258*. British Standards Institute, London.
13 Anon. (1990) *Method for delimitation of the containment value of laboratory fume cupboards, BS DD191*. British Standards Institute, London.
14 Anon. (1983) Guidelines for the handling of cytotoxic drugs – working party report. *Pharm. J.* **230**, 230–1.
15 Anon. (1983) *The safe handling of cytotoxic drugs*. ASTMS, Health and Safety Office, Special Report.
16 Anon. (1987) *Sterile hypodermic syringes and needles, Part 1 Specification of sterile hypodermic syringes for single use, BS 5081*. British Standards Institute, London.
17 Anon. (1984) *Sterile hypodermic syringes for single use, ISO 7886*. (Available through the Standards Institute of the relevant country.)
18 Petersen MC *et al.* (1981) Leaching of 2-(2-hydroxyethylmercapto)benzothiazole into contents of disposable syringes. *J. Pharm. Sci.* **70**, 1139–43.
19 Reepmeyer JC, Juhl YH (1983) Contamination of injectable solutions with 2-mercaptobenzothiazole leached from rubber closures. *J. Pharm. Sci.* **72**, 1302–5.
20 Parkinson R *et al.* (1989) Stability of low-dose heparin in pre-filled syringes. *Brit. J. Pharm. Prac.* **11**, 34–6.
21 Forrest SC (1984) Vepesid injection. *Pharm. J.* **232**, 88.

22 Anon. (1996) Controlling occupational exposure to hazardous drugs. *Am. J. Health-Syst. Pharm.* **52**, 1669–85.

23 Wilson JP, Solimando DA (1981) Aseptic technique as a safety precaution in the preparation of antineoplastic agents. *Hosp. Pharm.* **16**, 575–81.

3

Health and safety aspects of cytotoxic services

INTRODUCTION

It is now well recognized that most anticancer drugs are potentially hazardous substances, since they are mutagenic, teratogenic and/or carcinogenic.[1,2] There is also substantial evidence to show that patients may develop secondary neoplasms as a result of treatment with cancer chemotherapeutic agents,[3-6] indicating the potential threat to the health of any persons exposed to this class of drugs.

Such risks may be acceptable for patients with life-threatening diseases. They are clearly not acceptable to hospital personnel who are exposed to such chemicals in the workplace. There is now a large body of evidence to show that health care personnel involved in the preparation and manipulation of anticancer drugs can, if not adequately protected, absorb potentially harmful quantities of such compounds. Much of the evidence comes from epidemiological studies on such diverse groups as nurses, pharmacists and pharmacy technicians and has been extensively reviewed.[6-9] There is also recent evidence that not only workers involved directly with the cytotoxic drugs, but also workers in adjacent areas may absorb potentially hazardous amounts of the drugs.[10,11]

The potential dangers are, therefore, well established. Studies have, for example, shown the association between spontaneous abortions and malformations in the offspring of nurses with occupational exposure to cytotoxic agents.[12-16] Nurses handling these drugs have often shown increased mutagenic activity in their urine as compared with unexposed personnel.[17-19] Similar patterns have also been reported in the serum of oncology nurses.[20-22] Pharmacists and technicians who regularly handle cytotoxic drugs have also shown some evidence for an excess of acute adverse effects including chronic throat irritations and diarrhoea.[23] Physicians who regularly handle antineoplastic drugs appear to be at increased risk of leukaemia and lymphoma,[24] while antineoplastic drugs were suggested as causal in the development of bladder cancer in a pharmacist.[9] These and other studies indicate the potential high level of risk to staff working with anticancer drugs.

A number of relevant safety measures have been introduced, many as a result of regulatory requirements, to protect health care personnel who prepare or administer cytotoxic drugs. A number of studies have now been reported highlighting the fact that such improvements can substantially reduce staff exposure levels. For example, improved care in handling has been shown to reduce mutagenic activity detected in nurses' urine.[8,25] Cooke[26] reported that blood samples from pharmacy staff handling anticancer agents in purpose-designed cytotoxic units showed no greater evidence of mutagenicity than unexposed controls. In a comparative study, Kolmodin-Hedman et al.[27] showed that the provision of adequate safety precautions reduced significantly the mutagenic activity in the urine taken from staff working in oncology units and pharmacies.

Ferguson et al.[28,29] reported that a group of pharmacists working in a fully-protected environment preparing cytotoxic injections did not show evidence of drug absorption, although it was noted that an occasional individual did show evidence of exposure. It has been confirmed that pharmacy staff preparing cytotoxics in a vertical laminar flow cabinet (biological safety cabinet Type 2b) with 30% recirculation and wearing gloves and arm protection, did not show any evidence of increased urine mutagenic activity.[30] The use of a more sensitive technique, however, revealed that cytotoxic drugs are still being absorbed under these conditions, albeit at reduced levels.[10,31]

It can be concluded that there is now sufficient evidence to indicate that staff working in pharmacies who prepare cytotoxic injections for administration, or nurses who work in oncology departments either preparing drugs for administration, or dealing with patients' urine or other contaminated fluids, are potentially at risk. This risk is sufficient to indicate, unequivocally, that all necessary measures should be adopted to protect these staff from occupational exposure. It is not possible to establish maximum safe exposure levels. Therefore, all recognized steps need to be taken to prevent, or at least reduce to a minimum, exposure to these hazardous substances in the workplace. As all approaches available are, by the nature of the problem, of an indirect form, many different aspects of service operation must be included to ensure adequate, state-of-the-art staff protection. These should include the following.

▼ Provision of adequate protective environments (suitable safety cabinet, isolators or hoods) and suitable protective clothing.
▼ Regular staff monitoring by occupational health services.
▼ Effective written procedures and on-going staff training.
▼ Regular application of service audits.
▼ Adequate procedures for dealing with spillages and disposal of all contaminated materials.

Another key question to be addressed by pharmacy managers is whether to rotate staff through this service and other departmental activities. A number of factors need to be considered in making such a judgement. The advantages of employing staff specifically to work in the cytotoxic service include assurance that a high level of expertise is established, that speed and efficiency of operations are optimized and such personnel can also fulfil training roles. The disadvantages are that the same staff are exposed to the hazards associated with cytotoxic drug handling over longer periods and it is more difficult to cover for staff absences. Finally, boredom from carrying out the same activities over long periods can lead to lowering of performance.

If a rotational scheme is operated, this ensures that a maximum number of staff are trained and the levels of exposure to potentially harmful substances are reduced. However, it is likely that the overall level of competence is lower and a greater level of supervision and monitoring may be deemed necessary.

STAFF MONITORING

It is essential to maintain a system of health surveillance for staff directly involved in handling cytotoxic agents on a routine basis. This may comprise regular general health screening together with the use of specific biochemical, mutagenic and/or cytogenetic tests to determine if an individual has been exposed to harmful levels of mutagenic substances.

1 Health surveillance

Four data-gathering elements have been identified as contributing to a medical surveillance programme for staff working with cytotoxic drugs.[32]

1.1 Medical history

The employee's medical and occupational history is rightly the prerogative of the occupational health department. Its staff have a key role to play in record-keeping and counselling. The concept of an individual exposure record has been postulated as an attempt to quantify the drug 'burden' to which the individual has been exposed. A record of length of time handling hazardous materials is logistically simpler to produce and arguably more valid than a cumulative record of doses prepared. The scientific case for such records remains unproven and the problems of data interpretation are vast. Individual agents vary in their acute toxicity, particularly with regard to irritant effects, but differentiating between exposure to different drugs on a chronic basis is unlikely to be possible.

1.2 Physical examinations

These should be routine pre-employment practice. For staff involved in cytotoxic drug handling, these should be repeated at regular intervals, in order to identify symptoms that could be associated with acute exposure (for example, irritation of mucous membranes, dizziness, light-headedness).[32,33] Documentation of untoward events such as spills and accidents, together with estimations of potential exposure 'doses' will form a part of the individual health surveillance record. One aim should be to determine whether abnormal findings or test results are associated with longer handling times.

1.3 Laboratory tests

Full blood and differential white cell counts are performed routinely in many centres. Such data give little information accept in the case of a high amount of exposure, and must be interpreted with care. Tests for changes in liver and renal function have also been advocated[32] in the light of the toxicity profiles of many cytotoxic drugs. There is also some evidence to link any such changes with adverse effects reported in health care workers handling cytotoxic drugs without adequate protection.[23,33]

1.4 Biological monitoring

The measurement of concentrations of specific cytotoxic agents in body fluids (for example in blood and urine) has been reported for certain drugs or their known metabolites.[10,11,31,34,35] The value of monitoring such levels is, however, limited due to the increasing range of potential agents, and the likelihood that the extremely low concentrations of drug anticipated in an occupational exposure setting will be below the limits of sensitivity of many assay procedures.

Nevertheless, the measurement of individual drugs such as cyclophosphamide, using highly sensitive gas chromatography methods has proved informative in recent studies.[10,11,31] An alternative approach estimates accumulative effects at either the DNA or chromosomal level on body tissues such as buccal cells, sperm or blood.[36]

1.5 Health surveillance in practice

In practice, the cornerstone of an occupational health monitoring process is to give all new staff working with cytotoxic drugs a confidential interview, which is designed to review their medical history, and a physical examination. Simple laboratory tests, such as blood counts and differential white cell counts, together with urine and liver function tests, may also be performed, to confirm their current state of good health.

This interview should also be used as the opportunity for a staff member to discuss any fears they may have concerning work with such agents. In this way, all new staff can be educated about the risks involved. This should reinforce information imparted during the training programme. This interview should be repeated at suitable intervals when the employee's exposure record can also be updated. Such interviews are usually recommended on an annual basis.

The exposure record is an essential part of staff surveillance programmes. It should include a record of times spent by each staff member working with cytotoxic agents, together with a specific record of involvement with accidental spillages or other occurrence which could increase that person's exposure. In addition, all incidents involving accidental exposure, such as gross spillages or needle stick incidents, must be reported to the occupational health department. Following such incidents, blood testing and a physical examination should be undertaken to identify signs of acute toxicity to skin, mucous membranes, eyes etc.

Records should be maintained centrally, ideally by occupational health or personnel departments. Computerization of records allows for rapid data entry and recall, especially if linked to the pharmacy system used in the operation of the service. Exposure and incident records should be retained with the employee's personal record. A copy should be available on request to any employee who leaves the service or transfers to another hospital. If a local occupational health policy exists, this should be made available to general practitioners whose patients include such staff, for reference.

Many authorities now recommend that staff who are pregnant or contemplating pregnancy, or are breastfeeding, should be excluded from duties involving the preparation or administration of cytotoxic drugs.

In addition to professional and technical staff, other grades may be involved in handling cytotoxic drugs. These can include porters, storekeepers etc. They need to be educated to an appropriate level in relation to their responsibilities, and provided with appropriate health screening and advice.

2 Biological monitoring of staff

The need to monitor staff for specific biological evidence of enhanced exposure to cytotoxic drugs is controversial.[37] While such a system of staff surveillance offers, in theory, a sensitive means of monitoring the real biological risks to staff, in terms of indices of mutagenicity, there is some question as to whether test methods currently available can offer adequate assurance of their ability to identify the real risk.[5,6,8,32] Methods may either be insufficiently sensitive or poorly validated.

The following tests are available and, in theory at least, offer a monitoring test for staff. These have been assessed in the context of hospital staff exposure to cytotoxic drugs by Ferguson et al.[28,29] and Kaijser et al.[8] and for environmental exposure to mutagens and carcinogens, by the ICPEMC.[7] More recently, the significance of chromosomal aberrations in circulating lymphocytes as predictors of cancer incidence has been confirmed in prospective studies from two different centres within Europe.[38,39]

2.1 Tests for urine mutagenicity

The Salmonella/mammalian microsome mutagenicity test (Ames' test) can be used as a routine method to measure mutagenic activity in urine.[17] The test relies on the measurement of mutations in bacterial cells caused by carcinogenic agents. This test, while relatively simple and cheap to perform, lacks both sensitivity and specificity as a means of measuring staff exposure to cytotoxic agents in normal practice.[8] It is now considered unsuitable for staff monitoring.

2.2 Tests for DNA damage and cytogenetic changes

These tests are designed to identify biological changes which may have been caused by cellular exposure to mutagenic agents. These can be either chemical (e.g. chemical carcinogens) or physical (e.g. ionizing radiation) agents. The tests employ biological markers to detect various endpoints including chromosomal aberrations, or DNA interchange between chromatids.

2.3 ^{32}P-postlabelling and other assays to detect altered DNA bases

The alkylating anticancer drugs act through the formation of DNA adducts. These can be detected in the DNA of blood cells taken from cancer patients, using a highly sensitive postlabelling method.[40] Other authors have estimated the specific accumulation of O_6-methylguanine in similar samples, using different methodologies.[41] These methods are highly sensitive and have been suggested to be applicable to biomonitoring of oncology personnel. However, they have the following disadvantages:

▼ they are specific to alkylating agents
▼ they vary in quantitation between different laboratories
▼ their predictive powers are not yet well established.

2.4 Assays for DNA breakage

Many, if not most, anticancer drugs in common use are effective DNA-breaking agents. Highly sensitive assays which can measure DNA breaks include alkaline elution[42] and the comet assay.[43] Both have been applied to various studies with anticancer drugs and the alkaline elution assay has been recently used to demonstrate the effectiveness of protective clothing and procedures in reducing anticancer drug absorption by oncology nurses.[42] Although holding considerable promise, these assays are currently insufficiently validated for routine use in these situations.

2.5 Assay for chromosome aberrations

This method offers the most direct estimate of heritable changes, but is relatively insensitive and laborious to perform. Its main importance lies in the fact that it measures long-lasting lesions and, therefore, provides an index of cumulative damage. It is also the only one of these assays which has been validated as a long-term predictor of cancer incidence.[38,39] If the test indicates that a particular individual does show an increase in chromosomal aberrations with time, this probably indicates that hazardous substances are being absorbed and urgent preventative measures are required.

2.6 Micronucleus assay

This method provides a more indirect method of detecting exposure to cytotoxic substances. It is less time-consuming to perform than chromosomal aberration tests, and does not require the same high level of technical skill. It is, however, too variable to identify real differences in individuals[28] but it may be useful when applied to sufficiently large groups of workers to identify differences between populations or between working conditions. It may be improved by the use of the cytochalasin block method.[29]

2.7 Sister chromatid exchange (SCE)

This method detects reciprocal exchanges between chromatids. It is a sensitive method and detects changes that could be caused by very low levels of mutagenic compounds. However, it must be realized that SCE lesions are short-lived and decline substantially within a few days. The test must be performed immediately after the sample has been collected. It clearly will have relevance to testing personnel while working with cytotoxic drugs. It has no retrospective value.

3 Should blood tests be used to monitor staff?

Whether or not routine testing of staff for evidence of exposure to mutagenic substances should be conducted remains controversial.[37] Many official guidelines suggest that these tests are not sensitive enough and not yet sufficiently validated to provide meaningful information concerning the levels of risk to which staff have been exposed.[8,32] Although recent validation studies have confirmed the value of estimating chromosomal aberrations, these tests need to be applied with care.[44] In particular, the study design requires close consideration.[45] Ferguson et al.[28] argue that a monitoring programme would provide a means of assessing whether a relationship may exist between consistent detection of abnormalities and occupational exposure to cytotoxic agents. Such testing may also provide a warning of equipment failure, poor technique practised by an individual or inadequacies in protective clothing.[37]

The knowledge base relating to oncology staff testing remains insufficient to offer firm guidance on the value or the necessity for such testing. McDairmid[32] warns that, since it is not yet possible to interpret the results of these various tests accurately or link any single 'positive' result to occupational exposure, such a 'positive' result may provoke unjustifiable anxiety in individuals for whom its importance cannot be adequately explained. Ferguson et al.[29] suggest that the cytokinesis-blocked micronucleus test is most readily applied to testing personnel actively working in cytotoxic services. However, if tests are only performed as a routine on all staff, irrespective of their current duties, the chromosomal aberrations test may be the most appropriate method.

It has been suggested that the analysis of blood or urine for the presence of specific cytotoxic drugs, or metabolites, could be an alternative or additional valuable tool for monitoring staff exposure.[10,11,31] Both chromatographic and spectrophotometric methods have been investigated. These analytical methods have shown minor amounts of cyclophosphamide in urine of pharmacy nurses and technicians, even where they were handling drugs under special safety precautions. Sorsa et al.[46] calculate an increased cancer risk of 1×10^{-5} in these circumstances.

CONTROL OF EXPOSURE

1 Regulations controlling exposure of staff to hazardous substances

Many countries now have statutory controls concerning the protection of staff working with potentially hazardous substances. Specific examples include:

▼ UK – Control of Substances Hazardous to Health (COSHH) Regulations (1988)[47]
▼ US – Federal Occupational Health and Safety Administration (OHSA).

Such regulations require employers to prevent or control exposure of their employees (or of visitors to their premises) to any substance potentially or actually hazardous to health.

2 The working environment

All aseptic preparative work involving the handling of cytotoxics must be conducted within a suitable safety cabinet or isolator. A review of equipment options appears in Chapter 2. Cabinets, including isolators, should ideally be situated within a dedicated area, with access restricted to authorized personnel, to prevent the possible spread of contamination to other working areas. Standard operating procedures, such as those listed within the section on audit (*see* later) need to be in place. Strict adherence to these procedures ensures maximum operator protection.

3 Monitoring of the working environment

Practical experience in basic aseptic technique is essential before staff are involved in cytotoxic manipulation. All staff who reconstitute cytotoxics should understand the theory behind their use in the treatment of cancer, and the risks associated with drug handling. Handling techniques should be taught and assessed using non-hazardous materials until the operator's technique has been validated. Particular attention should be paid to pressure equalization techniques. The following standard tests exist for such validation.

▼ A 1% quinine hydrochloride solution can be used in aseptic transfers. This will fluoresce under UV light, indicating spilt material and poor cleaning technique.
▼ The transfer of dye solutions such as amaranth or methylene blue between pressurized vials is a useful method of demonstrating aerosol formation.

However, despite rigorous validation procedures, there is always a possibility that cytotoxic spillage can occur during preparation or administration with resultant contamination of the working environment. In addition, there may be a need to confirm the absence of contamination on equipment prior to disposal.

Work has been carried out on the development of techniques for identifying spilt materials and validating cleaning and inactivation procedures; this includes direct fluorescence measurement[48,49] and the bioluminescent estimation of residual mutagenic activity.[50]

In the UK, two relatively simple methods for monitoring the working environment have been developed and validated in a number of laboratories.[51] In looking for a monitoring method certain important criteria were identified. The methods needed to:

▼ detect cytotoxics prepared routinely or regularly. Such products could be used as markers to, at a minimum, give a yes/no indication of whether residues have been deposited
▼ detect products at normal handling concentrations
▼ use simple and reproducible laboratory methods.

The two methods are described below. Both methods are sufficiently simple that any quality assurance laboratory with basic equipment and experienced staff should be able to carry them out.

The environmental sampling and extraction stages are common to both methods.

3.1 Environmental sampling

1 Decide on the area of the working environment to be sampled and divide into 10 cm squares.
2 Swab each square with a separate Steret IPA swab. Place each swab in a test tube.
3 Include an unused Steret as a control.

3.2 Extraction

1 Add 0.5 ml methanol to each test tube.
2 To extract, agitate with a clean glass rod for 30 seconds.

3.3 Thin layer chromatography (TLC) method

1 Set up a TLC tank using a freshly prepared mobile phase of chloroform; methanol; glacial acetic acid 75 : 20 : 5.
2 Prepare fresh standard solutions as follows: vincristine 1 mg/10 ml; cyclophosphamide 500 mg/25 ml and methotrexate 5 mg/2 ml.
3 Use silica gel plates. Condition by heating at 110°C for 1 hour. Cool.
4 Apply 10 µl spots for each sample, each standard and the control. Allow to dry.
5 Run the chromatogram for 10 cm, dry and spray with potassium iodobismuthate solution BP.

3.4 Spot method

1 Prepare fresh standard solutions as follows: vincristine 1 mg/10 ml; cyclophosphamide 500 mg/25 ml and methotrexate 5 mg/2 ml.
2 Use either a silica gel TLC plate or a fine filter paper.
3 Apply 10 µl spots for each sample, each standard and the control. Allow to dry.
4 Spray with potassium iodobismuthate solution BP.

3.5 Interpretation of results

1 For either method, note the colour and intensity of any spots. For the TLC method also record the position of each spot, and calculate the R_f value.
2 Compare any spots from samples with those of the standard solutions.
3 Refer to the sampling plan and for each square record whether or not contamination is detected.
4 If spots are detected appropriate action should be agreed. This should include identification of the substance detected, examination and revalidation of the premises and equipment and examination of the operating procedures.
5 Results and actions should be fully documented and a full report kept on file.

Experience from using the methods: Spot colours are yellow-brown; with methotrexate giving the most intense colour. Vincristine is not detected on filter paper but should be detected on silica gel plates. No spot colour is found with the control. Use of the TLC method enables spot colours and R_f values to be used in identification.

R_f 100 values are:

▼ vincristine approximately 70–75 (with benzyl alcohol, approximately 90)
▼ cyclophosphamide approximately 85–95
▼ methotrexate approximately 10–20.

The method can also be used for fluorouracil. Yellow-brown spot colours are obtained and the R_f 100 value is approximately 60–70.

The detection limit of the methods is approximately a 10 µl spot of each of the standard solutions. Sensitivity can be increased by using repeat spot applications.

4 Handling precautions

Exposure to cytotoxic materials may arise as a result of ingestion, inhalation, absorption through the skin or direct splashing, e.g. into the eye.

The safe handling of cytotoxic materials is dependent on attention to a number of factors. These are:

▼ appropriate protective clothing
▼ adequate containment facilities for the scale of the operation, properly maintained and monitored
▼ extensive training and regular assessment of technical competence
▼ clearly defined, written procedures for all stages of operation, from goods receipt to the disposal of cytotoxic wastes.

A breakdown in any one of these areas will compromise safe working practice. It should be stressed that failure to perform in a safe and competent manner by a member of the team will create a potential risk, not only for that person, but also for the other staff working in the same unit.

In addition to professional and technical staff, other staff grades will be involved in cytotoxic drug handling, e.g. storekeepers, porters etc. They require education and training to an appropriate level in relation to their responsibilities.

4.1 Handling guidelines for non-parenteral cytotoxics

Chemotherapy regimens frequently include oral cytotoxic preparations, and topical formulations containing cytotoxic drugs may occasionally be prescribed. Clinical staff are often unaware that these preparations pose a potential health hazard if handled carelessly.

Requests for extemporaneous preparation of medicines may arise whenever a dose regimen falls outside commercially provided dose forms. This is particularly true of paediatric doses. There may also be demands for liquid formulations if patients have difficulty in swallowing standard dosage forms.

The extemporaneous preparation of medicines containing cytotoxic drugs should be avoided wherever possible. If unavoidable, any manipulation of dosage forms, such as attempting to divide tablets must be restricted to a controlled environment within the pharmacy department. Such activities, which may cause release of drugs into the atmosphere, should be discouraged at ward level.

Recommendations for the preparation and dispensing of non-injectable cytotoxic drugs have been promulgated by the American Society of Hospital Pharmacists.[6]

All cytotoxic drugs dispensed for inpatient use should carry a warning label to alert nursing staff to the need for special handling precautions. Ward staff should be trained to examine all containers before opening and report signs of tablet/capsule deterioration to the pharmacist. Patients or their carers should be given appropriate advice on handling cytotoxic drugs.

Precautions in the pharmacy should include the following.

▼ Staff should wear gloves when handling products containing cytotoxics or equipment used to manipulate them.
▼ All counting of tablets/capsules must be undertaken using designated equipment. Automated tablet counting machines should not be used for cytotoxic preparations.
▼ Procedures should be developed to avoid the release of aerosolized powder or liquid into the working environment.
▼ Containment cabinets must have airflow characteristics which prevent the dispersal of powders. Fume cupboards with external ducting and fitted with a HEPA filter may be acceptable for some levels of activity (see Chapter 2).
▼ Isolators or cabinets used for aseptic preparation should not be employed for non-sterile work.
▼ Solutions of drugs are easier to handle than powders, and should be used whenever possible. If tablets need to be crushed, they should first be placed in a small, sealable plastic bag.

Guidelines for the use of protective clothing, labelling, transport, disposal and dealing with spillages are the same as those used for parenteral cytotoxic preparations.

4.2 Spillage procedures

In the event of accidental spillage, personnel should be aware of clear written procedures for dealing promptly with the problem and should be appropriately trained. Separate procedures are required for:

▼ spillage within the cytotoxic reconstitution area
▼ spillage within the wider environs of the pharmacy department
▼ spillage within the ward/clinic areas of the hospital. This necessitates discussion with nursing, clinical and administrative staff, plus health and safety representatives.

General procedures for dealing with spillages are covered comprehensively by the latest ASHP technical assistance bulletin (TAB) on handling cytotoxic and hazardous drugs.[6]

In summary, the key elements are:

▼ adequate protective clothing for all individuals involved in the cleaning operation
▼ containment of the spillage as far as is possible
▼ prompt action to remove the hazard
▼ adequate, clearly labelled containers for the disposal of waste associated with the clean-up operation
▼ the provision of emergency 'spill-kits' at appropriate locations
▼ documentation of all significant spillages; a report should be forwarded to the occupational health department if individuals have been exposed to risk, e.g. of skin absorption.

The novel techniques for monitoring the efficiency of spill cleaning procedures by visualization methods[48–51] described on page 41 may in the future enable a more quantitative approach to estimating exposure risk from spillage incidents.

4.3 Handling of waste from patients receiving cytotoxic drugs

The excreta from patients receiving cytotoxic chemotherapy may contain potentially hazardous amounts of cytotoxic drugs, or, in some cases, their active metabolites. These are mostly eliminated by renal or faecal excretion.[52–54]

The period over which staff handling patient waste are at risk depends on:

▼ the particular drug involved
▼ pharmacodynamic factors: dose, route of administration, duration of therapy, renal and/or hepatic function
▼ concomitant drug therapy, which may influence elimination rates.

Guidance on the potential hazard from patient excreta has been collated in Table 3.1, which summarizes the time over which additional protective measures are required for specific drugs.[53,54]

Table 3.1: *Details of drugs requiring extended precautionary periods for handling excreta after chemotherapy*[54]

Drug	Route	Duration (days) after completion of therapy for which precautions are necessary when handling:	
		Urine	Faeces
Bleomycin	inj.	3	?
Cisplatin	IV	7	?
Cyclophosphamide	any	3	5
Dactinomycin	IV	5	7
Daunorubicin	IV	2	7
Doxorubicin	IV	6	7
Epirubicin	IV	7	5
Etoposide	any	4	7
Melphalan	oral	2	7
Mercaptopurine	oral	3	?
Methotrexate	any	3	7
Mitoxantrone	IV	6	7
Thiotepa	inj.	3	?
Vinca alkaloids	IV	4	7

?: no information.

As a general rule, the excreta from patients receiving cytotoxic drugs should be assumed to be hazardous for at least 48 hours after the completion of treatment.[54] Such patients should be clearly identified to ward staff.

PROTECTIVE CLOTHING

Protective clothing should be worn at all times when handling cytotoxics. The degree of protection required will depend on the perceived exposure risk to the operator/handler and should be based on local or nationally agreed guidelines, if available.

Table 3.2 summarizes the minimum requirements for the handling of cytotoxic drugs in various situations.

Table 3.2: *Minimum requirements to protect staff when handling cytotoxic drugs in various situations*

Activity	Protective measures
Preparation	
Controlled environment	Sterile/non-sterile gown, suit or laboratory overall
	Gloves of a suitable quality
	Non-absorbent armlets, except in isolators
Uncontrolled environment	As above, plus:
	Plastic apron or non-absorbent overall
	Eye protection
	Dust or respirator mask
Checking	No special protection is required provided appropriate procedures are in place to prevent the risk of contamination to the individual. Otherwise laboratory overall or long-sleeved uniform and gloves of a suitable quality should be worn
Transport	No special protection required provided drugs are transported in a suitable transport container and the messenger is aware of the potential hazards
Dealing with spills	Non-absorbent overall or laboratory overall and plastic apron
	Heavy duty gloves
	Eye protection
	Dust or respirator mask
Administration/ handling patient waste	Non-absorbent armlets
	Plastic apron
	Gloves of a suitable quality
	Eye protection, where appropriate

1 Gowns, cleanroom suits and armlets

In general these should be:

▼ lightweight
▼ low-linting
▼ of a low permeability, disposable or conventional fabric.

Gowns and suits should have:

▼ a solid front with covered fastenings
▼ long sleeves, cuffed at the wrists.

Most commercially available fabrics for use in aseptic preparation areas are permeable to cytotoxic drugs and additional protection is required if gowns/suits made of these materials are worn.

Laidlaw *et al.*[55] investigated the permeability of four disposable protective clothing materials to seven antineoplastic drugs over a four hour period. The materials tested were Saranex-laminated Tyvek, polyethylene-coated Tyvek and non-porous Tyvek and Kaycel.

All of the materials evaluated afforded protection from occupational exposure to antineoplastic drugs, whereas laboratory coats and disposable isolation gowns were completely absorbent. Saranex-laminated Tyvek and polyethylene-coated Tyvek afforded almost complete protection from the drugs. Non-porous Tyvek and Kaycel did allow some drug permeation, although the maximum permeation over a four hour exposure time was 3.3% of the applied drug dose.

As a general recommendation it is suggested that Saranex-laminated or polyethylene-coated Tyvek armlets be worn over standard cleanroom clothing for preparation of cytotoxics in a downward displacement, laminar air flow, cytotoxic cabinet where the arms of the operator are exposed throughout. These armlets may also be worn when preparing drugs in an isolator cabinet, as some rubber sleeves may not protect the operator from gross contamination.

Where disposable gowns are used, these should be made of Saranex-laminated Tyvek or polyethylene-coated Tyvek for maximum operator protection. However, these materials allow little airflow and tend to be uncomfortable to wear for an extended period of time. Non-porous Tyvek or Kaycel garments are more comfortable to wear but operators should be made aware of the lower degree of protection. Non-porous Tyvek armlets are suitable for all administration and waste disposal procedures.

2 Masks

Standard surgeons' masks are suitable for most procedures carried out in a 'contained environment'. If there is a possibility of inhalation and a drug is not handled in a 'contained environment' a suitable dust mask should be worn, e.g. a disposable 'bra cup' type to BS 6016.[56] A respirator mask may be required for dealing with largescale spills or contamination.

3 Eye protection

Eye protection to BS 2092C[56] is required for handling cytotoxic drugs if the material is not being handled in a suitable cabinet. Goggles should fully enclose the eyes to protect against dust and splashes.

4 Aprons

These provide a protective, water-resistant barrier to accidental spills or sprays. They can be ethylene oxide sterilized if required. Saranex-laminated or Tyvek aprons provide added protection for use in an uncontrolled environment.

5 Gloves

Disposable gloves should be worn at all times when preparing, checking and administering cytotoxic drugs.

The suitability of a wide range of commercially available gloves for cytotoxic handling has been investigated.[57–63] However, there is no consensus about which glove material offers the best protection.

A variety of techniques for determining permeation have been employed including a spectrophotometric method,[58] radiolabelling,[59] mutagenicity testing[60] and chromatographic analysis.[62] Permeation under static and flexed conditions has also been determined.[63] None of the studies considered the effect of solubility of the drug in the collection medium, yet Ehntholt *et al.*,[64] in an evaluation of protective glove materials in agricultural pesticide operations, found the collection medium to be a significant determinant of degree of breakthrough measured.

Several of these studies also determined the inter- and intra-batch variability in glove thickness and the surface characteristics.[58,65] Thomas and Fenton-May,[58] found that glove thickness varied considerably, with a tenfold difference between the extremes in the range. Variation in thickness within the same batch was also considerable for some manufacturers. Kotilainen *et al.*[65] used scanning electron microscopy to examine the surfaces of both PVC and latex gloves. They found that the surface was extremely irregular with multiple pits and defects, some up to 10 μ in width.

On the basis of these studies, it can be concluded that no glove material is completely impermeable to every cytotoxic agent. Although glove thickness is a major factor affecting drug permeation, molecular weight of the drug, lipophilicity, nature of the solvent in which the cytotoxic is dissolved, and glove material composition all affect permeation rates.

When selecting gloves for use with cytotoxics, the user must be assured that the glove material is of a suitable thickness and integrity to maximize protection whilst maintaining manual dexterity. Manufacturers should be asked to supply information on material composition, thickness (both mean and variation in) and durability. The use of poor quality, low-cost gloves is neither safe nor cost-effective because multiple glove changes are required to ensure integrity.

The practice of double-gloving should be unnecessary provided gloves with appropriate qualities are used and the gloves are changed regularly during each work session, or immediately following known contact with a cytotoxic, or if punctured.

Industrial thickness gloves (>0.45 mm thick) made from latex with neoprene, nitrile synthetic rubber or similar materials should be used to clean up largescale spills.

6 Recommended precautions for staff/relatives caring for patients[52–54]

▼ Protective clothing should be worn by staff dealing with blood or vomit from patients who have received cytotoxic drugs within the previous 48 hours, or longer if appropriate (*see* Table 3.1).

▼ All protective clothing should be treated as hazardous and disposed of accordingly.

▼ If contamination of skin, eyes or mucous membranes is suspected, the area should be rinsed thoroughly with large amounts of water and then washed with soap and water.

▼ Double sluicing of bedpans, vomit bowls and other items heavily contaminated with waste materials should be carried out. Disposable items are preferable, and should be treated as hazardous clinical waste and disposed of accordingly.

▼ Patients and staff should utilize different toilet facilities.

▼ Contaminated linen/uniforms may pose a threat to laundry staff. Lightly contaminated linen may be treated as 'infected waste' and dealt with by the normal laundry process. Heavily contaminated items may need to be incinerated.

Soaking of linen in sodium hypochlorite solution has been recommended for drugs such as doxorubicin.[52]

TRANSPORT OF CYTOTOXICS

Packaging and transport systems for cytotoxics must provide adequate physical, chemical and light protection during storage and transportation, be relatively impervious to the atmosphere, robust, and tamperproof, provide adequate protection to the handler(s), contain any leaked solution and allow easy identification of the contained drugs throughout.

All cytotoxic preparations should be packed in leakproof containers after preparation. Polythene tubing that can be heat-sealed to give an air/water tight seal and which can be cut to enclose any size or shape of container is recommended.

For transportation around the hospital, standard delivery containers may be utilized provided they fulfil the above criteria. Cytotoxics should not be transported in the same container as other drugs, and the nature of the contained material should be clearly indicated on the outer container.

Transportation to other clinical settings outside the hospital may necessitate more stringent, possibly custom-designed packaging.

DISPOSAL OF CYTOTOXIC DRUGS AND CYTOTOXIC-CONTAMINATED MATERIALS

Each institution should have a policy on the safe handling and disposal of cytotoxic drugs and materials contaminated with them. Clear and concise procedures for the collection, segregation and disposal of waste should be established; all staff involved, including non-pharmacy staff, should be trained in their use. Procedures should be updated at regular intervals and there should be a system of audit to ensure compliance with the procedures at all times.

Suitable containers, clearly labelled and reserved solely for cytotoxic waste, should be available in all areas where the drugs are handled. They should be brightly coloured with space to indicate the nature of the contents both during use and whilst awaiting disposal. 'Sharps' containers should be robust enough to contain any sharps and leaked solution. They should be constructed of plastic (not lined cardboard), with tightly fitting lids which can be sealed when the container is full. Absorbent material (paper or absorbent granules) should be placed in the bottom of the container to mop up any leaked solution. It is essential to carry out quality assurance on all disposal containers to check they are suitable for use and can be disposed of safely and in the appropriate manner.

Facilities for the storage of the cytotoxic waste awaiting destruction must safeguard the integrity of the packaging and not expose personnel to any risk. Waste should not be allowed to accumulate in either clinical or storage areas.

In the UK, prescription-only medicines are listed in Schedule 1 of the Control of Pollution (Special Waste) Regulations (1980)[66] as substances which are to be regarded as special waste. There is no specific reference to cytotoxics in these regulations, but their disposal will be subject to the general controls set out therein.

The risks associated with pharmaceutical wastes which might enter the water cycle have been discussed in detail in a review by Richardson and Bowron.[67] They calculated that the major source of pharmaceutical chemicals as contaminants in potable water would be from domestic sources, including homes and hospitals, with only a marginal contribution to the load from industry. The authors concluded, from analytical and biodegradation data, that few drugs were likely to survive treatment in sewage works, river retention, reservoir retention and waterworks. Such drugs that did survive would be unlikely to pose a health risk at the concentrations likely to be found in water supplies. It can be concluded, therefore, that disposal to sewer may be used for small quantities of pharmaceuticals.

Disposal via the domestic sewerage system should not be used for large quantities of pharmaceutical waste. The Royal Pharmaceutical Society of Great Britain, in their guidelines, recommend pharmacists to use their professional judgement when deciding on the disposal of substances which may be particularly toxic, insidious or persistent.[68]

The relationship between hazard and the quantities of any particular cytotoxic substance requiring disposal is not generally addressed. However, in the US, this issue is covered by regulations from the Environmental Protection Agency. These were recently summarized by Gallelli.[69] The relevant 'rules' are described as the '3%' and the 'mixture' rules. The former states that all empty containers that contain not more than 3% of cytotoxics by weight in relation to the total capacity of the container, need not be disposed of as hazardous waste. The 'mixture' rule states that if any amount of a listed waste is mixed with any other, the entire mixture is considered hazardous. This is to prevent the deliberate dilution of cytotoxic waste to avoid disposal regulations.

Many cytotoxics can be disposed of by chemical destruction. Details of recommended methods are summarized in Part 2 of this Handbook. Other important sources of information on chemical destruction of cytotoxics are recommended.[70,71]

The method recommended for disposal of cytotoxic drugs is incineration. Disposal into waste which might subsequently be tipped into a landfill site must not, under any circumstances, be used for cytotoxic drugs or materials contaminated with them. Several manufacturers recommend a temperature of 1000°C for the complete destruction of cytotoxic drugs.[72] Opinion differs as to the need for this, but until adequate research work has been carried out, this should be regarded as an ideal to be attained if possible. Perhaps of more importance than the actual temperature is the presence of an after-burner on the incinerator to be used. There is a possible risk of a solution containing a cytotoxic being aerosolized when passed into the incinerator. This may result in undegraded cytotoxic drug being emitted from the incinerator chimney. In the absence of a suitable incinerator, the services of a specialist waste disposal contractor should be employed.

REFERENCES

1 Sieber SM, Adamson RH (1975) Toxicity of antineoplastic agents in man: chromosomal aberrations, antifertility effects, congenital malformations and carcinogenic potential. *Adv. Cancer Res.* **22**, 57–155.

2 Ferguson LR (1995) Mutagenic properties of anticancer drugs. In: (Waring MJ, Ponder B eds), *The Genetics of Cancer.* Kluwer Academic Publishers, Lancaster, UK, pp. 177–216.

3 Kaldor JM *et al.* (1988) Quantifying the carcinogenicity of antineoplastic drugs. *Eur. J. Cancer Clin. Oncol.* **24**, 703–11.

4 Hawkins MM *et al.* (1992) Epipodophyllotoxins, alkylating agents, and radiation and risk of secondary leukemia after childhood cancer. *Br. Med. J.* **304**, 951–8.

5 Anon. (1986) OSHA work-practice guidelines for personnel dealing with cytotoxic (antineoplastic) drugs. *Am. J. Hosp. Pharm.* **43**, 1193–204.

6 Anon. (1990) AHSP technical assistance bulletin on handling cytotoxic and hazardous drugs. *Am. J. Hosp. Pharm.* **47**, 1033–49.

7 Carrano AV, Natarajan AT (1988) ICPEMC Publication No. 14: Considerations for population monitoring using cytogenetic techniques. *Mutation Res.* **204**, 379–406.

8 Kaijser GP *et al.* (1990) The risks of handling cytotoxic drugs. 1. Methods of testing exposure. *Pharm. Weekbl. Sci. Ed.* **12**, 212–27.

9 Levin LI *et al.* (1993). Bladder cancer in a 39-year-old female pharmacist. *J. Natl. Cancer Inst.* **85**, 1089–91.

10 Sessink PJ *et al.* (1994) Environmental contamination and assessment of exposure to antineoplastic agents by determination of cyclophosphamide in urine of exposed pharmacy technicians: is skin absorption an important exposure route? *Arch. Environ. Health,* **49**, 165–9.

11 Sessink PJ *et al.* (1993) Occupational exposure of animal caretakers to cyclophosphamide. *J. Occup. Med.* **35**, 47–52.

12 Selevan SG *et al.* (1985) A study of occupational exposure to antineoplastic drugs and fetal losses in nurses. *N. Engl. J. Med.* **313**, 1173–8.

13 Hemminki K *et al.* (1985) Spontaneous abortions and malformations in the offspring of nurses exposed to anaesthetic gases, cytotoxic drugs and other potential hazards in hospitals, based on registered information of outcome. *J. Epidemiol. Community Health* **39**, 141–7.

14 McDonald AD *et al.* (1988) Congenital defects and work in pregnancy. *Br. J. Ind. Med.* **45**, 581–8.

15 Taskinen HK (1990) Effects of parental occupational exposures on spontaneous abortion and congenital malformation. *Scand J. Work Environ. Health* **16**, 297–314.

16 Stucker I *et al.* (1990) Risk of spontaneous abortion among nurses handling antineoplastic drugs. *Scand. J. Work Environ. Health* **16**, 102–7.

17 Falck K *et al.* (1979) Mutagenicity in urine of nurses handling cytotoxic drugs. *Lancet* **i**, 1250–1.

18 Andersson RW *et al.* (1982) Risks of handling injectable antineoplastic drugs. *Am. J. Hosp. Pharm.* **39**, 1881–7.

19 Benhamou S *et al.* (1986) Mutagenicity in urine from nurses handling cytotoxic drugs. *Eur. J. Cancer Clin. Oncol.* **22**, 1489–93.

20 Norppa H *et al.* (1980) Increased sister chromatid exchange frequencies in lymphocytes of nurses handling cytotoxic drugs. *Scand. J. Work Environ. Health* **6**, 299–303.

21 Sorsa M *et al.* (1982) Induction of sister chromatid exchanges (SCEs) among nurses handling cytotoxic drugs. *Banbury Proc.* Vol. 14. Cold Spring Harbor Laboratory, New York.

22 Nikula E *et al.* (1984) Chromosomal aberrations in lymphocytes of nurses handling cytotoxic drugs. *Scand. J. Work Environ. Health* **10**, 71–4.

23 Valanis BG *et al.* (1993) Association of antineoplastic drug handling with acute adverse effects in pharmacy personnel. *Am. J. Hosp. Pharm.* **50**, 455–62.

24 Skov T *et al.* (1990) Risks for physicians handling antineoplastic drugs. *Lancet* **336**, 1446.

25 Vainio H (1982) Mutagenicity in urine of workers occupationally exposed to mutagens and carcinogens. In: (Aito, A *et al.* eds), *Biological monitoring and health surveillance of workers exposed to chemicals.* Hemisphere Publishing, Washington DC, pp. 324–30.

26 Cooke J (1987) Environmental monitoring of personnel who handle cytotoxic drugs. *Pharm. J.* **239**, R2.

27 Kolmodin-Hedman B *et al.* (1983) Occupational handling of cytotoxic drugs. *Arch. Toxicol.* **54**, 25–33.

28 Ferguson LR *et al.* (1988) The use within New Zealand of cytogenetic approaches to monitoring of hospital pharmacists for exposure to cytotoxic drugs: report of a pilot study in Auckland. *Aust. J. Hosp. Pharm.* **18**, 228–33.

29 Ferguson LR *et al.* (1990) Monitoring of drug absorption by pharmacists and oncology nurses in four New Zealand Hospitals using estimation of cytokinesis-blocked micronuclei. *Aust. J. Hosp. Pharm.* **20**, 212–21.

30 Guinee EP *et al.* (1991). Evaluation of genotoxic risk of handling cytostatic drugs in clinical pharmacy practice. *Pharm. Weekbl. Sci. Ed.* **13**, 78–82.

31 Ensslin AS (1993) Biological monitoring of cyclophosphamide and ifosfamide in urine of hospital personnel occupationally exposed to cytostatic drugs. *Occup. Environ. Med.* **51**, 229–33.

32 McDairmid MA (1990) Medical surveillance for antineoplastic handlers. *Am. J. Hosp. Pharm.* **47**, 1061–6.

33 Stellman JM, Zoloth SR (1986) Cancer chemotherapeutic agents as occupational hazards: A literature review. *Cancer Invest.* **4**, 127–35.

34 Venitt S *et al.* (1984) Monitoring exposure of nursing and pharmacy personnel to cytotoxic drugs: Urinary mutation assays and urinary platinum as markers of absorption. *Lancet* **i**, 777.

35 Hirst M *et al.* (1984) Occupational exposure to cyclophosphamide. *Lancet* **i**, 186–8.

36 Knudsen LE, Sorsa M (1993) Human biological monitoring of occupational genotoxic exposures. *Pharmacol. Toxicol.* **72** (Suppl. 1), 86–92.

37 Ferguson LR (1995) Occupational Health and staff monitoring: a genetic toxicologist's viewpoint. *J. Oncol. Pharmacy Pract.* **3**, 49–54.

38 Hagmar L *et al.* (1994) Cancer risk in humans predicted by increased levels of chromosomal aberrations in lymphocytes: Nordic study group on the health risk of chromosome damage. *Cancer Res.* **54**, 2919–22.

39 Bonassi S *et al.* (1995) Are chromosomal aberrations in circulating lymphocytes predictive of future cancer onset in humans? Preliminary results of an Italian cohort study. *Cancer Genet. Cytogenet.* **79**, 133–5.

40 Mustonen R *et al.* (1991) Measurement by ^{32}P-post-labelling of 7-methylguanine levels in white blood cell DNA of healthy individuals and cancer patients treated with dacarbazine and procarbazine. Human data and method development for 7-alkylguanines. *Carcinogenesis* **12**, 1423–33.

41 Kyrtopoulos SA *et al.* (1993) Accumulation of O6-methylguanine in human DNA after therapeutic exposure to methylating agents and its relationship with biological effects. *Environ. Health Perspect.* **99**, 143–7.

42 Fuchs J *et al.* (1995) DNA damage in nurses handling antineoplastic agents. *Mutation Res.* **342**, 17–23.

43 Fairbairn DW *et al.* (1995) The comet assay: a comprehensive review. *Mutation Res.* **339**, 37–59.

44 Sorsa M *et al.* (1992) Human cytogenetic damage as a predictor of cancer risk. *IARC Sci. Publ.* **116**, 543–54.

45 Bonassi S *et al.* (1994) Multiple regression analysis of cytogenetic human data. *Mutation Res.* **313**, 69–80.

46 Sorsa M *et al.* (1995) Biomonitoring of genotoxic anticancer drugs as a tool for improving work hygiene. *J. Oncol. Pharmacy Pract.* ISOPP IV Symposium issue.

47 Anon. (1988) *The control of substances hazardous to health regulations.* HMSO, London.

48 Van Raalte J *et al.* (1990) Visible-light system for detecting doxorubicin contamination on skin and surfaces. *Am. J. Hosp. Pharm.* **47**, 1067–74.

49 Dixon T (1990) Location of cytotoxic drug spillages using ultraviolet light. *Aust. J. Hosp. Pharm.* **20**, 469–70.

50 Wren AE *et al.* (1991) A novel technique for the validation of cytotoxic decontamination procedures. *Int. Pharm.* **5**, 119.

51 Personal communication (1995) M Douch, Quality Assurance Pharmacist, Pharmacy Support Unit, Colchester General Hospital, UK.

52 Harris J, Dodds LJ (1985) Handling of waste from patients receiving cytotoxic drugs. *Pharm. J.* **235**, 289–91.

53 Anon. (1986) OHSA work-practice guidelines for personnel dealing with cytotoxic (antineoplastic) drugs. *Am. J. Hosp. Pharm.* **43**, 1193–203.

54 Cass Y, Musgrave CF (1992) Guidelines for the safe handling of excreta contaminated by cytotoxic agents. *Am. J. Hosp. Pharm.* **49**, 1957–8.

55 Laidlaw JL *et al.* (1985) Permeability of four disposable protective-clothing materials to seven antineoplastic drugs. *Am. J. Hosp. Pharm.* **42**, 2449–54.

56 Glass DC *et al.* (1989) *The control of substances hazardous to health. Guidance for the initial assessment in hospitals.* HMSO, London.

57 Oldcorne MA *et al.* (1987) Handling cytotoxic drugs. *Pharm. J.* **238**, 488.

58 Thomas PH, Fenton-May V (1987) Protection offered by various gloves to carmustine exposure. *Pharm. J.* **238**, 775–7.

59 Slevin ML *et al.* (1984) The efficiency of protective gloves used in the handling of cytotoxic drugs. *Cancer Chemother. Pharmacol.* **12**, 151–3.

60 Laidlaw JL *et al.* (1984) Permeability of latex and polyvinyl chloride gloves to 20 antineoplastic drugs. *Am. J. Hosp. Pharm.* **41**, 2618–23.

61 Anon. (1987) Working Party Report – Guidelines for the handling of cytotoxic drugs: amendment. *Pharm. J.* **238**, 414.

62 Corlett SA *et al.* (1991) Permeation of ifosfamide through gloves and cadaver skin. *Pharm. J.* **247**, R39.

63 Colligan SA, Horstman SW (1990) Permeation of cancer chemotherapeutic drugs through glove materials under static and flexed conditions. *Appl. Occup. Environ. Hyg.* **5**, 848–52.

64 Ehntholt DJ *et al.* (1990) A test method for the evaluation of protective glove materials used in agricultural pesticide operations. *Am. Ind. Hyg. Assoc. J.* **51**, 462–8.

65 Kotilainen HR *et al.* (1989) Latex and vinyl examination gloves. Quality control procedures and implications for healthcare workers. *Arch. Intern. Med.* **149**, 2749–53.

66 Anon. (1980) *Joint circular from Department of Environment/Welsh Office, Control of Pollution (Special Waste) regulations.* HMSO, London.

67 Richardson ML, Bowron GM (1985) The fate of pharmaceutical chemicals in the aquatic environment. *J. Pharm. Pharmacol.* **37**, 1–12.

68 Appleby GE (1988) Disposal of pharmaceutical waste. *Pharm. J.* **240**, 100.

69 Gallelli JF (1988) Chemical destruction and disposal of antineoplastic drugs. In: *Proceedings of international symposium on oncology pharmacy practice*, Rotorua, New Zealand. New Zealand Hospital Pharmacists Association, Wellington, pp. 240–51.

70 Castegnaro M *et al.* (1985) *Laboratory decontamination and destruction of carcinogens in laboratory wastes.* International Agency for Research on Cancer, Scientific Publications No. 73, Oxford University Press, Fair Lane (NJ).

71 Armour MA *et al.* (1986) *Potentially carcinogenic chemicals: information and disposal guide*, University of Alberta. Terochem Laboratories Ltd, Edmonton.

72 Garner S *et al.* (1988) Disposal of waste cytotoxics. *Pharm. J.* **241**, Hospital Supplement 32.

4

Aspects of service operation

DOCUMENTATION

Adequate and efficient documentation is an essential aspect of a pharmacy-operated cytotoxic service. The design of documentation is clearly of importance in ensuring the maintenance of safe procedures and good records of service operation. Furthermore, the use of pharmacy-based documentation, such as patient treatment records, is a vital support to the pharmacist's professional role in ensuring optimal patient care and minimizing the risks of adverse events associated with chemotherapy. The range of documents used, their design, reproduction and updating aspects will vary widely between hospitals. They will be governed by local circumstances such as the scale of operation, the grades of staff involved and the extent to which computers are used.

It may be considered that for some services, documents can be combined or contain superfluous information. However, in this text all those aspects that require consideration have been indicated. Local circumstances then dictate whether or not they are included in the user documentation.

Most records are now computerized. However, the basic needs of documentation remain the same, whatever information system is utilized.

1 Documentation needs

The various aspects of cytotoxic services requiring documents for safe, reliable and cost-effective operation are shown in Figure 4.1. The actual document needs are summarized under each of the main categories depicted in the figure.

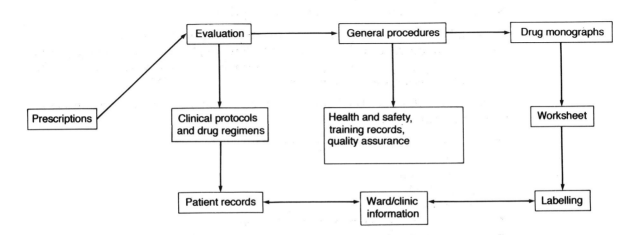

Figure 4.1: *Documentation required for cytotoxic services*

1.1 Prescriptions

There are several options regarding the ordering of chemotherapy.

- ▼ The patient's prescription may be sent to the pharmacy department.
- ▼ The patient's prescription may be transcribed at ward or clinic level by the visiting pharmacist.
- ▼ A specially designed order form completed by the clinician may be supplied to the pharmacy. This may have a worksheet incorporated in its design.
- ▼ Visual display units or fax machines may be used with terminals at ward, clinic and pharmacy level.

Where a prescription is used, it must fulfil the minimum legal requirements of a prescription for any cytotoxic medicine.

Local hospital or state policy may deem additional information necessary (e.g. patient diagnosis, chemotherapy regimen being used in concise terms, patient details (surface area, height, weight), cycle or pulse number, etc.).

An appropriate design must adequately satisfy the requirements of medical, nursing and pharmacy staff, and a degree of compromise may need to be negotiated.

1.2 Evaluation

Clinical protocols and drug regimens: Chemotherapy regimens are divided mainly into two groups:

- ▼ protocols that are part of a formal clinical trial
- ▼ regimens based on experience and subject to the clinician's expertise and judgement, many of them being standard first-line treatments.

Clinical trial protocols are often complex and subject to randomization. For quick reference it may be appropriate to summarize the pharmaceutical aspects in a card or file system, which details:

- ▼ schedules (induction, consolidation, maintenance, etc.)
- ▼ drug
- ▼ dose (/m² or /kg)
- ▼ how given (route, volume, equipment)
- ▼ timings (pulses, cycles, etc.)
- ▼ dosage reductions (when and how appropriate).

For standard treatment regimens, compilations of similar data from reference or from clinical sources can also be prepared. However, these are more likely to need updating frequently and hospital drug information units may be the appropriate means of gathering such information.

Prescription verification: The following checklist covers the key components of prescription verification:

- ▼ sufficient patient details are provided:
    full name
    hospital number
    date of birth
    diagnosis
- ▼ recognition of the regimen/protocol (reference source)
- ▼ the therapy prescribed is correct and complies with the reference source
- ▼ drug doses are calculated correctly against surface area/height/weight on prescription

- ▼ drug doses (single pulses within the cycle, stat doses, etc.) are time and date scheduled according to the protocol
- ▼ the form of administration: (route, diluent, volume, infusion rate) is acceptable and appropriate; for unlicensed drugs/routes of administration, a reference source should be provided by the prescriber, and the appropriate disclaimer documentation signed to accept liability
- ▼ patient record scrutiny will ensure that treatment progress through the protocol is appropriately timed; cycle delays, dose changes, protocol modifications, etc. should be documented within the pharmacy patient record.

Prescription checking: The checking process should be a separate stage between verification and final release of the product. A procedure based on a checklist such as the following should be implemented:

- ▼ the drug prepared is as stated on the label and as requested on the prescription
- ▼ the dose prepared is as stated on the label and as requested on the prescription
- ▼ diluents used are compatible with the drug
- ▼ infusion fluids are compatible with both drug and diluent used
- ▼ stability of the prepared drug is appropriate
- ▼ the storage conditions on the prepared drug label are appropriate
- ▼ the label details are correct
- ▼ all ingredients are batch number and expiry date checked and appropriate for use
- ▼ the intended route of administration is acceptable and appropriate.

1.3 General procedures

These should be clear, informative and comprehensive, covering all aspects of the pharmacy service. They should be readily accessible, comprehensible to all staff employed in the service and subject to regular review and updating.

Procedures covering the areas listed below are of particular importance:

- ▼ management structure
- ▼ receipt and storage of materials
- ▼ record keeping
- ▼ health and safety including:
    disposal of waste
    COSHH requirements
    handling
    spillage
    staff health monitoring
- ▼ preparation:
    general
    checking and labelling
    packing and distribution
    computer programs
- ▼ use of cabinet/isolator, including routine performance tests
- ▼ changing, including glove policies
- ▼ cleaning
- ▼ returned cytotoxics
- ▼ quality assurance standard operating procedures (SOPs) including:
    settle plates
    viable counts

finger dabs
surface sampling – swabs/contact plates
particle counting
di-octyl-phthalate (DOP) testing
process validation (broth transfers)
reading manometers.

For unlicensed products, advice and further information should be sought from the supplier. Such information should be documented for reference and reviewed regularly.

1.4 Worksheets

A general worksheet may be used for all drugs, or specific worksheets may be prepared for particular regimens. Prescription details can be transcribed on to the worksheet or the worksheet can be an integral part of the prescription.
Worksheets should include:

▼ name of the drug(s)
▼ presentation (physical form, quantity, strength, etc.)
▼ reconstituting solutions/diluents (identification and quantities to be added)
▼ resultant solutions (quantity in volume)
▼ compatible infusion solutions (where appropriate)
▼ storage details
▼ stability
▼ labelling details or sample label
▼ pertinent 'special precautions' (e.g. carmustine vials should be inspected before use for signs of decomposition of the drug).

They should allow the following to be recorded:

▼ batch numbers of all ingredients used
▼ the number of containers used
▼ the quantities of solutions to be drawn up or removed
▼ label duplicate
▼ identification of personnel involved in the preparation stages (formulation, assembly of ingredients, reconstitution, etc.)
▼ identification of personnel involved in the checking procedures.

1.5 Labelling

Labels should comply with national regulations and should state the:

▼ intended route of administration **(particular attention must be paid to identifying clearly preparations intended for intrathecal or regional administration; these must be distinguished from the 'standard' intravenous preparations to reduce the potential for administrative error)**
▼ name of the drug
▼ quantity of the drug
▼ vehicle containing the drug (infusion solution as appropriate)
▼ final volume
▼ batch number allocated to the product
▼ expiry date
▼ storage conditions that ensure stability, etc.

▼ patient's name and location (ward, etc.)
▼ name and address of the cytotoxic dispensary.

Outer packs for transport should also state clearly details of the contained items and any possible handling hazards.

1.6 Information documents for ward/clinic staff

These should comprise the elements listed below. The detail required will depend on local circumstances.

General introduction detailing local policies: These may include:

▼ designated areas on ward/clinic for the preparation of cytotoxic agents
▼ personnel (i.e. groups of staff appropriate to undertake reconstitution/ administration)
▼ protective garments that should be worn
▼ equipment that may be used
▼ extravasation policies
▼ disposal of waste.

Drug monographs: These will obviously be much less detailed than those required in pharmacy.

▼ Presentation.
▼ Reconstitution.
▼ Compatible solutions.
▼ Methods of administration.
▼ Special precautions (operator safety, extravasation, etc.).
▼ Stability.
▼ Accidental spillage (what to do in the event of).

Arrangements for the supply of cytotoxics from the pharmacy: These include:

▼ procedure for the agreed method of service operation at ward level (e.g. how and when to order)
▼ communication access (personnel to contact, telephone numbers, etc.)
▼ agreed presentations and possible alternatives for each drug.

QUALITY AUDIT SCHEMES FOR CYTOTOXICS RECONSTITUTION SERVICES

The activities which lead to the provision of a cytotoxic reconstitution service must be safe, effective and accord with the various standards and guidelines described in this Handbook and otherwise promulgated nationally and locally. These will be continually changing as new ideas emerge and improvements are proposed. It is therefore important that practices are frequently reviewed to ensure that standards are maintained. Even if services are subject to an accreditation process (e.g. by the UK Medicines Control Agency) the principle of self-inspection is commended, and professional audit is now well established in hospital pharmacy. Also, a systematic critique of process hazards should be undertaken as part of a risk management programme.

The audit process is based on peer review, it is therefore undertaken by colleagues who are well respected and fully conversant with the requirements of a cytotoxic reconstitution service. It is essential that the recommendations for change are, as far as possible, acted on and the 'acceptance criteria' are constantly reviewed to reflect current practice. The audit 'cycle' is not complete until change has been implemented and the effects of change have been assessed.

The following audit scheme provides a systematic approach to examining the structure and process aspects of a cytotoxic reconstitution service. The main objectives of the audit process are:

▼ to identify shortcomings and loopholes in procedures and processes
▼ to determine whether procedures are being followed and processes are being carried out effectively by competent staff
▼ to determine whether the facilities, equipment and environment comply with relevant standards
▼ to monitor quality trends and assess the effectiveness of management action to remedy perceived deficiencies
▼ to motivate staff to provide a safe, efficient and cost-effective service.

The audit form (Table 4.1, *see* Appendix, page 64) incorporates a rating scale for level of compliance and also guidance on the means of assessment for each acceptance criterion.

This audit scheme is not proffered as a definitive statement applicable to all situations; it is intended to be a model which can be adapted to local circumstances. It should also be regarded as one of a number of quality assurance mechanisms that can be applied. It does not, for instance, attempt to address the outcomes of the patient's treatment.

1 Guidance notes for using quality audit forms

Result ratings

1 Substantial compliance with acceptance criteria.
2 Significant compliance with acceptance criteria.
3 Partial compliance with acceptance criteria.
4 Minimal compliance with acceptance criteria.
5 Noncompliance with acceptance criteria.
NA Not applicable.

Glossary of terms used in connection with the checks required for each criterion.

Assess	requires the auditor(s) to use their professional judgement in attributing a compliance rating.
Data	generally relates to validation studies and evidence taken from the literature.
Examine	generally relates to procedures and/or materials which need to be examined, for content and validity.
Observe	generally relates to activities which can be observed by auditor(s) and are representative of normal work practices. In some situations it may be appropriate to do this covertly.
Procedure	relates to written procedures which should be assessed for appropriateness and compliance with official guidelines (e.g. by good manufacturing practice). They should have been recently appraised, signed and, where appropriate, countersigned (e.g. by quality control staff).
Records	generally relates to requirements for documentary evidence. These should be inspected at the auditor(s) discretion.
Test	applies to situations where the auditor(s) obtain their own evidence by test.

EDUCATION AND TRAINING

All staff employed to handle cytotoxic materials should receive education and training appropriate to their level of involvement in the handling, preparation or administration of the drugs.

A training programme should include practical experience, one-to-one teaching, learning exercises which may be tested and information on health and safety. A more advanced programme will also include clinical and theoretical training.

In some countries basic training for technical staff is by competency assessment. In the UK this is known as National Vocational Qualification (NVQ). National Vocational Qualifications are based on national occupational standards and have two arms:

▼ performance criteria, assessed by observation
▼ underpinning knowledge, assessed by questioning and written assignments.

These standards could be used as a baseline in the assessment of all staff and would highlight any training needs.

THE TRAINING CHECKLIST

A checklist is a good starting point for a formal or informal training programme. Staff may use the list simply as a guide to the areas that should be covered, or a more extensive programme may be written around the headings in a checklist.

The aim of the checklist (*see* Table 4.2) is that staff acquire knowledge of, and competence in, aseptic procedures, cytotoxic reconstitution, local procedures, current awareness, active information, management and research and development. These are intended as broad guidelines for training. Local variations will exist depending upon circumstance.

The degree of training required in each section depends on the level of involvement of different groups of staff in the provision of chemotherapy. The staff groups are indicated at the top of each column in Table 4.2.

Level 1 – Full time and rotational technicians involved with the provision of a cytotoxic reconstitution service.
Level 2 – Pre-registration pharmacists, junior/rotational pharmacists and senior pharmacists from other specialties.
Level 3 – Senior pharmacists and technical staff managing a sterile preparation or cytotoxic reconstitution service.

The checklist attempts to differentiate between activities that comprise a fundamental part of the individual's job and those where information only is required. In the former, competence must be demonstrated against the standards defined by the manager of the unit. The latter may be covered by directed reading/open learning programmes. Smaller units may require external support to cover some areas.

Table 4.2: *Education and training checklist*

	Level 1	Level 2	Level 3
ASEPTIC TECHNIQUE			
What it is	A	A	A
Why it is needed	A	A	A
How it is achieved	A	A	A
Test for ensuring and maintaining it	A	A	A
How to realize it has failed	A	A	A
What to do when it fails	A	A	A
CYTOTOXIC RECONSTITUTION			
What are cytotoxics	A	A	A
Why are they a hazard	A	A	A
How aerosols are generated	A	A	A
How aerosols are prevented	A	A	A
Other possible routes of exposure/contamination	A	A	A
General reconstitution techniques	A	A	A
Special reconstitution techniques	A	A	A
Use of special equipment	A	A	A
Correct documentation	A	A	A
Expiry and storage	A	A	A
Tests for ensuring, and maintaining, good technique	A	A	A
LOCAL PROCEDURES			
For aseptic technique	A	A	A
For cytotoxic reconstitution	A	A	A
USE OF EQUIPMENT			
Special reconstitution devices	A	A	A
Special administration devices	I	I	I
Evaluation of new equipment	A	A	A
CLINICAL DATA/PHARMACEUTICAL DATA			
Clinical notes	I	A	A
Laboratory tests	I	A	A
Disease evaluation tests	I	I	A
Clinical/nursing procedures	I	I	A
Administration procedures	I	A	A
Practical pharmacokinetics	I	A	A
EVALUATION OF INFORMATION			
Publications	I	A	A
Protocols	I	I	A
Basic statistics	A	A	A
Drug representatives	I	A	A
Promotional material	I	I	A
Spoken communications	A	A	A
OBTAINING DRUG/CLINICAL INFORMATION			
In-house	A	A	A
Reading list	I	A	A
Library	I	A	A

Key: A (activity) – trainee required to demonstrate competence in this area
  I (information) – trainee requires information only

Table 4.2: *Continued*

	Level 1	Level 2	Level 3
Oral communications	A	A	A
On-line via drug information centre	I	I	A
DATA HANDLING			
Protocols	A	A	A
Documentation	A	A	A
Workload statistics	A	I	A
Records	A	I	A
Clinical data	I	I	A
Adverse reaction reporting	I	I	A
Extravasation procedure	I	A	A
Mechanism of action	I	A	A
Overdose	I	A	A
Interactions with other drugs	I	A	A
Kinetics	I	I	A
Disposal	A	A	A
Legal and ethical considerations	A	A	A
HEALTH AND SAFETY REGULATIONS			
Nationally	A	I	A
Locally	A	A	A
Staff screening	A	I	A
Accident reporting	A	A	A
Accident procedure	A	A	A
HEALTH SERVICE BACKGROUND			
National framework for the provision of cytotoxic services	I	I	I
Current awareness	A	A	A
ACTIVE INFORMATION			
Bulletins	I	I	A
Seminars	I	I	A
Lectures	I	I	A
MANAGEMENT			
Education/training of appropriate pharmaceutical, nursing and medical staff	–	–	A
Monitoring of service quality	A	A	A
Work planning	A	A	A
Committee skills	–	–	I
Finance/budgeting	–	–	A
Interviewing	–	–	A
Guidelines for protocol submission, preparation and evaluation	–	–	A
RESEARCH AND DEVELOPMENT			
Service development	–	–	A
Technique evaluation	–	–	A
Drug evaluation	–	–	A
Publication	–	–	A

Key: A (activity) – trainee required to demonstrate competence in this area
I (information) – trainee requires information only

APPENDIX

Table 4.1: *Quality audit for cytotoxic reconstitutions*

HOSPITAL: DATE:

No.	Attribute	Acceptance criteria	Check required	Audit result	Comments and action to be taken
001	Medicines Act and Section 10 Exemptions (UK only)	The activities are carried out under the terms of a manufacturing licence; otherwise, the following conditions are met: 1 the preparation is done by, or under the supervision of, a pharmacist 2 the preparation uses 'closed' systems 3 products have an expiry date of no more than one week.	Assess Assess Records	Yes/No Yes/No Yes/No	
002	Facilities	Facilities are appropriate size for the activities undertaken	Assess	1 2 3 4 5 NA	
003		Facilities incorporate appropriate design features in terms of current GMP, ergonomics, security, work flow, ease of cleaning etc.	Assess	1 2 3 4 5 NA	
004		Facilities include sufficient shelves, cupboards, benches etc. for the activities undertaken	Assess	1 2 3 4 5 NA	
005		Walls, floors, ceilings, fixtures and fittings are in good decorative order and maintained to appropriate standards	Assess	1 2 3 4 5 NA	
006		Temperature, humidity control, lighting and noise levels provide comfortable working conditions for staff at all times of year	Assess	1 2 3 4 5 NA	
	Environmental acceptability (product protection)	(A) Applicable to use of a Modified Class 2 (BS 5726) microbiological safety cabinet			
007		Room used complies with Grade B air and tested at the designated frequencies	Records	1 2 3 4 5 NA	
008		Safety cabinet complies with Grade A air and tested at the designated frequencies	Records	1 2 3 4 5 NA	

Table 4.1: *Continued*

No.	Attribute	Acceptance criteria	Check required	Audit result	Comments and action to be taken
009		The direction of the air-flow air is inwards over the whole area of the work aperture (smoke test confirmation)	Records/ Test	1 2 3 4 5 NA	
010		The velocity of the down-flow air is in accordance with the requirements of BS 5726 (0.25–0.50 m/s)	Records	1 2 3 4 5 NA	
011		Safety cabinet/surrounding environment, changing areas, prep. rooms and personnel comply with standards for microorganisms	Records	1 2 3 4 5 NA	
012		Sterile cleanroom garments/face mask/ gloves used each session	Observe/ Procedure	1 2 3 4 5 NA	
013		Cleaning records comply with schedule and the cleaning procedures are appropriate	Records/ Assess	1 2 3 4 5 NA	
014		Manometer readings show adequate differential pressure and are recorded daily	Records	1 2 3 4 5 NA	
015		All items are swabbed with spore-free 70% v/v IMS/ IPA before entering the room and again before transfer into the safety cabinet, and the process has been validated	Observe/ Procedure/ Records	1 2 3 4 5 NA	
		(B) Applicable to use of negative pressure isolator system			
016		Air in controlled work space complies with Grade A air in the non-operational state and tested at the designated frequencies	Records	1 2 3 4 5 NA	
017		Background environment complies with appropriate standard for air quality according to the design of the isolator and transfer device used and tested at the designated frequencies	Records	1 2 3 4 5 NA	

Table 4.1: *Continued*

No.	Attribute	Acceptance criteria	Check required	Audit result	Comments and action to be taken
018		Cleaning records comply with schedule (including gaseous sterilization of the inside of the cabinet when applicable), and the cleaning procedures are appropriate	Records	1 2 3 4 5 NA	
019		Air pressure and filter status within the isolator are monitored continuously. An alarm indicates when these fall outside defined limits	Assess	1 2 3 4 5 NA	
020		Before preparation starts, pressure drops across filters, isolator pressure differentials and airflow rates are checked to confirm they are within limits, and no alarm condition is indicated	Examine	1 2 3 4 5 NA	
021		The transfer device allows transfer of items into the controlled work space without compromising the Grade A environment, and the process has been validated	Assess/ Records	1 2 3 4 5 NA	
022		Dedicated clothing is worn by isolator operators which is appropriate to the background environment	Assess	1 2 3 4 5 NA	
023		Gloves/garments comply with the limits for perforations specified in BS 4005; 1984 (sterile latex surgeons' gloves)	Examine	1 2 3 4 5 NA	
024		The procedure for changing gloves prevents a risk to the integrity of the isolator system and the process has been validated	Assess/ Data	1 2 3 4 5 NA	
025		All items are sprayed/ swabbed with 70% v/v IMS/IPA before entering the transfer hatch and, again, before entering the controlled work space	Observe/ Procedure/ Records	1 2 3 4 5 NA	
026	Environmental acceptability operator protection	Safety cabinet complies with KI discus test and tested within one year (not applicable for isolators)	Records	1 2 3 4 5 NA	

Table 4.1: *Continued*

No.	Attribute	Acceptance criteria	Check required	Audit result	Comments and action to be taken
027		Systems prevent disturbance of air currents during use of cabinet, including opening/closing of door to room (not applicable for isolators)	Procedure/ Assess	1 2 3 4 5 NA	
028		Appropriate type of garments, including gloves, used by staff	Assess	1 2 3 4 5 NA	
029		The glove/sleeve system allows adequate dexterity in use and gloves are replaced as necessary (isolators only)	Assess	1 2 3 4 5 NA	
030		Luer-lock syringes and large-bore needles used during manipulations	Observe/ Procedure	1 2 3 4 5 NA	
031		Appropriate air-venting of vials occurs to prevent pressure differentials	Observe/ Procedure	1 2 3 4 5 NA	
032	Health and safety	All personnel are aware of and comply with the local health and safety policy on handling of cytotoxic materials	Assess	1 2 3 4 5 NA	
033		Acceptable procedure for dealing with spillage in existence	Examine	1 2 3 4 5 NA	
034		Appropriate receptacles for contaminated liquids, 'sharps' and other consumables available	Assess	1 2 3 4 5 NA	
035		Appropriate procedure for disposal of contaminated waste available	Examine	1 2 3 4 5 NA	
036		Occupational health arrangements include regular monitoring of all staff working with cytotoxic drugs	Records	1 2 3 4 5 NA	
037	Documentation (general)	All documentation is subject to a system of control which includes regular review, the maintenance of an audit trail and, for computerized systems, a means of restricting access to authorized staff only	Assess	1 2 3 4 5 NA	

Table 4.1: *Continued*

No.	Attribute	Acceptance criteria	Check required	Audit result	Comments and action to be taken
038		Satisfactory standard operating procedures have been written/approved for all items of equipment	Examine	1 2 3 4 5 NA	
039		Worksheets for all different cytotoxic preparations have been written/approved	Examine	1 2 3 4 5 NA	
040		Satisfactory procedures have been written, signed and dated on the following:			
		a) changing and hand-sanitation prior to entry into preparation area (and is displayed)	Examine/ Observe	1 2 3 4 5 NA	
		b) cleaning and maintenance	Examine	1 2 3 4 5 NA	
		c) environmental and microbiological control	Examine	1 2 3 4 5 NA	
		d) other routine quality control testing	Examine	1 2 3 4 5 NA	
		e) health and safety policy	Examine	1 2 3 4 5 NA	
041	Prescription verification	The prescribed cytotoxics are in accordance with chemotherapy regimen/ protocol and prescription is explicit in terms of dose, route/rate of administration, time frequency and duration of treatment	Examine	1 2 3 4 5 NA	
042		The prescriptions are signed by authorized medical staff	Examine	1 2 3 4 5 NA	
043		The prescriptions can be related to current patient data including diagnosis, age, sex, body weight, height, surface area, haematology and renal function, as appropriate	Examine	1 2 3 4 5 NA	
044		Doses that have been calculated by the prescriber are checked independently	Procedure Assess	1 2 3 4 5 NA	
045	Compounding	Documentary evidence of correct reconstitution	Records	1 2 3 4 5 NA	
046		Evidence to show that the product is stable and an appropriate shelf-life in the container has been assigned	Data	1 2 3 4 5 NA	
047		Other documentary evidence completed and satisfactory	Records	1 2 3 4 5 NA	

Table 4.1: *Continued*

No.	Attribute	Acceptance criteria	Check required	Audit result	Comments and action to be taken
048		Evidence to show that correct solutions incorporated into syringe/bag	Observe	1 2 3 4 5 NA	
049	Presentation	Label has acceptable legibility	Examine Sample	1 2 3 4 5 NA	
050		Label indicates route of injection and includes appropriate hazard warnings (note special warnings for vinca alkaloids)	Examine Sample	1 2 3 4 5 NA	
051		Label bears unambiguous expression of ingredients/ quantities	Examine Sample	1 2 3 4 5 NA	
052		Label shows correct expiry date/time	Examine Sample	1 2 3 4 5 NA	
053		Label shows correct storage conditions if other than room temperature	Examine Sample	1 2 3 4 5 NA	
054		Outer packaging is properly sealed and prevents contents leaking during transit	Examine Sample	1 2 3 4 5 NA	
055		Contents clear, and free from visible particles	Examine Sample	1 2 3 4 5 NA	
056	Personnel	An agreed and defined management structure	Assess	1 2 3 4 5 NA	
057		Written training and education manual	Examine	1 2 3 4 5 NA	
058		Training records are maintained	Examine	1 2 3 4 5 NA	
059		Appropriately trained and, where appropriate, super-vised pharmacists/pharmacy technicians undertake the manipulations	Assess	1 2 3 4 5 NA	
060		Staff perform satisfactory process validations at defined intervals e.g. three-monthly	Records	1 2 3 4 5 NA	
061	Effective use of resources	Notification of pharmacy by ward/clinic allows convenient scheduling	Assess	1 2 3 4 5 NA	
062		Most cost-effective grade(s) of staff are used	Assess	1 2 3 4 5 NA	

Table 4.1: *Continued*

No.	Attribute	Acceptance criteria	Check required	Audit result	Comments and action to be taken
063		Choice of units of ingredients minimizes wastage	Assess	1 2 3 4 5 NA	
064		The ingredients carry the nearest expiry date of stock	Examine	1 2 3 4 5 NA	
065		The wastage of disposables used is minimal	Observe	1 2 3 4 5 NA	
066	Storage/ distribution and administration	Contents are suitably protected against heat/light etc.	Examine	1 2 3 4 5 NA	
067		Where products are refrigerated, the fridge temperatures are in the appropriate temperature range and are monitored	Examine Records	1 2 3 4 5 NA	
068		Syringes/bags are suitably protected for transport to ward/clinic	Examine	1 2 3 4 5 NA	
069		Bags can be delivered to ward/clinic by intended time of administration	Assess	1 2 3 4 5 NA	
070		Syringes/bags are appropriately stored on the ward if not to be used immediately and do not exceed their expiry date	Assess	1 2 3 4 5 NA	

	NAME:	JOB TITLE:	SIGNATURE:	DATE:

Auditor 1:

Auditor 2:

Auditor 3:

Other staff present:

Copies sent to:

Next audit date:

5

Administration of chemotherapy

INTRODUCTION

This chapter brings together many of the issues which need to be considered when preparing for, or administering, chemotherapy. By its very nature it covers a wide diversity of issues, both practical and theoretical, starting with the physical environment and location. This Handbook reflects the growing trend in the oncology community away from long inpatient stays that inflict considerable morbidity on both the patient and their carers and family, towards outpatient and day-care chemotherapy, as well as the broadening horizons for community and/or home-based chemotherapy.

The physical, pharmacological advantages and disadvantages of this type of therapy, as well as the educational, documentational and safety aspects are discussed. Finally, the chapter gives some consideration to the advantages and disadvantages of the vast variety of alternative routes of administration for chemotherapy which are increasingly entering routine clinical use, and presents a wide variety of issues both in terms of stability in new delivery systems or fluids, and from a practical point of view with regard to preparing and monitoring 'old' drugs in new environments.

NON-HOME ENVIRONMENT

Despite enormous research effort into determining the value of different cytotoxic drugs and combinations in the treatment of malignancies, and the development of protocols for the safe prescription and administration of chemotherapy by most hospitals and oncology departments, relatively little attention has been paid to the environment in which treatment is given. In the UK, only a few of the newest centres have accommodation designed specifically for the administration of chemotherapy. Often this activity is carried out in whatever ward or clinic area the oncology department has occupied for the last few decades, with little concession to the increasing number of patients receiving chemotherapy and the increasing complexity of their treatments.

Consideration of the facilities required for the safe administration of chemotherapy in the community and at home, where an increasing number of patients are being treated, has also been scant. Some of the factors that must be considered in creating a pleasant and safe environment for chemotherapy administration are discussed below.

1 Inpatient chemotherapy

At present, many patients receiving routine chemotherapy are admitted to wards attempting to cater for a broad cross-section of oncology patients. This may be inappropriate given the different needs of patients receiving active treatment and those receiving palliative care after the exhaustion of active treatment options. It also creates problems for staff trying to balance the need to expedite the treatment of short-stay chemotherapy patients, who are in a hurry to get on with their treatment, with the sometimes less urgent – but equally as important – physical, spiritual and emotional needs of chronic patients. One solution to this conflict is to have separate nursing teams looking after these two patient populations.

The physical environment on most medical wards is satisfactory for the administration of chemotherapy, though small bed clusters of two, four or at maximum six beds, with an appropriate balance of side or single bedrooms within the total ward or unit area may be more appropriate than traditional open wards for patients whose intravenous therapy requires regular attention during the night, when nursing intervention may disturb neighbouring patients, and whose disease and treatment require a very careful balance between privacy and camaraderie.

Bathroom facilities on wards with large numbers of chemotherapy recipients may also need to be expanded. Many patients will receive large quantities of intravenous fluid and some will also suffer gastrointestinal upset resulting in frequent visits to the toilet.

If chemotherapy is being administered on a ward, cytotoxic-contaminated waste will be produced and proper facilities need to be available for the safe storage of such material prior to disposal. Any storage area should be readily cleaned in the event of any spillage.

As important as the ward layout is its communication with other key departments, notably pathology and pharmacy. Chemotherapy cannot proceed until blood counts and, often, blood biochemistry have been checked, nor until pharmacy-prepared cytotoxic doses are available on the ward. Similarly, patient discharge is dependent upon the delivery to the ward of any discharge medication dispensed by pharmacy. Therefore, an oncology ward should, ideally, be situated very close to both pathology and pharmacy departments and either adequate provision made for portering between ward and departments or investment made in vacuum line technology.

In a busy oncology unit, consideration should be given to establishing a satellite pharmacy unit at ward level. If such a unit is planned, this must be done with input from sufficiently experienced pharmacy staff to ensure that it will be of an adequate size and specification to meet the demands that are likely to be placed upon it.

2 Day-patient chemotherapy

An increasing number of patients who would formerly have been treated as inpatients are now receiving chemotherapy in day-case units. This approach has obvious cost advantages to the treatment centre and is, in general, preferred by patients. The facilities needed for the administration of prolonged and complex chemotherapy regimens in this way are more akin to those needed on an oncology ward than those traditionally provided in a medical outpatient clinic. For example, patients need access to beds so that they can lie down if they feel tired or unwell, or are being subjected to procedures, like intrathecal drug therapy, which require it. Beds should be in an area that affords an appropriate degree of privacy. There should be refreshment facilities and, ideally, a social area with television etc. to help patients pass the time and to provide distraction.

Nursing staff also need adequate facilities for storing drugs, dressings and other disposables correctly, and for the preparation of non-cytotoxic drug doses in a clean, calm and quiet environment where interruptions are kept to a minimum in order to reduce the risk of mistakes.

As with ward areas (*see* previous page) consideration needs to be given to the provision of facilities for the storage of cytotoxic waste, adequate toilet facilities, and to the proximity of day-treatment areas to the departments of pharmacy and pathology. In addition, facilities must be available, close at hand, for dealing with patients who become acutely unwell during treatment and require overnight hospitalization.

Very few therapies need to be performed as an inpatient stay. This is due to the increasing sophistication of support therapies (e.g. antiemetics). With careful education and selection of patients, even cisplatinum-based therapy can be performed on a day-case basis.

3 Outpatient chemotherapy

Outpatients will continue to be the largest group of chemotherapy recipients in the foreseeable future, and their numbers are increasing rapidly in the UK. Unfortunately, the chemotherapy they receive is still, too often, administered in inadequate facilities.

Problems often begin upon arrival in clinic when patients are kept waiting long periods to see a doctor, to have blood samples taken and processed, to have their chemotherapy prepared and administered and, finally, for any take-home medication to be prepared by pharmacy.

Such delays are, at best, unpleasant, but disastrous for patients experiencing anticipatory, or post-chemotherapy nausea and vomiting. Many delays reported are the result of inadequate resourcing, particularly when patient throughput is increased without a corresponding expansion in the support staff looking after them, but others can be kept to a minimum by good organization.[1]

Almost all of the organizational and operational systems discussed with regard to day-case chemotherapy facilities apply equally well to outpatient treatment. However, the functional links between the chemotherapy clinic and the pharmacy and pathology departments are even more critical given the need to minimize patient delays. Indeed, in any large and busy clinic, the arguments for an on-site pharmacy become compelling.

HOME ENVIRONMENT

1 Potential benefits of home chemotherapy

Traditionally, a considerable proportion of patients have been admitted to hospital as inpatients or as day-case patients to receive their chemotherapy. This may be socially, geographically or psychologically difficult for either the patient or their carer(s); and despite the best facilities, staff and supportive therapies available in a designated treatment centre, it is the desire of most patients to be able to remain at home and to live as normal a life-style as possible.[2] Demand for home-based treatment combined with developments in drug administration technology has resulted in the emergence of domiciliary chemotherapy programmes, where the patient is able to receive parenteral chemotherapy in their home.

Home-based chemotherapy not only reduces the stress and inconvenience of attending hospital but also enables the patient to take an active role in their treatment.

Home chemotherapy enables the patient to enjoy greater independence, particularly if the chemotherapy is self-administered. The active involvement of patients in their treatment tends to encourage a more positive attitude to chemotherapy. Drug-related adverse effects may be more readily tolerated if patients are able to remain at home with their families in familiar surroundings.

Families of cancer patients often experience a feeling of helplessness and inadequacy and home-based treatment provides an opportunity for families and close friends to give assistance and support with treatment. All of these factors can contribute to increased morale of patients and their families.

Psychological studies[3] on both domiciliary and hospitalized patients receiving similar chemotherapy regimens have demonstrated an improved quality of life and a greater sense of well-being in home-based patients. Evidence suggests that quality of life is also schedule-dependent and favours patients receiving chemotherapy by continuous infusion.[4] Home treatment also reduces the potential exposure of immunocompromised cancer patients to hospital infections.[2]

A properly managed, home chemotherapy programme can reduce costs associated with hospitalization and increase treatment availability. In a randomized study of inpatient versus outpatient continuous infusion chemotherapy for patients with locally advanced head and neck cancer, Vokes et al.[5] estimated a reduction in daily costs of $366 per patient for domiciliary chemotherapy.

2 Limitations of home chemotherapy

In the home setting, professional assistance is not readily available to the patient. Acute drug-related toxicity, equipment failure, extravasation of the drug infusion, thrombus formation, blockage, and/or infection of the central venous catheter are difficulties which may cause patients severe distress. Acute toxicity can be kept to a minimum by:

▼ using adequate supportive medication
▼ continuous ambulatory infusions for drug delivery
▼ pharmacodynamic individualization of drug dosage.

It is essential that patients are given thorough training in how to react in cases of equipment failure and that this is supported by written instructions and a 24 hour telephone number to enable home-based patients to contact a member of the oncology team. Most complications can be anticipated and dealing with them forms an integral part of the patient training programme. With experienced home care oncology teams, complications are rare and catheter infection rates of less than 1% are obtainable.[6] Furthermore, the health care team must expect and anticipate either new or alternative manifestations of drug toxicities.

Some patients are incapable of maintaining their treatment at home. This may be because they are unable to understand basic instructions relating to their treatment or because of a physical disability (e.g. arthritis) that would prevent them from handling the infusion device and other equipment. In some cases support from family or friends may not be available and communications with the hospital-based oncology team may be difficult (e.g. the patient may not have access to a telephone). Some patients may prefer the security of a hospital and are unwilling to take on the responsibility of home-based treatment. Careful patient selection is essential and will exert a profound influence on the outcome of home chemotherapy.

The economics of home chemotherapy may not always be viewed in a favourable light, largely because health care financial systems are inflexible and geared to inpatient treatment. Although home chemotherapy may release hospital beds, costs will increase if these are subsequently occupied by other patients. At best, home-based treatment provides hospital managers with a choice to:

▼ either reduce the number of oncology beds and save money
▼ or re-occupy released beds with other patients (not necessarily cancer patients) and reduce the waiting lists.

In addition, savings made at ward level may be difficult to transfer to the budgets of those departments (e.g. pharmacy) where expenditure is increased as a result of home chemotherapy.

3 Patient selection

Careful patient selection is crucial to the success of a home chemotherapy programme. Before the option of domiciliary treatment is offered, the clinician must establish that the patient is well motivated, physically capable of managing their medication syringes, infusion pump or other equipment and that they are able to understand the detailed instructions. Normally, patients should have a reasonable performance status (Karnofsky score of at least 60) and should be capable of enjoying a satisfactory quality of life during home treatment. Ideally, support should be available from family and friends who are able to adjust their own routines in order to help care for the patient. The availability of transport to and from the oncology outpatient clinic must be considered and although it is possible to offer home chemotherapy to patients who live some distance from their hospital, access to a telephone is essential.

Patients with a wide range of cancers, including leukaemias (during remission) and solid tumours can be treated in the domiciliary setting.[6-8] In many cases, home patients are receiving palliative treatment for recurrent disease following surgery or radiotherapy and the disease may be at an advanced stage. Patients in the last stages of disease or with fistulae, internal bleeding, ascites, systemic infection or severe nutritional deficiency are clearly not suitable for home treatment. Similarly, those patients who are unable to cope with the psychological and emotional stress associated with cancer should be offered the professional care available in the hospital or hospice system.

4 The home oncology team

The success of home-based chemotherapy is dependent upon a team approach towards patient care. The team would typically include:

▼ consultant oncologist
▼ oncology nurse
▼ oncology pharmacist.

Chemotherapy by continuous infusion using ambulatory pumps may be placed by a surgeon or anaesthetist, or if peripherally inserted, can be placed by trained nurses. If home-based patients are receiving ambulatory chemotherapy at least one member of the team (usually the pharmacist or nurse) should be available

24 hours a day to deal with any problems that may arise with infusion pumps or the central venous catheter.

The team should also be able to call upon the resources of other departments, such as microbiology and medical electronics (for testing and calibration of infusion pumps). If home chemotherapy is to be based on nurse-administered bolus or short infusion schedules, the team should contain a fully trained oncology nurse. It is, of course, essential that the patient's general practitioner is informed of the treatment. If it becomes necessary to switch from chemotherapy to pain control, the venous access system used for chemotherapy can then be used for the infusion of opiates. In these cases, hospice nurses may become involved in the preparation and administration of opiate or other analgesic/antiemetic infusions.

5 Patient procedures

Although based on the experience of a UK home treatment centre[6,9] the patient procedures described below represent a typical approach common to other home oncology centres.

Suitable patients are introduced to the concept of home chemotherapy (and prolonged continuous infusion, if appropriate) by a senior member of the medical team. If a patient decides to accept the option of home-based treatment they may then be referred to the oncology pharmacist for a more detailed explanation of the treatment. In some centres the patient is invited to view a video presentation, together with the oncology pharmacist, in which health care professionals discuss various aspects of home chemotherapy with previously treated patients and their relatives. The video would normally deal with specific issues of interest to the patient, including insertion of the central venous catheter, changing of medication reservoirs, management of the infusion pump or venous access port, and care of the dressing at the site of catheter entry. The video presentation may also include previously treated patients discussing their treatment, their life-style, and any difficulties they encountered with the infusion pump. This often prompts the prospective patient to raise questions about the treatment and provides an opportunity for any anxieties or fears to be raised. In some institutions the oncology pharmacist is required to take on the role of counsellor; a role that will be developed with each new patient as they attend the oncology outpatient clinic for routine assessment.

Normally the patient is admitted to the oncology ward for insertion of the central venous catheter. This is an aseptic procedure and is carried out under local anaesthetic by an experienced anaesthetist. Prior to discharge from hospital, the patient is trained in the management of their treatment by the oncology pharmacist. The patient is taught how to operate the infusion pump, how to recognize and respond to any warning alarms the pump may have, how to store medication reservoirs and change them in the pump when necessary. Instruction is given in the safe disposal of cytotoxic waste and used medication reservoirs. Often potential problems can be anticipated and dealt with before they arise. For example, patients are often concerned by the presence of a small bubble of air in the infusion catheter. This is not clinically significant and the patient can be reassured before they even experience the problem themselves. Occasionally the patient forgets to close the tap on the catheter before disconnecting the medication reservoir, resulting in venous blood flowing out through the catheter. Difficulties of this nature and the necessary action to take are always discussed with the patients before they leave the hospital. The patient remains on the ward until the pharmacist is satisfied that they are fully competent. This usually takes 24 to 48 hours.

In some cases it may be advisable to train patients' relatives in the relevant techniques so that they are able to offer constructive support to the patient. As a back-up to the training programme, patients also receive concise written instructions and are given telephone numbers which may be used to contact oncology nurses or the oncology pharmacist, 24 hours a day. With the development of peripherally inserted central venous catheters there may be less need to hospitalize patients for catheter insertion. It is important, however, to ensure that adequate time is made available for patient training.

On discharge from hospital, the patient is supplied with pre-filled syringes or a medication reservoir for ambulatory pump use, or with pre-filled syringes for bolus injection. Where drug stability permits, the patient is supplied with sufficient medication for 14 days of treatment (or if the treatment schedule is based on a period of less than 14 days, sufficient medication to complete the course). During breaks in chemotherapy, to permit bone marrow recovery, heparinized saline is supplied to ensure that the subclavian catheter remains patent.

The patient is also given supplies of consumables to take home. These include spare batteries for infusion pumps, protective gloves, sterile wipes for absorbing any minor spillage and burn-bins for disposing cytotoxic waste and used syringes/medication reservoirs. To help protect other members of the patient's household from inadvertent cytotoxic drug contamination, home-based patients should be supplied with a small, locking drug refrigerator (complete with thermometer) for storage of their medication and a spillage clean-up kit to contain and decontaminate accidental drug spillages (*see* page 91).

Patients attend the oncology outpatient clinic usually every two weeks where they are seen by the consultant oncologist who monitors the patient's clinical condition. The dressing at the site of catheter entry is changed by the oncology nurse. Outpatient visits also present an opportunity for the oncology pharmacist to deal with any infusion pump-related problems or queries concerning adverse effects from medication. During these fortnightly visits, patients collect further supplies of consumables from the outpatient clinic and further supplies of medication from the hospital pharmacy.

Some patients participating in home chemotherapy programmes will be entered into controlled clinical trials, usually of a phase II or phase III nature. Visits to the outpatient clinic provide the clinician with an opportunity to monitor the patient extensively and to determine the quality of life enjoyed by the patient during treatment. If pharmacokinetic studies also form part of the trial, it is preferable for blood samples to be taken by a visiting oncology nurse (or pharmacist trained in phlebotomy), rather than subject the patient to repeated hospital visits.

6 Preparation of medication for home chemotherapy patients

The introduction of a home chemotherapy programme is likely to affect the workload of the hospital pharmacy department in several areas. Consideration should be given to resource and funding implications before a home chemotherapy programme is implemented.

Unless the number of hospital-based oncology beds is reduced, the introduction of home chemotherapy may result in an increased patient throughput. This would be reflected by increased demands for the preparation of cytotoxic infusions and increased expenditure on the drugs budget. The preparation of pre-filled medication reservoirs for ambulatory infusion pumps will require additional staff training.

In the case of home chemotherapy it must be recognized that even pre-filled syringes for bolus medication may be stored in the patient's refrigerator for several weeks before use. Drug infusions delivered by ambulatory pumps are not only stored for long periods (up to 14 days) under refrigerated conditions before use but are also subjected to temperatures of 35–37°C in the pump reservoir worn under the patient's clothing. It is, therefore, essential to determine the physical and chemical stability of infusions used in home chemotherapy regimens when under storage (4–8°C) and in use (35–37°C). Exposure time will vary according to the type of infusion pump used. Pre-filled syringes used in the Graseby syringe driver usually contain a maximum of 24 hours supply of medication and are changed daily by the patient. If it is proposed to give a full 14 days supply of medication, stability studies should be carried out under storage conditions (4–8°C) over 14 days and under in-use conditions (35–37°C) over 24 hours. In the case of infusion pumps with large-volume cassettes or pouch-type medication reservoirs which contain sufficient infusion for five to 14 days treatment (depending on the regimen), drug stability under in-use conditions (35–37°C) should be determined over the treatment period. Since medication cassettes/pouches are normally connected to the infusion pump within 24 hours of preparation, stability studies under storage conditions (4–8°C) need only be continued over 24 hours. If, however, two pre-filled medicated cassettes/pouches are supplied to give a total of 14 days treatment, drug stability would be determined over seven days under both storage and in-use conditions. It is advisable to monitor the temperature of the drug refrigerator supplied to each patient to ensure that medication is stored at the correct temperature.

Stability data for drug infusions in ambulatory infusion devices (where applicable) are given in the individual drug monographs on pages 181 to 391.

Provision of several days or weeks supply of medication to home patients necessitates a marked deviation from the 'ideal' practice of commencing drug administration within 24 hours of preparation. The chemical and physical stability of the drug infusion must be established and the microbiological aspects of long-term supply must also be considered. It cannot be assumed that cytotoxic infusions are bactericidal[10] and it is, therefore, essential that all equipment associated with the aseptic preparation of medication for home patients is carefully monitored, and that all procedures are thoroughly validated. In the UK recent guidelines issued by the Department of Health[11] preclude the assignment of a shelf-life of more than seven days to any aseptically dispersed product, irrespective of data that would support a longer expiry period.

This guidance will largely restrict the preparation of medication supplies for home use to those centres licensed for the manufacture of aseptic 'specials' by the UK Medicines Control Agency where longer, more practical shelf-lives are permitted, providing stability and aseptic procedures have been validated.

COMMUNITY CHEMOTHERAPY

Community or outreach chemotherapy represents the latest and perhaps most logical development for day care, outpatient and home-based chemotherapy. Either a mobile unit or specified partially-dedicated community facility (e.g. a treatment room in a large general practitioner practice) is established, and staffed or visited on a timetabled basis. The mobile unit or outreach centre is staffed by a combination of primary and secondary health care workers, thus giving a much better balance of expertise and 'trusted friend', bridging the health care interface and so delivering seamless care to the cancer patient.

The centre actively delivers chemotherapy at predetermined times but is also available as a 'drop-in' centre to deal with physical or psychological problems on an extended 'full-time' basis.

Outreach centres are a co-ordinating cancer centre in that they will screen potential patients, establish care plans and act as a safety and communication bridge for the network. One centre or mobile unit can cover a population of 100 000 to 150 000 and is thus sized to be viable whilst still being able to cater to the needs of local patients. The outreach centres suit urban and inner-city areas, whilst mobile centres suit rural communities.

Patients utilizing the service can receive either bolus or continuous infusion chemotherapy and can use one or more of the centres with prior arrangement (e.g. the one nearest to their home and work). They can use any one of the outreach posts or centres in case of emergency. This has been facilitated by one-press 'Help' buttoned autodial mobile telephones, a simple safety procedure with direct 24 hour hospital contact and access backup and 'smart' cards with patients' relevant medical histories.[12]

AMBULATORY INFUSION PUMPS FOR CYTOTOXIC THERAPY

Introduction

Traditionally, cytotoxic chemotherapy has been administered in single or combined regimens designed to maximize cell-kill whilst minimizing toxicity. However, in practice, these high dose, 'pulsed' regimens are not always ideal because of the need to hospitalize patients and the high incidence of side-effects which can delay further therapy.

Evidence has shown that continuous infusion of a low dose of a cytotoxic drug achieves equivalent or higher tumour concentrations over a longer period than bolus, pulsed therapy,[13] and that clinical benefits, particularly in terms of reduced toxicity[14] and improved quality of life,[4] may be achieved.

In response to the demand for this method of administration, there have been rapid advances in pump technology. A wide variety of ambulatory infusion pumps is now available, ranging in complexity from external syringe drivers to implantable, programmable pumps. Some of the more recent introductions offer particularly advanced electronic features, including the ability to print out an infusion history for clinical audit purposes and programming facilities to emulate circadian drug delivery to exploit the perceived advantages of chronotherapy in cancer treatment.[15]

In many ways the pace of ambulatory infusion device development has increased the difficulties of device selection. Studies that compare the different ambulatory infusion pumps available have defined some of the clinical, economic and pharmaceutical parameters of relevance to the selection process.[16,17] Pump selection influences the clinical outcome of ambulatory treatment and also the quality of life experienced by the patient.[18] It is essential that health care professionals involved in ambulatory care have a detailed knowledge of infusion devices to facilitate appropriate device selection. For this and other reasons (training, spare-parts inventory etc.) it is preferable that the number of different devices used within an institution is limited and that they are selected by objective evaluation, rather than by individual preference.

The pumps described below represent a selection of those available in the UK and US and are by no means intended to be comprehensive. Ambulatory pumps using new technologies such as *in situ* gas generation (e.g. Smart-dose device) are not included because these have been developed for infusion of non-cytotoxic drugs and the range of flow rates and reservoir sizes are, as yet, not suited to the administration of chemotherapy.

A larger range of pumps is available worldwide and readers are directed to the literature available in their own country for details of additional types of pump which have been used for the administration of cytotoxic chemotherapy.

SYRINGE PUMPS

Models: Braun Medical, Perfusor M (Figure 5.1); Perfusor ME; Graseby Medical, MS16A (Figure 5.2) and MS26; Critikon, Syringe Minder 2

Syringe pumps are pocket-sized, usually battery-operated and are simple in design with only a few alarms, e.g. low battery, end of infusion and occlusion pressure. They use a range of syringes from 1 ml to 35 ml, although individual models may be limited to a narrower range.

The drug reservoir is a pre-filled syringe firmly clamped on to the pump. The pump is driven by a small battery-powered motor or, in the case of the Braun, Perfusor M, by a clockwork mechanism. A rotating lead screw (or drive shaft)

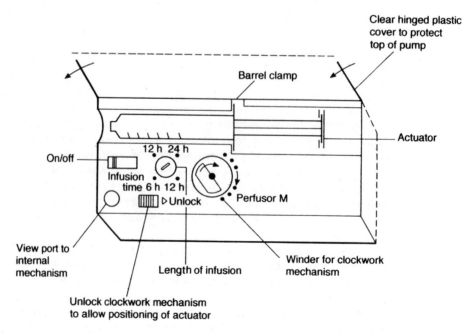

Figure 5.1: *Braun Medical Perfusor M pump*

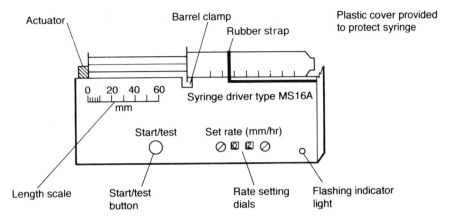

Figure 5.2: *Gaseby MS16A pump*

moves the actuator (or drive nut) down the device at a constant rate, pushing the syringe plunger into the syringe barrel. The delivery rate of the drug is determined by the diameter of the syringe and the speed at which the lead screw rotates. The Perfusor ME is identical to the Perfusor M but is fitted with an alarm to indicate the end of the infusion.

Syringe pumps have been used successfully for self-administration of cytotoxic agents.[6,19] They can be used with variable flow rates to a high level of accuracy (± 2% to 5%). Due to the pressure generated, the pump can be used for both intra-arterial and intravenous infusions. Syringe size is a limiting factor and, if large volumes are required, it is necessary to replace the syringe reservoir several times during treatment. This can be an advantage in the case of infusions with poor stability since the infusion is exposed to in-use operating temperatures (33–37°C) for relatively short periods.

To set up the pumps, the administration line is primed either manually, before putting the syringe in the pump, or by a venting mechanism, if included in the pump. Priming should be carried out prior to rate setting in pumps that use the mm/h or mm/day system, since at low infusion rates the dead volume of the tubing could alter the final infusion time by several hours. The syringe is placed into the pump and fixed in position. The actuator should be placed as close to the plunger as possible, so that there is little slack to take up in the lead screw when the pump is started. If the priming procedure or positioning of the actuator is not performed correctly, then, at low infusion rates, this could result in no drug being delivered for up to an hour and the patency of the venous access may be compromised.

The infusion rates are calculated in mm/hr for the Graseby, MS16A and Syringe Minder 2 pumps or mm/day for the Graseby, MS26 pump. Errors can occur when changing the pump setting if the patient or user does not understand the concept of mm/h instead of ml/h; or alternatively, confuses hours with days. The Syringe Minder 2 pump has preset rates of travel, 1, 2, 3, 4, 5, 6, 8, 10, 11, 12 mm/h. The Graseby, MS16A and MS26 have continuously variable rates which are set as required. The Braun, Perfusor M has three preset rates of travel which deliver the contents of a 10 ml syringe in 6, 12, or 24 h. Setting of infusion rates is straightforward for all those syringe drivers available in the UK. However, this simplicity also makes them easy to tamper with, which may be a disadvantage in some circumstances.

All of the pumps have a fixed occlusion pressure which causes the pump to alarm or stop. However, due to the need to overcome the build-up of pressure when infusing viscous fluids, the pressure at which the pump will alarm can be high. At low flow rates there is a considerable delay before the alarm is activated. This problem has been overcome in larger infusion pumps by positioning a pressure sensing device in the extension set rather than in the pump, but this feature is not yet available on the ambulatory pumps.

Patient education and training are required to ensure correct rate setting, mounting of syringe and priming of the set. Patients and their carers need to be aware of the various alarms and how to deal with resulting malfunctions. Some knowledge is required of the mechanism of the syringe pumps. Regular checks must be kept on the batteries.

Despite their lack of sophistication, syringe drivers have several advantages as drug delivery systems. They are relatively cheap to purchase and the disposables associated with their use are cheap and readily available from several sources (excepting those devices dedicated to a certain brand of syringe). The simplicity of syringe drivers may make them less intimidating to patients and the necessity to change syringes frequently allows the patient to gain confidence rapidly in their mastery of the machine. The low weight and bulk of several of these devices is very popular with patients, who consider this a very important feature.[16] A further advantage of the syringe driver to the pharmacist is the large amount of published data on the stability of drugs in plastic syringes. There is a paucity of such information for the dedicated reservoirs of many other ambulatory pumps. The disadvantage of syringe drivers, apart from the susceptibility to tampering already alluded to, is the large number of syringes that have to be filled to provide a course of treatment, normally at least one per day. This can make them considerably more labour-intensive than pumps with larger drug reservoirs.

ELASTOMERIC PUMPS

Model: Baxter Infusor (Figure 5.3)

This group of disposable, single-use pumps employs elastomer technology for drug delivery. The balloon, which acts as both drug reservoir and the pump, is made from an inert polyisoprene rubber material. This gives it elastic properties enabling the reservoir, once expanded, to contract to its original shape and size.

The operating principle of the pump is the Hagen-Poiseville Law[20] which states that flow through a tube is a function of pressure difference (P), radius of the lumen (r), length of the tube (l), and viscosity of the liquid (v).

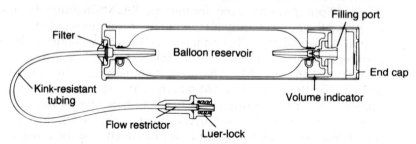

Figure 5.3: *Baxter infusor pump*

The law is represented by the equation:

$$F = \frac{P \times \pi r^4}{8 \times v \times l}$$

The variable function viscosity will be affected by vehicle and temperature. The effects of the vehicle are known if glucose or 0.9% sodium chloride solution is used[21] and temperature fluctuations are kept to a minimum by wearing the infusor close to the skin. High concentrations of drugs occasionally affect viscosity.

An increasing range of infusors is being made available by Baxter. These infuse their contents over periods of up to seven days.

Infusors are filled by connecting a luer-lock syringe, filled with drug solution, to the valve assembly in the infusor, and forcing liquid into the elastomer reservoir. This requires significant force and can be tiring, especially if many infusors are to be filled. Once filled, the microbore administration set primes automatically in about 15 minutes.

The patient removes the winged luer cap from the administration set and attaches the infusor to the venous access device. The drug is delivered via a 10 µm filter at a constant rate, which depends upon the infusor model and the diluent solution. The duration of infusion can be altered by adjusting the volume filled and dose rate can be altered by choice of infusor model and by adjusting the volume filled or drug concentration. The infusor can be used by the intra-arterial or intravenous route.

Infusors are intended for single use and are not designed to be refilled or resterilized for repeat use. Therefore, although there is no capital cost involved in the pump, since it cannot be re-used, revenue costs are high. However, the ongoing introduction of infusor models with longer discharge times may make them competitive with electromechanical pumps requiring dedicated disposables. Infusors are lightweight, small, comfortable in use and silent in operation. They are provided with a fabric holder which is pinned inside the patient's clothes.

The infusor has been studied in 18 patients who received 52 treatment courses, representing 247 patient–days of treatment at home rather than in hospital. During this period there was no known failure to infuse and no reported flow rate or administration difficulties. There was one report of a leaking unit.[21]

The infusor has been used to administer a wide range of drug infusions including antibiotic, analgesic and cytotoxic. There is little published data on stability or compatibility of these injections in the devices. However, research has been conducted by Baxter Healthcare Ltd on the stability of a variety of drugs in infusors; data are available from the company. Unfortunately, the parameters by which stability is considered to be satisfactory have not been fully described. This information should, therefore, be considered for guidance purposes only. Where appropriate it has been included in the relevant drug monographs (see pages 181 to 391).

Patients need to be educated about storage, infusion rates, monitoring the infusion and care of their central line after completion of the infusion. The infusor is popular with patients in comparison with more sophisticated pumps[13] because they do not have to be concerned with battery checks, setting of infusion rates or monitoring for mechanical malfunction of the pump. In addition, as the unit is disposable, they do not have equipment to return to the hospital at the end of treatment.

As well as constant rate infusors, Baxter now market a variety of infusors with additional flow controls which make them suitable for pulsatile or 'basal-bolus' drug delivery. Although primarily intended for antibiotic administration and patient-controlled analgesia, these devices are likely to be useful to those attempting to transfer more complex chemotherapy regimens from the hospital to the domiciliary setting.

PERISTALTIC PUMPS

Models: Pharmacia/Deltec, CADD-1 (Figure 5.4), CADD-PCA, CADD-PLUS

These pumps employ a motorized rotating drum powered by a battery, which rolls over a silicone tube. The drug reservoir is a 50 ml or 100 ml disposable bag enclosed in a rigid plastic shell. These pumps can also be used to deliver the contents of conventional collapsible infusion containers via a special administration set. These devices are programmable and the infusion rate and drug dose can be varied. The CADD pumps have six alarms comprising internal malfunction, set-up review, pump stoppage, low residual volume in medication cassette, low battery and occlusion. There are a number of lock levels for varying patient involvement in the programming of the dose and rate of infusion. However, when used for chemotherapy, the patient is not normally involved in programming and the ability to 'lock' the pump memory against deliberate or accidental alteration is useful. Although these pumps are more sophisticated they aim to be user friendly, but still require a significant amount of training to ensure correct usage. With this in mind the company has prepared training programmes for operators. The pump is robust, but rather heavy and, with a 100 ml drug reservoir *in situ*, bulky $(19.5 \times 9 \times 2.8 \text{ cm})$.

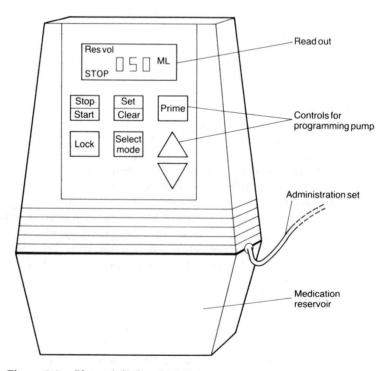

Figure 5.4: *Phamacia/Deltec CADD-1 pump*

The manufacturers of the Pharmacia pump will provide information on the stability of various cytotoxic drugs in Pharmacia cassettes. This information, which is incorporated in the relevant drug monographs, was obtained from unpublished studies conducted at Apotekseolaget AB Central Laboratories and Apotekseolaget AB Karolinska Pharmacy, Stockholm, Sweden.

As well as the CADD constant-rate pump, Pharmacia markets two other pumps which differ only in their programming characteristics. The CADD-PCA delivers a continuous base drug infusion which may be boosted by the user activating a bolus control, whilst the CADD-PLUS (which is intended for antibiotic administration) can give pulsatile infusions. Both of these pumps are also capable of continuous, constant rate infusion and may be attractive to the user involved in providing a range of drug administration services, since they offer flexibility of application.

Model: Medfusion Inc., INFU-MED 300 (Figure 5.5)

The INFU-MED 300 is a linear peristaltic pump that delivers drug solutions from soft PVC reservoirs of 65, 150 or 250 ml via a silicone tubing administration set which is acted upon by the pump mechanism. Additionally, a special 'spike set' makes it possible to use the pump to infuse the contents of conventional collapsible infusion bags. The 65 ml drug reservoir will fit entirely within the pump's rigid plastic cover. Larger reservoirs are carried separately in the pump's fabric carrying pouch. The infusion rate is set by means of an infusion rate setting dial. This is simple to operate, but also easily tampered with, accidentally or deliberately.

The INFU-MED 300 is simple to use, reasonably compact, and offers a comprehensive range of reservoir sizes, but is neither as small nor as lightweight as certain other devices and is, therefore, less popular with some patients. Although no longer in production and superseded by the Walk Med pumps described overleaf, there are many still in use.

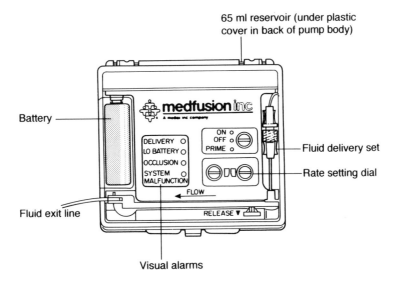

Figure 5.5: *Medfusion INFU-MED 300*

Models: Medfusion Inc., Walk Med 350, 410c, Walk Med 420i/c, Walk Med 430pca, Walk Med 440pic

The Walk Med pumps share their pumping mechanisms and chassis construction with the INFU-MED 300 pump described previously. However, flow control is achieved by programming the pump via an electronic keypad which can be locked in a similar way to that of the Pharmacia pump to prevent unauthorized tampering. Flow parameters are displayed on an LCD display.

The Walk Med 350 is the most basic pump for continuous, steady rate, drug infusion. The other three pumps in the range are all capable of fulfilling this task, and also function as devices for the delivery of patient-controlled analgesia (430pca), intermittent drug infusion (420i/c) or both (440pic) and their flexibility may be attractive to the pharmacist involved in operating a range of services. No data are available on the stability of drugs in INFU-MED reservoirs, either from the distributors of the pump or from other published sources. This information will be required before the pump can be accepted for routine use.

Model: Graseby Medical 9000 series (9100, 9200, 9300, 9400)

The Graseby Medical 9000 series devices are based on a common pump body and a set of four 'smart cards' which slot into the front of the device and give the user a choice of either continuous infusion (9100), intermittent infusion (9200), patient-controlled analgesia (9300) or non-zero order (circadian) programming (9400). The facility that enables an infusion history to be downloaded to a computer printer is particularly attractive in the case of cytotoxic drugs. Medication reservoir volumes range from 50–250 ml and are enclosed in a rigid plastic case for protection. A spike adapter is also available to allow the use of virtually any collapsible infusion bag with this device. Graseby Medical is able to supply stability data on most of the commonly used cytotoxic drug infusions, including some drug admixtures. Some of this information has been published in abstract form.[22]

Model: Baxter APII

This peristaltic device can be used for continuous, PCA or combination PCA/basal-rate infusions. The APII pump may be worn in a holster or waist-bag, or alternatively can be mounted on a pole adjacent to the patient. Reservoirs of 100 ml and 250 ml volume are available and the fluid delivery set incorporates an anti-syphon device.

A spike set is also offered for use with this device which enables virtually any collapsible infusion bag to serve as a medication reservoir. An infusion history display or printout option is also available with this device. All pump alarms are identified on the device screen and once a malfunction has been cleared the pump re-starts without the need to reset the device.

IMPLANTABLE PUMP SYSTEMS

Implantable pump systems have been developed for drug delivery, offering the patient a more normal life-style, since there is no externalized portion of the system to be seen or to be managed. Additional advantages of the implantable pump system are a reduction in the potential for microbial infections and improved patient compliance with therapy. These advantages are of particular benefit to the ambulatory patient receiving long-term therapy. The primary disadvantages of the implantable pump systems are the small volume capacity of the pump reservoirs, and the high cost of the pump and surgical implantation of the system.

Implanted in a subcutaneous pocket, the pump can easily be felt through the skin. The silicone injection septum is accessed through the skin using a special Huber-type needle for up to 1000 punctures, depending on needle size.

Two commercially available implanted pump systems are the Pfizer Infusaid implantable pump and the Medtronic SynchroMed pump.

Model: Pfizer Infusaid implantable pump (Figure 5.6)

The Infusaid pump is made of titanium, is approximately 90 mm in diameter, 28 mm thick, weighs slightly more than 200 g, and has a reservoir capacity of approximately 50 ml. The operating mechanism of the pump utilizes a non-electronic metal bellows concept. The pump consists of two chambers, separated by flexible metal bellows, and is attached to a silicone rubber catheter placed into the delivery site. The outer chamber contains a fluorocarbon charging fluid, and the inner chamber serves as a drug reservoir. When the drug chamber is filled, the charging fluid is compressed. Expansion of the charging fluid exerts a vapour pressure which compresses the drug chamber, forcing drug from the reservoir through the flow restrictor and into the delivery catheter. Because there is no electromechanical component, the energy of the charging fluid is limitless, not requiring replenishment.

Flow rate is controlled by a restricted capillary tube which cannot be changed after implantation. Flow rate is affected by a number of variables, including fluid viscosity, patient temperature and altitude. The Infusaid pump is supplied by the manufacturer with a specific capillary tube to deliver a specific drug at a specific flow rate for normal body temperature and at the geographical location of the patient. Increased temperatures, for example as experienced by a patient in a hot bath, will increase the flow rate of the pump by approximately 10–13% for each 1°C rise in temperature. Higher altitudes will also cause the pump to flow faster. An infusion pump calibrated for sea level will flow approximately 45% faster at an altitude of 2000 metres. After implantation, slight alterations in flow rate can

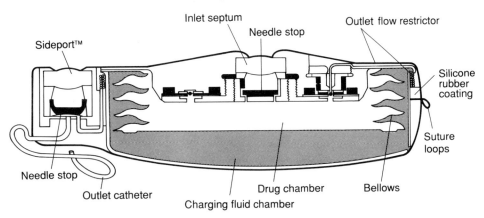

Figure 5.6: *Infusaid Model 400 implantable pump*

be achieved by varying the concentration or viscosity of the fluid. Only one model of the Infusaid pump is commercially available, Model 400, although there is both a single catheter and a dual catheter version. The use of the sideport allows direct access to the catheter, bypassing the pump mechanism, for bolus doses, if required.

A programmable version of the Infusaid pump, Model 1000, is not yet commercially available, but is now in clinical trials. The pump uses telemetry via an external programme to change delivery rates after implantation.

Model: Medtronic SynchroMed pump (Figure 5.7)

This pump can be reprogrammed for delivery rate changes (0.1 to 18 ml/day) after implantation using an external programmer. Approximately 70 mm in diameter, 27 mm thick, and 200 g in weight, the pump has a usable capacity of 18 ml. The operating mechanism of the SynchroMed pump is a rotary peristaltic system that is powered by an internal lithium battery, improving delivery accuracy and eliminating the dependence on temperature, viscosity and pressure characteristic of the Infusaid pump. The typical life of the battery is approximately three to four years at a flow rate of 0.5 ml/day. Two models of the pump are commercially available, Model 8611H and Model 8615. Model 8615 has a sideport access site to bypass the pumping mechanism for bolus doses. The pump can be programmed to deliver continuous, intermittent and complex circadian administrations using the external programmer and a radiotelemetry link via the programming wand.

The use of implantable pumps has been primarily restricted to regional deliveries, e.g. intra-arterial and intrathecal, although the pumps are also being used for systemic applications.[23–25]

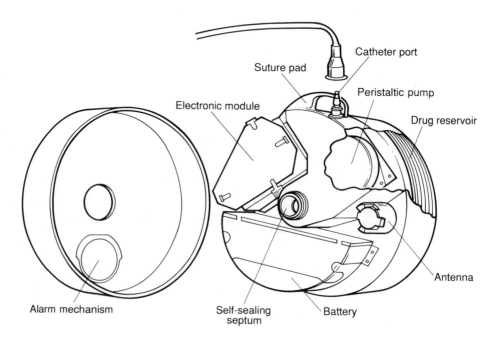

Figure 5.7: *SynchroMed implantable pump*

CONCLUSION

A summary of the features of the ambulatory pumps discussed is contained in Table 5.1 (*see* Appendix, page 102).

Ambulatory pumps have made the concept of continuous infusion attainable, with all the concurrent benefits mentioned previously. All the pumps provide accurate dosing and are portable. Pumps differ in the number of features available, which may include flexible administration rates, variable reservoir sizes and a range of alarms. With all these devices, not only the capital cost of the pump, but also the cost of disposables required must be considered.

For successful home treatment with ambulatory pumps, the patient must feel confident and be proficient in the use of the unit. Patient (or carer) education is an important part of any ambulatory programme[6] and the level of knowledge required and staff time involved in training and providing a backup service for each type of pump should be carefully evaluated.

BOLUS AND SHORT-TERM INFUSIONS

Although it is possible to administer home chemotherapy in traditional bolus or short-term infusion schedules, this approach is not always appropriate for domiciliary patients. In the hospital setting it is possible to control the acute toxicity (such as nausea and vomiting) associated with conventional chemotherapy schedules. For domiciliary patients, such toxicity is more difficult to control and could be unacceptable, although this may be less of a problem with the introduction of symptomatic treatment such as the $5HT_3$ antagonist antiemetics. Conventional bolus or short-term infusion schedules would normally be administered by a community nurse. Some patients may feel that this restricts their freedom and independence, negating the advantages of home treatment over hospital day-case treatment.

In cases where experience has shown that bolus chemotherapy is well tolerated, it may be possible to offer patients the option of self-medication by using a venous access port (such as the Intraport device, Figure 5.8). The catheter is inserted into a central vein (usually the subclavian vein) and the medication port is implanted subcutaneously, usually in the anterior chest wall, with the silastic septum located just beneath the skin. However, for the self-administration of bolus injections some patients find it more convenient if the port is placed subcutaneously in the lower abdomen. The septum is designed for multiple puncture and when not in use the patency of the system is maintained by flushing with dilute heparinized saline at monthly intervals.[26]

Self-medication does however raise concerns about compliance and the accuracy that can be achieved in terms of dose, administration rate and dose intervals. An alternative to patient or nurse administration is to use a pre-programmed infusion pump capable of intermittent or pulsed infusions. The device can be programmed to deliver a defined volume of drug solution at a preset infusion rate at time intervals specified by the programmer. Examples of ambulatory infusion devices with intermittent infusion capacity include the CADD-PLUS (Pharmacia/Deltec) (*see* page 84) and the 9000 series (Graseby Medical) (*see* page 86). With the latter device it is possible to print a history of infusions delivered by the pump to audit both pump function and patient compliance.

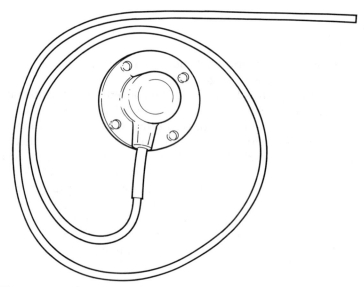

Figure 5.8: *Intraport venous access port*

Self-administration of small-volume subcutaneous injections may be appropriate for low-dose maintenance regimens providing that drug-related toxicity is minimal and the drug is non-vesicant (e.g. alpha-interferon). Homecare packs containing medication and the necessary syringes and needles are now available for this purpose. Devices used to aid the subcutaneous administration of insulin to diabetic patients may also be of benefit to leukaemia and cancer patients.

Finally, from the medico–legal view point, bolus or short-term infusions tend to be the licensed or recognized route of administration listed in the manufacturers' data sheets.

PROLONGED CONTINUOUS INFUSION

Among various attempts to improve the therapeutic index of antitumour drugs, one approach involves the replacement of traditional, rapid infusion schedules with prolonged continuous infusion regimens.[27] Developments in the design, operating capability and operational safety of ambulatory infusion pumps have facilitated continuous infusion chemotherapy in the domiciliary setting.

The rationale for continuous infusion chemotherapy is based on the pharmacokinetic characteristics of cytotoxic drugs and on the cytokinetic (growth cycle) profile of tumour cells.[27] Since many cytotoxic drugs exhibit short plasma half-lives, continuous infusion regimens prolong the exposure of tumour cells to the drug. As tumour cells progress through the cell cycle, a greater proportion of the tumour cell population is exposed to the drug during the sensitive phase(s) of the cell cycle.

An additional advantage with continuous infusion regimens in home chemotherapy programmes is that adverse effects associated with peak plasma levels are reduced or eliminated. For example, doxorubicin is less cardiotoxic[28] and fluorouracil less myelosuppressive[29] in continuous infusion regimens. There is evidence that nausea and vomiting associated with bolus doses of cisplatinum are significantly reduced when infusional regimens are used.[30] However, other toxicities, such as mucositis and hand–foot syndrome in the case of fluorouracil,[31] may occur more readily with prolonged infusions.

Controlled studies[4,14] indicate that, on balance, drug-related adverse effects are reduced with infusional regimens and quality of life for the patient is improved.

Continuous infusion is a technique which also lends itself to combined modality treatments. For example continuous infusion fluorouracil is now used on an adjuvant or neo-adjuvant basis with surgical resection in the treatment of colon cancer. In a recently reported study,[32] continuous infusion carboplatin was combined with synchronous radiation therapy. The carboplatin infusion was delivered from an ambulatory pump and, when appropriate, external-beam radiation was administered on an outpatient basis.

DOCUMENTATION AND SAFETY

Although the safety of home chemotherapy has been established over at least a decade, there is a need for continued vigilance, particularly as the number of patients treated in the domiciliary setting continues to increase, and the complexity of infusion regimens and ambulatory pumps is also increasing. The main safety issues focus on the potential risk of exposure of patients' relatives and carers to cytotoxic drugs used in the home or workplace, and the obvious requirement for accurate and reliable infusion delivery by the ambulatory infusion device.

1 Safe handling of cytotoxic drugs in the home

The importance of patient and carer training in the safe handling of cytotoxic drugs has already been stated (*see* page 76) and cannot be overemphasized. The most significant route of cytotoxic contamination appears to be dermal absorption.[33] It is therefore essential that surface contamination around the home or workplace is avoided. This requires the provision of dedicated refrigerators and sealed, leakproof polypropylene containers for the storage of pre-filled syringes or medication cassettes. A supply of gloves and absorbent preparation mats should be made available to the patient or carer together with a cytotoxics sharps bin for the safe disposal of cytotoxic waste. Ideally, these consumables should be provided together with the medication[34] (*see* page 77). Arrangements must also be made for the safe disposal of cytotoxic waste, usually through a regular collection service.

The possibility of a cytotoxic drug spillage in the home cannot be overlooked and patients should be provided with spillage kits designed for such an occurrence. These should contain the following equipment:

▼ protective gloves
▼ goggles
▼ overshoes and gowns to protect the individual dealing with the spillage
▼ booms to contain the spillage
▼ absorbent pads to mop up spilled liquid
▼ pre-labelled containers for the safe disposal of contaminated consumables from the spillage kit.

Although written instructions in the use of spillage kits should be included with the kit contents, this is not a substitute for thorough education and training in the use of kits.

Finally, it is always valuable to audit safe handling in the home so that any deficiencies can be identified and rectified. An audit tool with a section applicable to safe handling of cytotoxic drugs in the domiciliary setting has recently been developed in the UK.[35]

2 Documentation

2.1 Regimen protocols

Comprehensive control documentation is a key element in the provision of safe and effective home chemotherapy. A protocol should be prepared for each regimen used detailing:

▼ name and dose of each drug
▼ route of administration (e.g. central venous catheter)
▼ diluent
▼ normal concentration range
▼ infusion rate
▼ duration of infusion
▼ ambulatory device to be used
▼ shelf-life of infusion under storage and in-use conditions (appropriately referenced)
▼ details of any supportive therapy.

Each protocol should be approved by the clinician responsible and also by the oncology pharmacist.

2.2 Programming infusion devices

The programming of infusion devices is a major source of error and separate protocols for the uses, limitations and programming of each device in use should be prepared. These protocols should also be carefully validated and approved.

For each pump programming operation a pump programming pro-forma should be completed, detailing all pump settings which should be signed by the health care professional making or programming them. These settings should be checked and countersigned by a second individual with proven experience in the use of ambulatory devices and all pump settings should be checked against the original prescription and the relevant treatment protocol. Any deviations from the protocol must be recorded and approved by the clinician responsible for the patient.

Some of the more recently introduced ambulatory infusion devices (e.g. Graseby Medical 9000 series devices, see page 86) have the facility to retain a history of each course of treatment administered and can provide a printout when required. Such printouts are valuable for clinical audit purposes and after review these should be retained together with completed pump programming pro-formas and other documents relevant to the patient.

ALTERNATIVE ROUTES OF ADMINISTRATION

A brief summary of each alternative administration route for chemotherapy is provided, and the drugs specific to the route are listed.

1 Intravesical

1.1 Advantages

▼ Localized treatment to tumours confined to the bladder with limited systemic absorption, so that systemic toxicity is reduced or eliminated.
▼ High localized drug concentrations in contact with the tumour and surrounding mucosa for prolonged time periods.
▼ Reduced risk of tumour implantation following surgery.

1.2 Disadvantages

▼ Considerable local inflammation and pain.
▼ Inconvenient for patients – there is a retained catheter into the bladder and this is rotated during installation.
▼ Not suitable for drugs requiring systemic activation.

1.3 Drugs used in intravesical chemotherapy

A variety of anticancer drugs have been administered via the intravesical route and the list below represents the most widely used drugs only. Dosage, schedule, diluent volume instilled and residence time in the bladder are also subject to variation between treatment centres. The typical conditions and values are from the literature, and in most cases there is no evidence to suggest these are optimal. The information presented is intended for guidance only.

Doxorubicin

Dose and volume instilled: 50 mg in 50 ml.[36]

Schedule: Two doses in first week, then monthly for one year and three monthly for a further year.[37]

Diluent: Water for injection or 0.9% sodium chloride injection.[38]

Residence time in bladder: One hour, with rotation of patient.[36]

UK data sheet recommendation for intravesical use: Yes.[36]

Possible complications: Chemical cystitis, allergic reaction, haematuria, reduced bladder capacity, gastrointestinal effects and fever.[39]

Epirubicin

Dose and volume instilled: 50 mg in 50 ml.[36,40] In cases of chemical cystitis dose reduction to 30 mg is advised[40] while for carcinoma *in situ*, a dose of 80 mg is recommended.[36]

Schedule: One dose weekly for eight weeks. For prophylaxis after transurethral resection; one dose weekly for four weeks followed by one dose monthly for 11 months is recommended.[36]

Diluent: 0.9% sodium chloride injection.[40]

Residence time in bladder: One hour with rotation of patient.[36]

UK data sheet recommendation for intravesical use: Yes.[36]

Possible complications: Chemical cystitis, allergic reaction and other adverse effects similar to doxorubicin.[39] Systemic toxicity with epirubicin is rare.[39]

Mitomycin C

Dose and volume instilled: 20–40 mg in 20–40 ml.[41]

Schedule: Weekly or three times a week for a total of 20 doses.[41] A recent report[42] suggests that in cases of a solitary initial tumour with tumour recurrence at three months, or multiple initial tumours with no recurrence at three months, a single instillation followed by repeat doses at three monthly cystoscopies up to and including one year post-diagnosis should be used.

Diluent: Water for injections.[41]

Residence time in bladder: Minimum of one hour.[43]

UK data sheet recommendation for intravesical use: Yes.[41]

Possible complications: Chemical cystitis, allergic reactions, leukopenia, thrombo-cytopenia, reduced bladder capacity.[39]

Mitozantrone

Dose and volume: 5–10.5 mg in 30 ml.[44]

Schedule: Once a week for six weeks.[44]

Diluent: 0.9% sodium chloride injection.[44]

Residence time in bladder: Two hours.[44]

UK data sheet recommendation for intravesical use: Not recommended.[45]

Possible complications: At doses of 9 mg or less, minor bladder irritation.[39] At doses of 10 mg or more, moderate to severe bladder irritation including urothelial necrosis.[39]

Thiotepa

Dose and volume instilled: 30–60 mg in 60 ml for multiple instillation. 90 mg in 100 ml for single dose instillations in adjunctive prophylaxis with surgical resection.[46]

Schedule: Every two weeks for a total of 4–8 instillations starting at least one week after tumour resection. Maintenance therapy after the initial dose is given every 4–6 weeks for one year or longer.[46]

Diluent: Water for injection.

Residence time in bladder: Two hours, except for single dose adjunct to surgical resection where residence time is 30 minutes with alteration of patient position.[46]

UK data sheet recommendation for intravesical use: Yes.[47]

Possible complications: Leukopenia, thrombocytopenia, irritative voiding symp-toms.[39] The risk of drug-related toxicity is increased with patients who have received previous radiotherapy to the bladder.[46]

Bacillus Calmette-Guérin (BCG)

Although not a cytotoxic drug, BCG is included here because:

▼ it is widely used in the treatment of superficial bladder cancer

▼ many pharmacies prepare BCG bladder instillations
▼ there may be significant risks to the preparation environment associated with BCG.

Dose and volume instilled: 5×10^8 bacilli (live attenuated vaccine) in 50 ml.[43,47]

Schedule: Once a week for six weeks, with repeat courses for recurrent or persistent disease.[43]

Diluent: 0.9% sodium chloride injection.[43,47]

Residence time in bladder: One hour minimum.[43]

UK data sheet recommendation for intravesical use: No information.[48]

Possible complications: Bacterial cystitis (not BCG related), chemical cystitis, allergic reaction, fever, nausea, malaise, haematuria, prostatitis and epididymitis.[43] There is a potential risk that environmental contamination of pharmacy workstations occurring during the preparation of BCG instillations could result in the contamination of other infusions prepared in the same workstation. A recent report[49] describes two cases of meningitis resulting from iatrogenic BCG infection in two immunocompromised children receiving intrathecal chemotherapy for leukaemia.

2 Intraperitoneal

2.1 Advantages

▼ Tumours that spread by direct invasion of the omentum or peritoneal lining e.g. ovarian and colorectal cancers are sensitive to direct bathing of their often small volume, poorly vascularized bulk with proportionally high concentrations of drug.
▼ Therapy can be high dose, intermittent; or low dose, continuous. The latter is similar to peritoneal dialysis.

2.2 Disadvantages

▼ Difficulties with selection and placement of the catheter are a practical and fairly common problem because the peritoneum is invaded with tumour and 'overgrowth'. Consequent occlusion of the catheter is also a problem. An early manifestation of this problem is the formation of a 'one-way' proteinous/ fibrin/tumour flap.
▼ As a function of tumour growth the peritoneal cavity may fill with proteinous exudate. This ascites may contain malignant cells and/or high concentrations of protein. The high levels of protein can result in protein binding and in-activation of any chemotherapy instilled. Furthermore, the dilutional effects are difficult to quantify and if target concentrations were hoped for these may be difficult to obtain.
▼ Loculation, either due to previous intraperitoneal therapy, radiation fibrosis or tumour growth/regrowth again means that certain areas, or pockets, receive uniproportional exposure to the therapy.
▼ Peritonitis, either chemical or infective or both, can develop. It is often painful and can be fatal if allowed to progress to full peritonitis.

2.3 Drugs used in intraperitoneal chemotherapy

▼ bleomycin
▼ carboplatin

▼ cisplatin
▼ 5-fluorouracil
▼ mitomycin C
▼ mitozantrone
▼ paclitaxel.

3 Intrahepatic

3.1 Advantages

▼ This can be achieved either via the portal vein or via the hepatic artery. As the liver tissue acts like a sponge, high local concentrations of drug can be achieved. The relative advantage of hepatic infusions over intravenous infusions is described by the equation:

$$R_d = 1 + \frac{Cl_{TB}}{Q\,(1-E_H)}$$

Where R_d is the hepatic advantage
Cl_{TB} is the total body clearance of the drug
Q is arterial blood flow
E_H is the fraction of the drug extracted across the liver.

▼ It is estimated and increasingly proved in the literature that liver tissues can be exposed to two- to 400-fold the local drug concentration. It is also practical to have the liver act as a reservoir, spilling drug over into the peripheral circulation, leading to a 'standard' intravenous-type peripheral exposure to the cytotoxic.
▼ Metastatic disease in the liver is inevitably fatal and often unresponsive to systemic chemotherapy. Targeted high-dose chemotherapy appears highly effective.

3.2 Disadvantages

▼ Complications in catheterizing the appropriate veins or arteries.
▼ High pressures in the arterial circulation.
▼ Inflammation, infection and pain in the hepatic tissues.
▼ Hepatic artery thrombosis.
▼ Catheter displacement.
▼ Due to the cellular and vascular architecture of the liver drug delivery systems such as biodegradable, starch microspheres are an attractive method for increasing local drug concentrations.

3.3 Drugs used in intrahepatic chemotherapy

▼ carmustine
▼ cisplatinum
▼ 5-fluorouracil
▼ floxuridine
▼ mitomycin C.

4 Isolated limb/breast perfusion

4.1 Advantages

▼ Allows high local drug concentrations to be achieved with minimal systemic exposure.

4.2 Disadvantages

▼ Technically difficult, involves isolation of blood supply to affected part.
▼ Cannot be done on outpatient basis.
▼ Very invasive, may be distressing and uncomfortable for patient.
▼ Cytotoxic action limited to perfused area, no activity against metastatic disease elsewhere, therefore inappropriate for most large tumours.
▼ May require preparation of drugs in unusual perfusion fluids, at high (body) temperature and at concentrations for which few stability data are available.
▼ Not suitable for drugs that require systemic activation e.g. cyclophosphamide.
▼ Not of proven value in any condition, should be reserved for clinical trials only.

4.3 Drugs used in isolated limb/breast perfusion chemotherapy

▼ doxorubicin
▼ mitozantrone.

5 Intrathecal/intraventricular

5.1 Advantages

▼ Allows direct access to the CNS of drugs that normally cross the blood–brain barrier in very limited amounts.
▼ Of proven value in leukaemia and certain types of lymphoma, where the CNS provides a sanctuary site for tumour cells during systemic chemotherapy.

5.2 Disadvantages

▼ Unpleasant for the patient.
▼ Technically difficult requiring repeated lumbar punctures or placement of a suitable access device such as an Ommaya reservoir.
▼ Only applicable to a very limited range of non-irritant anticancer agents e.g. thiotepa, cytarabine, methotrexate and hydrocortisone.
▼ Has been associated with frequent, fatal drug errors in patients receiving concomitant intravenous therapy.
▼ Risks of CNS trauma or infection.
▼ Only formulations known to be suitable for intrathecal use (and preferably licensed for administration by this route) should be used. (Extremes of pH or osmotic strength, or the presence of preservatives may render other formulations unsuitable.)
▼ Of no proven value other than as a prophylactic measure in leukaemia or lymphoma.
▼ Has no place in the treatment of CNS metastases of solid tumours.

5.3 Drugs used in intrathecal/intraventricular chemotherapy

▼ cytarabine
▼ methotrexate.

6 Intra-arterial

6.1 Advantages

▼ With drugs where the level of extraction by the tissue of the target organ/ tumour is high, high tumour exposure with much reduced systemic exposure can be achieved e.g. fluoropyrimidines administered via the hepatic artery.

6.2 Disadvantages

▼ Very high drug levels in the perfused organ may result in excessive local tissue damage.
▼ Drug delivery system needs to work against a high back-pressure, this will activate excess-pressure alarms on some infusion pumps designed for intravenous infusion.
▼ Few drugs have a high enough tissue extraction ratio to make the procedure worthwhile.
▼ Displacement of arterial cannula results in excessive bleeding which can be difficult to stop and which is distressing to patients.
▼ Not of proven benefit, should only be used as part of a research protocol.

7 Intrapleural

7.1 Advantages

▼ Potential for delivering active agents to a site of poor systemic penetration, producing an anticancer effect against small-volume disease.
▼ Alleviates symptoms of plural disease which may occur in up to 80% of patients with certain malignancies e.g. lung or breast disease.

7.2 Disadvantages

▼ Systemic toxicity particularly to alkylating agents.
▼ Local inflammation and pain.
▼ Fever, particularly common with bleomycin.
▼ Partial sclerosing of the plural membrane leading to re-occurrence being loculated and even more difficult to treat.
▼ Highly variable success rates of 20–88%, perhaps reflecting the effect of incomplete drainage prior to instillation leading to dilution of the cytotoxic.
▼ Complicated technique.
▼ Cytotoxic instillation as effective.

7.3 Drugs used in intrapleural chemotherapy

▼ BCG
▼ bleomycin
▼ *Corynebacterium parvum*
▼ doxorubicin
▼ 5-fluorouracil
▼ mitozantrone
▼ mustine
▼ thiotepa.

8 Other local chemotherapies

Users of this Handbook should also be aware that a number of cytotoxics have also been, on a one-off basis, instilled into other cavities or directly into organs. These include:

▼ intraocular – 5-fluorouracil
▼ intrapancreatic – mitomycin C
▼ pericardially – CMF (cyclophosphamide, methotrexate and 5–fluorouracil), bleomycin, thiotepa
▼ topically – carmustine, 5-fluorouracil
▼ subcutaneously – ifosfamide, bleomycin, cytarabine.

REFERENCES

1 Constable SE *et al.* (1995) Reducing the wait for chemotherapy. *UFM Update* **15**, 10–11.
2 Bacovsky RA (1988) *Home parenteral chemotherapy programs*. Proceedings of 1st international symposium on oncology pharmacy practice. New Zealand Hospital Pharmacists' Association, New Zealand, pp. 294–300.
3 Payne S (1989) Quality of life in women with advanced breast cancer. PhD Thesis, Department of Psychology, University of Exeter.
4 Coates A *et al.* (1987) Improving the quality of life during chemotherapy for advanced breast cancer. A comparison of intermittent and continuous treatment strategies. *New Engl. J. Med.* **317**, 1490–5.
5 Vokes EE *et al.* (1989) A randomised study of in-patient versus out-patient continuous infusion chemotherapy for patients with locally advanced head and neck cancer. *Cancer* **63**, 30–6.
6 Sewell GJ *et al.* (1989) Home based cancer therapy by continuous infusion. *Pharm. J.* **243**, 139–41.
7 Ausman RK *et al.* (1982) Long-term, ambulatory, continuous intravenous infusion of 5-fluorouracil for the treatment of metastatic adenocarcinoma in the liver. *Wisc. Med. J.* **81**, 25–8.
8 Lokich JJ *et al.* (1982) The delivery of cancer chemotherapy by constant venous infusion: ambulatory management of venous access and portable pump. *Cancer* **50** (12), 2731–5.
9 Sewell GJ *et al.* (1987) HOPE for cancer. *J. Dist. Nur.* **April**, 4–6.
10 Kramer I, Williams DA (1995) Drug stability. *J. Oncol. Pharm. Pract.* **1** (ISOPP IV Symposium Issue), 26–7.
11 Department of Health (1995) *Aseptic Dispensing for NHS patients*. DoH, London.
12 Stanley AP (1996) Community Chemotherapy: The logical evolution of home based therapy. Submitted for publication *Eur. J. Cancer*.
13 Moody DG (1986) External ambulatory infusion devices and the oncology patient. *J. Pharm. Tech.* **2**, 160–5.
14 Lokich JJ *et al.* (1989) Prospective randomised comparison of continuous infusion fluorouracil with a conventional bolus schedule in metastatic colorectal carcinoma: a mid-Atlantic oncology program study. *J. Clin. Oncol.* **7**, 425–32.
15 Hrusesky W (1987) The rationale for non-zero order drug delivery using automatic computer based drug delivery systems (chronotherapy). *J. Biol. Resp. Modifiers* **6**, 587–98.

16 Summerhayes M *et al.* (1991) A comparison of two devices for the continuous infusion of cytotoxic drugs in non-hospitalized patients. *Int. J. Pharm. Pract.* **1**, 94–7.

17 Hardy EM, Williamson C, Sewell GJ (1995) An evaluation of six infusion devices for the continuous infusion of cytotoxic drugs in ambulatory patients. *J. Oncol. Pharm. Pract.* **1** (1), 15–22.

18 Williamson CA, Ridler C, Sewell GJ (1993) A study to determine the quality of life of patients receiving low-dose ambulatory chemotherapy. *Hosp. Pharm. Pract.* **3**, 197–204.

19 Adams PS *et al.* (1987) Pharmaceutical aspects of home infusion therapy for cancer patients. *Pharm. J.* **238**, 476–8.

20 Thomas M *et al.* (1985) Miniaturised continuous delivery systems for injectable solutions: individual patient control and physico-chemical properties. *Proc. of the Guild.* **19**, 3–37.

21 Akahoshi MP *et al.* (1987) Safety and reliability of the Travenol Infusor in administering chemotherapy in the home. *J. Pharm. Tech.* **3**, 65–8.

22 Sewell GJ, Priston MJ (1995) Stability and compatability studies on cytotoxic and analgesic infusions in a new multi-purpose ambulatory device *J. Oncol. Pharm. Pract.* **1** (ISOPP Symposium Issue), 15.

23 Kwan JW (1989) High technology IV infusion devices. *Am. J. Hosp. Pharm.* **46**, 320–35.

24 Kemeny N *et al.* (1987) Intrahepatic or systemic infusion of fluorodeoxyuridine in patients with liver metastases from colorectal carcinoma. *Ann. Intern. Med.* **107**, 459–65.

25 von Roemeling R *et al.* (1988) Progressive metastatic renal cell carcinoma controlled by continuous 5-fluoro-2-deoxyuridine infusion. *J. Urol.* **139**, 259–62.

26 Finley RS (1988) *Ambulatory infusion pumps and venous access devices.* Proceedings of 1st International Symposium on Oncology Pharmacy Practice. New Zealand Hospital Pharmacists Association, New Zealand, 279–93.

27 Lokich JJ (1987) Introduction to the concept and practice of infusion chemotherapy. In: (JJ Lokich ed.), *Cancer Chemotherapy by Infusion.* Precept Press Inc., Chicago, 3–11.

28 Legha SS *et al.* (1982) Reduction of doxorubicin cardiotoxicity by prolonged continuous intravenous infusion. *Ann. Intern. Med.* **96**, 133–9.

29 Seifert P *et al.* (1975) Comparison of continuously infused 5-fluorouracil with bolus injection in treatment of patients with colorectal adenocarcinoma. *Cancer* **36**, 123–8.

30 Thigpen JT (1989) A randomised comparison of a rapid prolonged (24hr) infusion of cisplatin therapy of squamous cell carcinoma of the uterine cervix: A gynecologic oncology study. *Gynecol. Oncol.* **32**, 198–202.

31 Mortimer J, Anderson I (1989) Managing the toxicities unique to high-dose leukovorin (CF) and fluorouracil (FU). *Proc. Am. Clin. Oncol.* **8**, 98.

32 Allsopp MA, Sewell GJ (1995) A pharmacokinetic – pharmacodynamic study on carboplatin administered in prolonged continuous infusion regimens with synchronous radiotherapy. *J. Oncol. Pharm. Pract.* **1** (3), 25–32.

33 Sessink P, van der Kerkhaf M, Anzion R *et al.* (1995) Biological and environmental monitoring of occupational exposure to cyclophosphamide in a hospital pharmacy department. *J. Oncol. Pharm. Pract.* **1** (ISOPP IV Symposium Issue), 25.

34 Shrubb D, Sewell GJ (1995) Home care, ambulatory chemotherapy, nursing and pharmaceutical issues. *J. Oncol. Pharm. Pract.,* **1** (ISOPP IV Symposium Issue), 14.

35 Sizer S, Sewell GJ (1996) Check exposure to cytotoxics: development and use of an audit for cytotoxic drug handling in pharmacy, clinical and domiciliary areas. *Pharm. Pract.* **6** (5), 153–6.

36 *ABPI Data Sheet Compendium 1995–1996* (1995) DataPharm Publications Ltd, London, p. 1262.

37 Schulman CC, Denis LJ, Oosterlinck W *et al.* (1983) Early adjuvant adriamycin in superficial bladder carcinoma. *Cancer Chemother. Pharmocol.* **11** (suppl), 532.

38 Barbuir PE, Bono AV, Gianno E *et al.* (1984) Intravesical doxorubicin for the prophylaxis of superficial bladder tumours: A multi-centre study: Binor Italian Cooperative Group. *Cancer* **54**, 756.

39 Thrasher JB, Crawford ED (1992) Complications of intravesical chemotherapy. *Urol. Clin. North Am.* **19** (3), 529–39.

40 Cumming JA, Kirk D, Newling DW *et al.* (1990) A multicentre phase II study of intravesical epirubicin in the treatment of superficial bladder tumour. *Eur. Urol.* **17**, 20.

41 *ABPI Data Sheet Compendium 1995–1996* (1995) DataPharm Publications Ltd, London, p. 760–1.

42 Hall RR, Parmar MKB, Richards AP *et al.* (1994) Proposal for changes in cystoscopic follow-up of patients with bladder cancer and adjuvant intravesical chemotherapy. *Br. Med. J.* **308**, 257–60.

43 Witjes JA, Meijden APM vd, Witjes WPJ *et al.* (1993) A randomised prospective study comparing intravesical instillations of mitomycin C, BCG Tice, and BCG-RIVM in pTa – pT1 tumours and primary carcinoma *in situ* of the urinary bladder. *Eur. J. Cancer* **29A** (12), 1672–6.

44 Stewart DJ, Green R, Futter N *et al.* (1990) Phase 1 and pharmacology study of intravesical mitozantrone for recurrent superficial bladder tumours. *J. Urol.* **143**, 714.

45 *ABPI Data Sheet Compendium 1995–1996* (1995) DataPharm Publications Ltd, London, p. 808–10.

46 *ABPI Data Sheet Compendium 1995–1996* (1995) DataPharm Publications Ltd, London, p. 818–9.

47 Debruyne FMJ, Van der Meijden PM, Witjes MD *et al.* (1992) Bacillus Calmette-Guerin versus mitomycin intravesical therapy in superficial bladder cancer. *Suppl. Urol.* **40** (1), 11–15.

48 *ABPI Data Sheet Compendium 1995–1996* (1995) DataPharm Publications Ltd, London, p. 560–1.

49 Stone MM, Vannier AM, Storch SK *et al.* (1995) Brief report: Meningitis due to iatrogenic BCG injection in two immunocompromised children. *New Engl. J. Med.* **333** (9), 561–3.

APPENDIX

Table 5.1: *Summary of pumps described*

Make/Model	Weight**	Dimensions***	Pump mechanism	Reservoir	Battery	Flow rate	Accuracy	Alarm*
Graseby Medical								
MS16A	275 g	16.5 × 2.3 × 5.3 cm	syringe pump electric	2 ml–35 ml syringe	9 V	0–99 mm/h variable	±5%	1,2,3
MS26	275 g	16.5 × 2.3 × 5.3 cm	syringe pump electric	2 ml–35 ml syringe	9 V	0–99 mm/day	±5%	1,2,3
Braun Medical								
Perfusor M	450 g	17 × 7.5 × 3.5 cm	syringe pump clockwork	10 ml Braun Omnifix syringe	none	10 ml in 6–24 h fixed	±5%	none
Critikon								
Syringe Minder 2	270 g	11.7 × 5 × 1 cm	syringe pump electric	2 ml–20 ml syringe	9 V	1–12 mm/h fixed intervals	±3%	1,2,3
Pharmacia/Deltec								
CADD-1	425 g	2.8 × 9 × 16 cm	peristaltic rotary programmable	50 ml/ 100 ml cassette	9 V	0–299 ml/day	theor. ±10% in studies ±3%	1,2,3 4,5,6
CADD-PCA	425 g	2.8 × 9 × 16 cm	peristaltic rotary programmable	50 ml/ 100 ml cassette	9 V	0–20 mm/h		1,2,3 4,5,6
CADD-PLUS	425 g	2.8 × 9 × 16 cm	peristaltic rotary programmable	50 ml/ 100 ml cassette	9 V	0–75 ml/day		1,2,3 4,5,6
Baxter								
Single day Infusor	100 g	16.5 × 3 cm dia.	elastomeric pressure	60 ml	none	2 ml/h	±5%	none
Multi day Infusor	100 g	16.5 × 3 cm dia.	elastomeric pressure	60 ml	none	0.5 ml/h	±5%	none
Seven day Infusor	150 g	25 × 3 cm dia.	elastomeric pressure	90 ml	none	0.5 ml/h	±5%	none
Medfusion								
INFU-MED 300	350 g	11.2 × 10.4 × 4.6 cm	linear peristaltic	65 ml/ 150 ml/ 250 ml collapsible reservoir	9 V	0.1–9.9 ml/h	±5%	2,3,4
WalkMed 410c	360 g	11.2 × 10.2 × 4.6 cm	linear peristaltic programmable	65 ml/ 150 ml/ 250 ml collapsible reservoir	9 V	0.01–30 ml/h	±5%	2,3, 4,5
WalkMed 420i/c	360 g	11.2 × 10.2 × 4.6 cm	linear peristaltic programmable	65 ml/ 150 ml/ 250 ml collapsible reservoir	9 V	0–9.9 ml/h	±5%	2,3 4,5

Table 5.1: *Continued*

Make/Model	Weight**	Dimensions***	Pump mechanism	Reservoir	Battery	Flow rate	Accuracy	Alarm*
WalkMed 430pca	360 g	11.2 × 10.2 × 4.6 cm	linear peristaltic programmable	65 ml/ 150 ml/ 250 ml collapsible reservoir	9 V		±5%	2,3 4,5
WalkMed 440pic	360 g	11.2 × 10.4 × 4.6 cm	linear peristaltic programmable	65 ml/ 150 ml/ 250 ml collapsible reservoir	9 V		±5%	2,3 4,5
Pfizer Infusaid 400	200 g	9 × 2.8 cm	non-electronic metal bellows concept	50 ml	none	flow rate affected by a number of variables		none
Medtronic SynchroMed 8611H	200 g	7 × 2.7 cm	rotary peristaltic system	18 ml	lithium	0.1–18 ml/day		none
SynchroMed 8615	200 g	7 × 2.7 cm	rotary peristaltic system	18 ml	lithium	0.1–18 ml/day		none
Baxter APII	454 g	12.4 × 4.6 × 8.6 cm	peristaltic programmable	100 ml/ 250 ml collapsible reservoir (also spike for IV bag)	9 V	0.1–49.9 ml/h	±10%	1,2,3,4
Graseby Medical 9000 series	316 g	16.8 × 10 × 2.7 cm	peristaltic programmable	50 ml 100 ml 250 ml cassette (also spike for IV bag)	9 V	0–100 ml/h	±10%	1,2,3, 4,5,7

* Alarms
1 – end of travel/infusion, 2 – low battery, 3 – occlusion, 4 – internal malfunction, 5 – lower residual volume in medication cassette, 6 – start-up review (power up), 7 – air in line.
** Includes batteries and smallest reservoir.
*** Includes smallest reservoir (empty) and protective cases for syringe pumps.

6

Managing complications of chemotherapy

INTRODUCTION

Cytotoxic drugs have, without exception, the potential to cause great harm if they are not prescribed, dispensed and administered safely and correctly. Cytotoxic drugs are taken to the very limit of, and often beyond, their toxic threshold. This is unlike most other drugs, which have a therapeutic dose set within the maximum and minimum tolerated doses.

It is important that all members of a multidisciplinary health care team play a part in safe administration, a process that begins with the writing of a prescription, and is followed by pharmaceutical dispensing, to end with chemotherapy nurses administering. Pharmacy is invested with being the gatekeeper of this process. The professional responsibilities of a pharmacist can be defined as the safe and appropriate administration of drugs. To fulfil this function of safe, accurate and appropriate dispensing a pharmacist needs to have a concise protocol referred to when dispensing each and every prescription. In broad terms the protocol should cover:

▼ is the patient fit and able to receive chemotherapy?
▼ is the chemotherapy being prescribed for the patient appropriate, protocolized and pharmaceutically sound?
▼ is the prescription written such that it can be dispensed safely and without question or doubt?
▼ has the patient been prescribed appropriate and effective support therapies in order to minimize trauma, physical or psychological, associated with the chemotherapy?

SUITABILITY OF THE PATIENT FOR CHEMOTHERAPY

In order to carry out all of these functions, a fairly comprehensive clinical knowledge of cytotoxic drugs is required. However, it is not the remit of this Handbook to consider all of these parameters.

However, a number of general issues are worth touching on. There must be checks made to confirm the patient is suitable for the chemotherapy prescribed for them. It is necessary to consider the patient's haematological status (if not dose-limiting, haematological suppression is a common toxicity of almost all chemotherapies). An assessment of the patient's general performance or well-being needs to be established as, again, fairly universally intravenous chemotherapy will debilitate and fatigue the patient. A number of more drug-specific checks should also be made which result as a function of specific drug toxicities. Particularly important are checks on renal function in patients destined to receive nephrotoxic agents e.g. cisplatin, or renally eliminated agents e.g. methotrexate. Checks of risk factors predisposing ifosfamide recipients to encephalopathy (low serum albumin, poor renal function, presence of a large pelvic mass) should be made and a check of adequate cardiac function in patients scheduled to start anthracycline treatment should also be made. The absence of third-space fluid accumulations in patients due to receive methotrexate should be confirmed.

SUITABILITY OF THE DOSE

A check must be made on the chemotherapy dose. Chemotherapy is peculiar in that rather than the dosage being a straight number of milligrams or, as in paediatric circles, mg/kg; the concept of body surface area (BSA) is used to try and individualize a dose to a patient. Here, through a consideration of weight and height and the application of the Du Bois formula (Equation 1) or more commonly the Graham and George modification (Equation 2) a BSA is calculated (in units of metres squared) for a patient. The patient's individualized dose can then be calculated by knowing the milligrams per metre squared for the individual doses in the drug regimen.

$$\text{Equation 1}\quad \text{BSA (cm}^2) = \text{weight}^{0.425} \times \text{height}^{0.725} \times 71.84$$

$$\text{Equation 2}\quad \text{BSA (m}^2) = \frac{\text{height (cm)} \times \text{weight (kg)}}{3600}$$

There is much debate about whether ideal or actual body weight should be used for such calculations, and whether body weight including such disease-related symptoms as effusions, particularly those of the peritoneum, should be corrected for, and whether maximum or minimum surface areas should be assigned. It is known that all the formulae are weak at the periphery of their calculations, usually considered to be where the BSA is less than $1.4\ m^2$ and/or greater than $2.1\ m^2$. In good clinical oncology practice, the dose in milligrams per metre squared should be defined in a treatment protocol outlining the dosage and the conditions which make it permissible to administer the chemotherapy. Not only is it important to consider the individual dose per treatment, but for a number of the cytotoxic drugs, there exists cumulative or maximum ceilings which should only be breached with sound clinical reasoning. Probably the most famous of these is vincristine, where the intravenous dose should not exceed 2 mg in any one administration, even though the protocol may specify $1.5\ mg/m^2$. Again, this threshold may be deliberately altered in a particular protocol aimed at a more susceptible group of the population. For example, because the elderly are more susceptible to vincristine-induced neuropathy the maximum dose per course may be 1.0 or 1.5 mg. Furthermore, cardiotoxic thresholds exist for all the anthracyclines and whilst it is possible and not fatal to administer beyond these doses, the patient's risk factor for cardiac complications magnifies considerably.

Whilst it is accepted that pharmacists do not prescribe, it is beholden upon them to intervene in the prescribing process if they think that the patient has passed either a dose per administration ceiling or accumulative dose ceiling, which is detrimental to their health or the safe administration of the chemotherapy.

SUITABILITY OF THE ADMINISTRATION ROUTE

An important part of a pharmaceutical protocol is to check the vehicle and schedule of the drug to be administered are suitable. The final generalized check is that the administration route is appropriate; this is of particular importance with subcutaneous routes and intrathecal routes. Whilst the subcutaneous (or even intramuscular) route is safe and often appropriate for drugs such as cytarabine, methotrexate and bleomycin, it is important to consider the total volume to be injected. Volumes of greater than 1 ml often cause unnecessary pain and suffering to the patient, however, whilst these drugs are safe, there is no indication for the administration of anthracyclines or platinum compounds subcutaneously.

The potentially fatal issue regarding a route of administration is that of the intrathecal route. It is perhaps safest if as a general principle no drug is given intrathecally – however, cytarabine and methotrexate have a valuable role in the treatment and prevention of CNS disease in lymphomas and leukaemias. They are therefore permissible by this route. But the vinca alkaloids should **never** be given intrathecally. So potentially devastating are the consequences of mis-administration of chemotherapeutic drugs through the wrong route, that institutions and individual pharmacists should derive practices which allow rapid identification of the abnormal, e.g. the use of fluorescent labels or coloured syringe caps to identify drugs to be given by an alternative route to the intravenous route. Those drugs intended for administration by an alternative route should **never** be presented to practitioners, whether medical or nursing, for administration at the same time as intravenous therapies.

INTRAVENOUS ADMINISTRATION AND EXTRAVASATION

The majority of cancer chemotherapy will be given by the intravenous (IV) route and therefore the remainder of this chapter will consider some of the issues surrounding IV administration. The most devastating consequence of inappropriate IV administration will be discussed first. This is the injury of extravasation.

Extravasation is the inappropriate or accidental administration of chemotherapy into the subcutaneous or subdermal tissues rather than into the intravenous compartment. The consequence of this action is often pain, erythema, inflammation and discomfort which, if left undiagnosed or inappropriately treated can lead to necrosis and functional loss of the tissue and limb concerned.

Extravasation injuries can therefore range from apparently insignificant erythematous reactions, through skin sloughing to severe necrosis. Whilst extravasation is possible with any IV injection, it is only considered problematic with those compounds that are known to be vesicant or irritant.

1 Occurrence

Whilst extravasation is a serious consequence of IV therapy, evidence exists to demonstrate that appropriately treated extravasation, dealt with within 24 hours causes no further problems to the patient.[1-4]

It is a condition that is often under-diagnosed, under-treated and unreported. A large number of articles and reviews of extravasation have been published over the past ten years.[5-11] Their relevance is difficult to assess, as they often refer to isolated incidents that may have been treated in a haphazard way, without incorporating the knowledge that may be gleaned from a wider view of the literature. There are, however, several retrospective reviews and clinical trials that go part of the way to offering evidence of the efficacy of various treatments.[12-15] However, much can be done to minimize extravasation by forethought, planning and improved prevention measures.

2 Risk factors associated with extravasation

The following factors contribute to extravasation injury:

▼ error associated with the administration technique i.e. the human angle
▼ error associated with the administration device
▼ factors associated with the patient
▼ the inherently physical properties of the drugs concerned.

2.1 The administration

The elimination of human error can be considered to be impossible. In excess of 100 000 doses of chemotherapy and over 1 000 000 IVs are in progress each day inevitably leading to some degree of human error. However, risk associated with these factors should be minimized by the use of good training and educational policy, not only as stand-alone courses, but, importantly, on a continuing educational basis. One of the greatest skills that individuals can bring to the administration of chemotherapy is the fact that it is for them routine. It is neither appropriate nor is it safe practice to administer chemotherapy on a 'when required' basis. It is a blind process where no two administrations will be similar, it is thus as much an art as a science.

2.2 The administration device

More-rigorous scientific thought can govern the selection of cannula; it inherently makes sense and has been demonstrated in a number of studies and through the National Extravasation Register that rigid steel cannulas lead to more problems than flexible Teflon or Silicone cannulas. The selection of device or cannula is also influenced by the competing issues of biology and physics.

Flexible cannulas are supplied in a variety of widths and lengths and the biology of veins means that the smaller and shorter the cannula the less the trauma associated with the cannulation process. However, the physics of short narrow pipes means that smaller diameter pipes increase the resistance and decrease the flow of the fluid through them. Or conversely, the pressure of delivery has to be increased.

The insertion of a cannula necessitates the puncture of the vein wall. This wall is relatively fragile. If the pressure of the flowing blood is greater than that of the fluid entering the vein via the cannula, there is a risk of back-flow into the cannula, or of rupture of the vein around the cannula edge, leading to leakage. Vein walls contain small holes and therefore the greater the pressure of the incoming fluid, the greater is the chance of wall rupture.

There needs to be a series of professional judgements. For example, if the quantity of the necessary chemotherapy to be administered is a 2 mg/2 ml dose of vincristine, then probably a small paediatric cannula is appropriate.

The science and technology of cannula have developed rapidly and there are now a number of high-technology developments, e.g. the Silicon/Teflon IV cannula, and the cannula materials that soften once exposed to the warmer internal body temperature of 37°C.

2.3 Location of cannulation site

Once the appropriate cannulation device has been selected, a site for cannulation has to be chosen. This must be a site where the cannula can be inserted easily and fastened securely, observed easily and one which will not come under stress if the patient or administrator moves. Taking these factors into account, the most appropriate site for location of a cannula is considered to be the forearm.

However, it has to be accepted that this is not always going to be an available site for cannulation. The vessels in the dorsum of the hand are probably the next most appropriate location for cannulation. Such sites as the antecubital fossa should be avoided. As a general rule joints and creases should be avoided as these often represent a 'small' anatomical space, with nerves and tendons (often with little 'covering') present.

2.4 Factors associated with the patient

Despite these theoretically correct sites for cannula location, a number of other patient factors come into play. Disease parameters such as lymphodema in breast disease, or other underlying physiological conditions, such as diabetes and peripheral circulatory diseases such as Raynard's disease; all can modify this theory. Patients who have had previous radiation therapy at the site of injection may develop severe local reactions from extravasated cytotoxic drugs. This is known as recall injury and has been noted in patients who have received doxorubicin.[16]

Cytotoxic drugs also have the potential to cause cutaneous abnormalities in areas that have been damaged previously by radiation, even if the areas are distant from the injection site. Furthermore, areas of previous surgery where the underlying tissue is likely to be fibrosed and toughened all dramatically increase the risk of extravasation.

Because of the toxic chemical nature of many cytotoxic drugs and because of the stress and trauma involved in the cannulation process, combined with the fact that chemotherapy is given over a number of cycles on a three-weekly or even weekly basis; it is thought by many that the sites of cannulation should be alternated. A final factor to be worked into this complicated equation is the patient's preference. Often patients do not wish to be cannulated in their dominant hand and, in fact, there is some evidence to suggest that this is a more complicated, more traumatic process anyway because the underlying muscular structures of the dominant hand or arm are better developed and therefore apply greater pressure to the vascular structures which they surround.

2.5 Factors associated with the drugs

Whilst pharmacists may be involved in the education and training of personnel and may be involved in the administration of chemotherapy, their influence over this and the choice of cannula and site of cannulation may be limited.

The most important input that pharmacy can have is by consideration of the drugs themselves and by characterizing their extravasation risk. It is now well documented that a number of physico-chemical factors influence, and usually increase, the extravasation risk of individual drugs. These are:

▼ the ability to bind directly to DNA (most cytotoxic drugs do this)
▼ an ability to kill replicating cells of which such drugs also include the cytotoxic and anti-viral agents
▼ an ability to cause tissue or vascular dilatation
▼ the pH, osmolarity and excipience in the formulation of the drug.

These parameters are more specifically defined as pH outside the range 5.5–8.5 and osmolarity greater than that of plasma, 290 mosmol/L and formulation components such as alcohol, polyethylene glycol and Tweens. Other formulation-related parameters include the concentration and volume of the solutions to be administered.

Unfortunately, these two parameters are contradictory to each other in so far as the smaller the volume the less the likelihood of extravasation but the greater the concentration, the higher the risk of extravasation, or the greater the damage should any extravasation be caused. As the commonest way to decrease the volume is to increase the concentration, juggling these two factors becomes more of an art than a science. Table 6.1 classifies the cytotoxic drugs with these factors in mind in three groups: vesicant, irritant and non-vesicant.

Table 6.1: *Classification of cytotoxic drugs according to their potential to cause serious necrosis when extravasated*

Vesicants: Group 1	Irritants: Group 2	Non-vesicants: Group 3
Aclarubicin	Carboplatin	Asparaginase
Amsacrine	Etoposide	Bleomycin
Carmustine	Lipsomal daunorubicin	Cladribine*
Cisplatinum	Methotrexate	Cyclophosphamide*
Dacarbazine	Mitozantrone	Cytarabine
Dactinomycin		Fludarabine
Daunorubicin		Fluorouracil*
Docetaxel		Gemcitabine
Doxorubicin		Ifosfamide*
Epirubicin		Melphalan
Idarubicin		Pentostatin
Mitomycin		Raltitrexed
Mustine		Thiotepa*
Paclitaxel		α Interferons
Plicamycin		Aldesleukin (IL-2)*
Treosulfan		
Vinblastine		
Vincristine		
Vindesine		

The classification of those drugs in Group 3 marked with an asterisk is controversial.[19] While being regarded by some as non-vesicant, others have argued that they represent an irritant hazard to subcutaneous tissues. Cox *et al.* have further suggested that a simple/non-vesicant classification would be more helpful as this is less confusing with regard to the significance of the extravasation. It is the view of this author that all extravasation is significant, but that the three-group classification can be helpful in individualizing treatment.

3   Prevalence

It is, however, encouraging that the occurrence of extravasation, certainly in the oncological population, is remarkably low. Many surveys, including the author's research work in Birmingham, has shown that the general rate of extravasation for intravenous therapy runs at between 20% and 30% and, in fact, some authors have proposed that if left long enough, any intravenous access will extravasate and that the time to extravasation will range from one to seven days, but at seven days 95% of all intravenous access sites will have extravasated, i.e. the cannula will have been displaced from the venous compartment into the surrounding tissues. Whilst this may be alarming, it must be remembered that other than some local and transient morbidity for the patient, the vast majority of these extravasation injuries are non-complicated. However, in at-risk populations extra care and highly educated administrative personnel means that the incidence rate falls to below 5% and often below 1%.

PREVENTION OR MINIMIZATION OF THE PROBLEMS OF EXTRAVASATION

The position, size and age of the venepuncture site are the factors which have greatest bearing on the likelihood of problems occurring. However, if the following points are borne in mind, the likelihood of extravasation can be significantly reduced.

▼ For slow infusion of high-risk drugs, a central line or drum catheter should be used.

▼ To ensure patency of a peripheral IV site, it is best to administer cytotoxics through a recently-sited cannula. Site the cannula so it cannot become dislodged; use the forearm and avoid, if possible, sites near joints.

▼ Administer vesicants by slow IV push into the side-arm port of a fast-running IV infusion of compatible solution. The most vesicant drug should be administered first.

▼ Assess a peripheral site continually for signs of redness or swelling.

▼ Verify patency of the IV site prior to vesicant infusion and regularly throughout; if there are any doubts, stop and investigate. Resite the cannula if the patency of the cannulation is still not entirely satisfactory.

▼ Ask the patient to report any sensations of burning or pain in the infusion site. Some investigators suggest delaying the administration of antiemetics until after vesicant administration. The sedative and anti-inflammatory effects of antiemetics often mask the early warning signs of extravasation and may impede the patient's ability to report any sensation at the infusion site.

▼ Never hurry. Administer drugs slowly to allow the drug to be diluted by the carrier solution and to allow careful assessment of the IV site.

▼ Document carefully the rate of administration, location and condition of site, verification of patency, and patient's responses, on giving any potentially extravasable drugs.

If vein diameter or vein collapse are a problem, then the use of glyceryl trinitrate patches distal to the cannula may be helpful.[17,18]

DIAGNOSIS OF EXTRAVASATION INJURY

It is important when diagnosing extravasation that a misdiagnosis is not made. This is because the treatment is physiologically traumatic to the body and may involve the administration of drugs which, in their own right, could cause or potentiate extravasation.

Early detection of extravasation is crucial. Common misdiagnoses are made because the observer is not differentiating discoloration reactions in the vein, venous shock, flare or phlebitis reactions of the vein wall and/or anaphylaxis. This is complicated further as some cytotoxics are highly coloured agents and if the vein in question is particularly superficial then a bright red solution injected into the vein may cause local discoloration. Furthermore, cytotoxics are often administered cool, at best at room temperature. They are then administered fairly rapidly into blood at a temperature of 37°C. The greater the thermal gradient between the drug solution and the blood the greater the stress on the vein and often contraction and/or venus spasm is observed due to thermal shock.

It is also important to differentiate extravasation from other intravenous phenomena such as phlebitis and/or anaphylaxis. Phlebitis (inflammation of the vein) occurs often as a result of correct administration due to the nature of some of the agents involved either because their formulation had an irritant component e.g. etoposide, or because the pH of the formulation is particularly acidic or alkaline e.g. doxorubicin and epirubicin. Here a transient, but well pronounced inflammation along the line of the vein will occur and this may track for some considerable distance. Anaphylaxis will have a central component of cardiovascular nature along with pulmonary complications, but often starts at the local site of injection. A less traumatic form of anaphylaxis is the hypersensitivity reaction. This was not well observed or recognized with the oncology drugs until the recent introduction of the taxains, both of these due to the nature of their formulation often cause local and/or central hypersensitivity. Once these alternative diagnoses have been considered, and excluded, the practitioner should go on to consider the diagnosis of extravasation.

SYMPTOMS OF EXTRAVASATION

Extravasation should be suspected when:

▼ the patient complains of burning, stinging, pain or any acute change at the injection site. The patient is often the first person to become aware that something is wrong with their IV therapy, so instruct them at the beginning of treatment to inform staff of any acute change during treatment. Explain the reason for this in a way which is not frightening but conveys the need for the patient's input and participation. Given reassurance that, if a leakage of drug should occur, it would probably not cause serious problems if the infusion is promptly stopped and the correct treatment instituted. Patients who are unable to communicate should be particularly closely observed

▼ induration, erythema, venous discoloration or swelling is observed at the site (discoloration alone may not indicate extravasation as doxorubicin, epirubicin and mitozantrone have been reported to produce this)

▼ no blood return is obtained. A lack of blood return from the cannula is commonly quoted as a sign that extravasation has occurred. It is however, the most misleading of all signs and has been implicated in a number of serious incidences. This occurs because although there has been extravasation injury and the cannula has become displaced, the act of trying to draw blood back to test for blood return moves the cannula back into the vein. Thus blood is returned, however, there is a hole in the vein wall in the proximity of the cannula tip. So when administration recommences, a larger and more significant extravasation injury ensues. Alternatively, the bevel of the needle can puncture the vein wall during venepuncture, allowing drug to escape into the tissue whilst the lumen of the needle may still remain in the blood vessel and allow adequate blood return

▼ the flow rate is reduced. A reduced rate may not be observed when using an infusion pump, so close observation is necessary

▼ increased resistance to the administration, once possible changes in the position of the body e.g. bending of wrist or elbow, or cannula support e.g. the bandaging, have been excluded as possible causes of the increased resistance, then a displaced cannula and hence extravasation are the next most likely causes. This is often one of the first signs of a problem or of pre-extravasation syndrome.

THE EXTRAVASATION SYNDROME

1 Pre-extravasation syndrome

In general, this is either pre-extravasation syndrome or a type I or type II extravasation injury. The pre-extravasation syndrome (PES) often involves little or no leakage, but particularly severe phlebitis and/or local hypersensitivity together with a number of other local risk factors e.g. difficult cannulation, one (but not multiple) patient symptoms, and is probably the easiest to treat by withdrawing IV therapy immediately to prevent further deterioration to a fullblown type I or type II extravasation. It should however, be remembered that if patients have shown a susceptibility towards pre-extravasation syndrome, further administrations should proceed with extreme caution and ideally in the contra-lateral limb to where the problem was diagnosed.

2 Type I extravasations

Type I extravasation injuries raise a bleb or blister and have a defined area of increased firmness around the injury site. Type I injuries are most commonly associated with rapid intravenous bolus-type injections where the pressure applied by the person administering the drugs causes fluid to collect around the injury site. Type I injuries also occur when IV infusions are administered through over-pressurized pumps.

3 Type II extravasations

Type II extravasation injuries are those characterized by soft, diffuse 'soggy' tissue-type injuries, where obvious dispersal into the intracellular space has occurred. This type of injury is most commonly associated with gravity-fed IV infusion, or a bolus injection given into the side-arm of a free-flowing IV infusion, which has become subtly or partially dislodged.

The treatment of both of these type of injuries is the same however, the success at different points in the treatment pathway can be dramatically different.

TREATMENT OF EXTRAVASATION – GENERAL

All extravasation injuries should be aspirated i.e. the removal or the attempted removal of the offending drug as this is probably the only viably successful way of preventing further injury. If the treatment can be delivered quickly, this process is often successful in type I injuries where the blister or bleb can be aspirated, but is notoriously unsuccessful in the diffused type II tissue infiltrated injuries. It is important during this treatment process not to remove the offending cannula as this is the key to locating the affected area, and the area around the cannula tip where the injury has occurred should be marked clearly on the skin surface so that its site and size at first diagnosis can be recalled.

Once the extravasation injury has been characterized in terms of size, volume and type; aspiration is attempted and then, traditionally steroids, either hydro-cortisone or dexamethasone, are administered locally by subcutaneous injection to the area or by central IV injection. These may be administered down the original cannula or subcutaneously into the area.

The function of steroids in the treatment of extravasation has no proven basis and there is, at best, only limited circumstantial evidence. The most convincing reason for their inclusion is the idea that the whole process of extravasation involves local tissue trauma. This trauma is made worse by the treatment process and as a consequence of this trauma, a local inflammatory cascade is started and therefore the applied steroids suppress or settle this cascade, making further treatment easier and improving its effectiveness and making any improvement easier to assess.

Once these two basic principles have been initiated, treatment can be characterized as either:

'Spread and dilute' using:

▼ normal saline
▼ hyaluronidase
▼ warm, continuous compression and elevation of limb.

or

'Localize and neutralize' using:

▼ antidote (if available)
▼ intermittent cold compression.

If these treatments are applied in the wrong order during treatment of an extravasation injury, the consequences can be catastrophic.

1 In summary

▼ It is vital to act promptly.
▼ There should be clear guidelines for prompt 'first aid' treatment.
▼ The extravasation kit should remain simple to avoid confusion but comprehensive enough to meet fully all reasonable needs.

▼ Comprehensive treatment and expert advice must be available as soon as possible. Ideally within ten minutes of the injury occurring, certainly within one hour and definitely within 24 hours. Post-24 hours the treatment philosophy is completely different and is no longer an active 'curative' treatment, but is a damage limitation exercise.

▼ There should be clear, easy to follow instructions.

▼ The emergency treatment should aim to remove as soon as possible, as much of the offending drug as is feasible from the subcutaneous tissue.

▼ The emergency treatment should not cause further tissue damage or, in the event of misdiagnosis, cause damage where extravasation has not occurred.

GENERAL PROCEDURE FOR MANAGEMENT OF EXTRAVASATION

▼ Seek experienced assistance from someone more used to looking at extravasation.

▼ Stop the infusion, disconnect the drip but DO NOT REMOVE THE CANNULA.

▼ Mark the extravasated area with a pen.

▼ Aspirate the extravasated drug, trying also to draw some blood back from the cannula. This may be facilitated by sc injection of either 0.9% sodium chloride, to dilute the drug, or 1500 units of hyaluronidase in 2 ml water for injection. (Hyaluronidase should NEVER be used with vesicant drugs, unless as a specific antidote.)

▼ Remove the cannula.

▼ Give 100 mg hydrocortisone IV. This should be administered via a new cannula, resited remotely from the extravasation area.

▼ Give 100 mg hydrocortisone (2 ml) as 0.1–0.2 ml sc injections at about six to eight points around the circumference of the extravasation site.

▼ Give sc injections of specific antidote where applicable.

▼ Apply 1% hydrocortisone cream to the area.

▼ Cover with sterile gauze and apply heat to disperse the extravasated drug or cool the area to localize the extravasation.

▼ Measure the area of the extravasation and document the treatment in the patient's notes. Complete a Green Card (*see* page 118). Photographing the area can be very helpful.

▼ Give antihistamine cover (terfenadine 60 mg, po, or chlorpheniramine 4 mg, po, once only).

▼ Provide analgesia if required (indomethacin 25 mg tds or dihydrocodeine has proved effective).

This general procedure can be refined, depending upon the type of extravasation provision that is required (*see* below). If this refinement is based on the 'group' classification (*see* page 110) of cytotoxics then the following general and specific procedures could be used.

1 Management of extravasation of a non-vesicant Group 3 drug

If a large volume has extravasated, aspirate as much fluid as possible. Dispersal of the extravasated drug may be facilitated by the use of subcutaneous hyaluronidase (1500 units in 2 ml water for injection, or 0.9% sodium chloride) injected around the area of the injury. Apply heat and compression to assist with natural dispersal of the drug. No further treatment should be required. Manage the situation symptomatically.

2 Management of extravasation of an irritant Group 2 drug

With the irritant group there exists the possibility of some local inflammation or necrosis, and/or some pain, particularly in sensitive individuals. Aspirate as much fluid as possible, give 100 mg hydrocortisone via the venflon, 100 mg sc hydrocortisone as 0.2 ml injections around the circumference of the affected area, apply topical hydrocortisone and cover the area with an ice pack. There are no specific antidotes for these drugs. Manage further symptoms symptomatically.

3 Management of extravasation of a vesicant Group 1 drug

Dactinomycin	Infiltrate the affected area with 1–3 ml of 3% sodium thiosulphate.
Aclarubicin Daunorubicin Doxorubicin Epirubicin Idarubicin Mitomycin	Paint dimethylsulphoxide (DMSO) topically to the extravasated area. This should be applied every two hours, followed by hydrocortisone cream and 30 minutes of cold compression, for the first 24 hours. Treatment for the next 14 days should consist of topical application of DMSO at six-hourly intervals, alternating with six-hourly applications of topical hydrocortisone cream, a preparation thus being applied every three hours on an alternate basis. Contact with good skin should be avoided. If blistering occurs, the DMSO should be stopped and further advice sought. (Sodium bicarbonate may have a role.*)
Cisplatinum	Infiltrate the area with 1–3 ml of 3% sodium thiosulphate, aspirate back, then given 1500 units of hyaluronidase around the area and apply heat and compression.
Carmustine Plicamycin Treosulfan	Infiltrate the area with 1–3 ml of 2.1% sodium bicarbonate, leave for two minutes and aspirate off again.*
Docetaxel Paclitaxel	Infiltrate the area with 1–3 ml of a mixture of 100 mg hydrocortisone and 4 mg chlorpheniramine in 10 ml, as 0.2 ml 'pin cushion' subcutaneous injections. Large-volume extravasations may need as much as 10 ml. This should be followed by 1500 units of hyaluronidase and warm compression. Warm compression should be alternated with the application of topical mepyramine (Anthisan) or any topical anti-histamine cream. The creams should be applied alternately for the following three days. In particularly severe cases, 1 g of oral sodium cromoglycate should be administered as soon as possible after the injury.
Mustine	Infiltrate the area with 1–3 ml of 3% sodium thiosulphate. Introduce a further 100 mg of hydrocortisone to the infiltrated area. Apply cold compression intermittently for 12 hours.

Vincristine Vinblastine Vindesine	Infiltrate the area with 1500 units of hyaluronidase, as 0.2 ml injections, over and around the circumference of the affected area. Apply heat and compression for the first 24 hours. On following days apply a topical non-steroidal anti-inflammatory cream to the affected area, four times a day for the subsequent seven days.

Note that 2.1% sodium bicarbonate is not commercially available but can be produced when required at the scene, by a double dilution of 8.4% ampoules. However, 2.1% sodium bicarbonate still represents an extravasation hazard and should be used **with extreme care**. The 3% sodium thiosulphate is obtained by diluting 1.2 ml of the commercially available 50% sodium thiosulphate injection up to 20 ml with sterile water for injections.[19-24] Dimethylsulphoxide topical can be between 50–99% pure, both BP and chemical Analar grades have and can be used.

*While many reports in the literature discuss the successful use of sodium bicarbonate – indeed this author has used it successfully himself – there has been an increase over the last three years in the number of reports involving sodium bicarbonate as the causative agent of extravasation injuries. Furthermore, at least four of these incidences reported via the National Extravasation Reporting Scheme have occurred as a consequence of using sodium bicarbonate as a treatment agent. While the overwhelming number of cases is concerned with the use of 8.4% sodium bicarbonate, it is the author's opinion that sodium bicarbonate should be taken out of the routine treatment of extravasation and only used by those extremely familiar with its potential consequences in cases of low pH (0–5) extravasation injuries, and only then used at dilution to give 2.1% or 1% strengths. If it is infiltrated into an area it should be introduced very sparingly into the 'body' of the injury – not the periphery – and aspiration to remove excess sodium bicarbonate should always be attempted.

PROVISION OF AN EMERGENCY POLICY AND EXTRAVASATION KIT

Both the emergency treatment policy and extravasation kit should be simple and, therefore, easy to use without the risk of further damage; or complete and comprehensive but with the consequent necessity for expertise and care.

Whichever option is chosen for the local situation at ward or patient level, it will be necessary to hold the complete set of antidotes and hot and cold facilities at one or several locations within the hospital. Considering the following points may help in deciding the answer to the question, 'Is a "simple" or a "comprehensive" set-up required?'

▼ Is it a department or ward routinely (i.e. more than 30% of the time) using potentially vesicant drugs?
▼ Are the staff particularly trained in the detection and treatment of extravasation?
▼ Does the treatment policy require a special antidote for any of these drugs?
▼ Are potentially hazardous treatments being carried out 24 hours a day?
▼ Is inpatient or outpatient treatment intended?

If the answer to the first four questions is 'yes', almost irrespective of the fifth, then a comprehensive set-up is required. The fifth question is to help assess the qualification and educational needs of the staff most likely to have to carry out the procedure. Outpatient areas are often staffed with a lower skill mix.

Appendix 1, page 124 details the contents of a complete/comprehensive extravasation kit as used in the St Chad's Oncology Unit, City Hospital, Dudley Road, Birmingham, UK. The kit also contains details of the local emergency policy which are contained on two plastic-covered cards within the box.

Appendix 2, page 124 details the contents of a simple extravasation kit which contains modified emergency cards giving 'first aid' treatment and directions indicating where full antidotes can be obtained.

DOCUMENTATION AND REPORTING OF EXTRAVASATION

It is important that a complete history of an extravasation event is documented, with diagrams and photographs, in the patient's notes. Observation and documentation of the injury should be on a daily basis for the first few days, extended then to weekly observation on a planned follow-up. (Figure 6.1 shows an ideal extravasation documentation slip.)

In an attempt to collate and analyse data on extravasation events in a large number of patients, a 'Green Card' scheme for reporting extravasation incidences, their treatment and outcome is being co-ordinated through the St Chad's Unit, City Hospital, Dudley Road, Birmingham, UK.

Extravasation Documentation Slip

Name: Date: Time: Location:

Drug sequence:

Needles size and type:

Technique:

Venepuncture site:

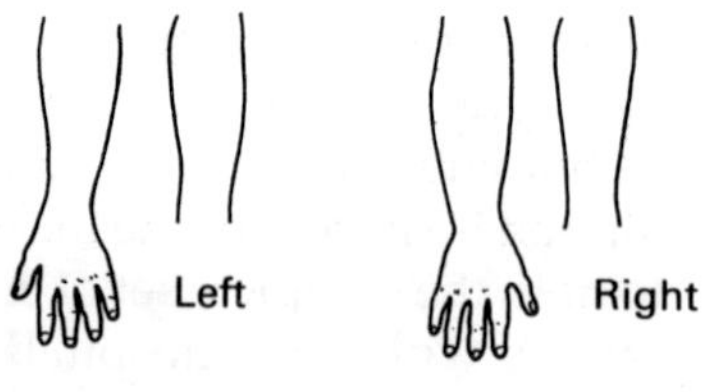

Approximate amount of extravasation:

Appearance:

Diameter of injured area:

Nursing management:

Patient's complaints and statements:

Signature:

Figure 6.1: *Extravasation documentation form*

1 Aims and objectives of the Green Card scheme

▼ To obtain accurate statistics on the number of incidents categorized by extravasating drug and type of treatment.
▼ To collect data on treatment methods and antidotes being used for extravasation incidents.
▼ To obtain accurate information on the outcome of incidents.
▼ To feedback information on treatments and their effectiveness.

2 What do Green Cards ask for?

▼ Drug(s) involved.
▼ Circumstances of detection.
▼ Extent of the problem.
▼ Drugs used in the treatment.
▼ Procedure for treatment.
▼ Type of cannulation.
▼ Location and extent of the extravasation.

The Green Cards are intended to be user-friendly. The information is strictly confidential and the reporting centre and patient remain anonymous.

The report cards are available from hospital pharmacy departments or oncology units in the UK or can be obtained direct from the Extravasation Report Co-ordinator, c/o St Chad's Unit, City Hospital, Dudley Road, Birmingham B18 7QH, UK.

An example of the Green Card is shown in Figure 6.2.

IN-CONFIDENCE REGISTER OF EXTRAVASATION AND ITS TREATMENT FOR THE REPORTING OF EXTRAVASATION FROM ANY THERAPEUTIC COMPOUND

Patient   Male*/Female*   Age _____   Height (m) _____   Weight (kg) _____

Drug causing extravasation was _____   Dose _____

Infused in* _____   Added to last running drip of* _____ /Stat*

Given Cannula/Butterfly (please state size) _____ over _____ mins/hr

The above drug formed part of course No. _____ in the following regimen

Drug	Total Dose	Infusion Fluid/Stat	Time	Already Given	Not Yet Given
				Yes/No*	Yes/No*
				Yes/No*	Yes/No*
				Yes/No*	Yes/No*
				Yes/No*	Yes/No*

Other drugs being given concurrently (oral + IVs) _____

Were the drugs being administered via a pump or syringe driver? | YES | NO |

If YES please indicate model _____

Please indicate SITE and cannulation and area of extravasation with measurements on the diagrams below

Front   Back   Left or Right Arm*

Other method of administration:

Central or long line*/Hickman line*/Portacath*/Drum catheter*

Other (please specify) _____

Location (please specify) _____

Details of extravasation treatment (Drug, Dose, Procedure)

_____

_____

Date of extravasation _____ Time of extravasation _____

Acute extravasation treatment started on _____ Stopped on _____

This section is not compulsory. Contact name for further details (Dr, nurse, pharmacist)   Name _____ Tel.No. _____

Additional comments _____

_____

_____

* Please delete or fill in as appropriate

_____

FOLLOW UP REPORT ON THE OUTCOME OF PREVIOUSLY REPORTED EXTRAVASATION INCIDENCE

Please detach this portion of the Green Card

Please give details of any chronic pharmacological treatment _____

_____

_____

Outcome (please tick one)

Resolved following acute treatment   ☐

Resolved using pharmacological treatment only   ☐

Extravasation untreated and required skin grafting   ☐

Patient lost to follow up   ☐

If the extravasation injury ulcerated, was there any functional loss in the affected limb? | YES | NO |

If yes, please give details _____

_____

If surgery was performed please give brief details _____

_____

_____

Figure 6.2: *Example of a Green Card*

ANAPHYLAXIS

An anaphylaxis reaction occurs as a result of an over-stimulation of the body's immune system. There are four types of hypersensitivity reactions documented. However, type I reactions are those most frequently associated with chemotherapy and are of the type where the body generates IgE antibodies to the foreign substance. This consequently means that there is often a sensitization period where a pre-anaphylaxis state occurs and during which the patient may report some of the more minor signs and symptoms associated with anaphylaxis. The site of administration may also demonstrate a flare-type reaction.

The signs and symptoms of an anaphylaxis are normally fairly rapid in onset and develop in general through the following course.

▼ Localized or generalized itching.
▼ Facial flushing leading to generalized flushing.
▼ Shortness of breath (sometimes with a wheeze).
▼ Uneasiness and agitation.
▼ Local oedema and then often facial oedema.
▼ Light-headed dizziness.
▼ Tightening of the chest.
▼ A tachycardic heartbeat.
▼ Falling blood pressure.
▼ 'Flu-like symptoms, often with quite violent shaking.

Whilst hypersensitivity is theoretically possible with any of the neoplastic agents, those that are more commonly associated with this phenomenon are asparaginase, bleomycin, cisplatin and carboplatin, cyclophosphamide and ifosfamide, daunorubicin, doxorubicin, epirubicin, mustine, methotrexate, melphalan, etoposide and teniposide.

The recent introduction of docetaxel and paclitaxel has seen a variation of the true anaphylaxis, called formulation-induced hypersensitivity. If untreated, the signs and symptoms as described above for anaphylaxis will result. However, careful prophylactic desensitization regimens can minimize, if not eliminate these types of hypersensitivity reactions. This usually involves giving high doses of steroids in the preceding 12 hours to administration, normally at approximately 12 hours and six hours prior to administration and the dose most commonly used is dexamethasone 20 mg orally. These drugs have fairly long half-lives and therefore, the timing is not critical within three hours. Because in the case of both docetaxel and paclitaxel the hypersensitivity is known to be associated with the release of histamine, immediately prior to administration both H_1 and H_2 type antihistamines should be administered. The author also has experience in particularly sensitive patients of using oral sodium cromoglycate 1 g one hour prior to administration in order to stabilize mast cells and so prevent the hypersensitivity cascade.

LEGAL ASPECTS OF ADMINISTRATION

Finally, some consideration should be given to the legal aspects of administration. This is most easily summarized with the four 'Cs':

▼ competency
▼ consent
▼ controls
▼ checks.

Both the institution and the individual have a duty of care to the patient and therefore must feel competent both in their own right and as a member of the institute, to deliver chemotherapy.

As we have seen previously in this chapter, the two most devastating outcomes of mis-administration, extravasation and anaphylaxis, are not wholly under the control of the operator and in the vast majority of cases will be due to intrinsic properties of the drugs.

However, the intravenous process does have an operator element to it and neglect in this area could be a neglect of duty of care, just as the administration of chemotherapy to known or suspected hypersensitive individuals would also represent a failure to deliver with due care and attention.

Whilst it is important not to increase the anxiety associated with the administration of chemotherapy, the patient is often the best and most accurate source for diagnosis of impending mishap, and therefore, before intravenous cannulation and administration is attempted, the patient should be informed and verbally consent to the process. This should therefore take the form of some brief outline as to what is to happen, what constitutes a successful outcome and signs and symptoms to report of early mishap.

The institution and individual should put in place controls so as to minimize and facilitate early detection of extravasation. This will include access to a documented extravasation and anaphylaxis policy as well as the individual concerned developing some sort of look and feel routine which they can adhere to during the administration of chemotherapy.

Only the person giving chemotherapy can exercise the honesty to acknowledge that extravasation may have occurred.

REFERENCES

1 Hecker JF (1990) Survival of intravenous chemotherapy infusion sites. *Br. J. Cancer* **62**, 660–2.
2 Bareford D (1985) Treatment of extravasation of vincristine with hydrocortisone and hyaluronidase. *Br. Med. J.* **291**, 1242.
3 Rudolph R (1978) Ulcers of the hand and wrist caused by doxorubicin hydrochloride. *Orthop. Rev.* **7**, 93–5.
4 Tsavaris NB *et al.* (1990) Conservative approach to the treatment of chemotherapy-induced extravasation. *J. Dermatol. Surg. Oncol.* **16**, 519–22.
5 Ignoffo RJ, Friedman MA (1980) Therapy of local toxicities caused by extravasation of cancer chemotherapeutic drugs. *Cancer Treat. Rev.* **7**, 17–27.
6 Banerjee A *et al.* (1987) Cancer chemotherapy agent-induced perivenous extravasation injuries. *Postgrad. Med. J.* **63**, 5–9.

7 Rudolph R, Larson DL (1987) Etiology and treatment of chemotherapeutic agent extravasation injuries: A review. *J. Clin. Oncol.* **5**, 1116–26.

8 Dorr RT (1981) Extravasation of vesicant antineoplastics. *Ariz. Med.* **28**, 271–5.

9 Cullen ML (1982) Current interventions for doxorubicin extravasations. *Oncol. Nurs. Forum* **9**, 52–3.

10 Linder RM *et al.* (1983) Management of extensive doxorubicin hydrochloride extravasation injuries. *J. Hand Surg.* **8**, 32–8.

11 Cohen MH (1979) Amelioration of adriamycin skin necrosis: An experimental study. *Cancer Treat. Rep.* **63**, 1003–4.

12 Hart LL, Middleton RK (eds) (1989) Treatment of doxorubicin extravasations. *DICP* **23**, 386–7.

13 Larson DL (1985) What is the appropriate management of tissue extravasation by antitumor agents? *Plast. Reconstr. Surg.* **75**, 397–405.

14 Coleman JJ *et al.* (1983) Treatment of adriamycin-induced skin ulcers: A prospective controlled study. *J. Surg. Oncol.* **22**, 129–35.

15 Olver IN *et al.* (1988) A prospective study of topical dimethyl sulfoxide for treating anthracycline extravasation. *J. Clin. Oncol.* **6**, 1732–5.

16 Donaldson SS *et al.* (1974) Adriamycin activity: A recall phenomenon after radiation therapy. *Ann. Intern. Med.* **81**, 407–8.

17 Khawaja HT *et al.* (1988) Effect of transdermal glyceryl trinitrate on the survival of peripheral intravenous infusions: A double-blind prospective clinical study. *Br. J. Surg.* **75**, 1212–15.

18 Wright A *et al.* (1985) Use of transdermal glyceryl trinitrate to reduce failure of intravenous infusion due to phlebitis and extravasation. *Lancet* **ii**, 1148–50.

19 Cox K *et al.* (1988) The management of cytotoxic drug extravasation: Guidelines drawn up by a working party for the Clinical Oncological Society of Australia. *Med. J. Aust.* **148**, 185–9.

20 Hirsh JD, Conlon PF (1983) Implementing guidelines for managing extravasation of antineoplastics. *Am. J. Hosp. Pharm.* **40**, 1516–19.

21 Schneider SM, Distelhorst CW (1989) Chemotherapy-induced emergencies. *Semin. Oncol.* **16**, 572–8.

22 Harwood KV, Aisner J (1984) Treatment of chemotherapy extravasation: Current status. *Cancer Treat. Rep.* **68**, 939–45.

23 McNeece J, Lightly J (1986) *Cytotoxic extravasation manual.* Pharmacy Department, Leeds General Infirmary, Leeds.

24 Smith R (1985) Prevention and treatment of extravasation. *Br. J. Parenter. Ther.* **6**, 114–18.

APPENDIX 1

Contents of a 'comprehensive' extravasation box:

▼ dimethylsulphoxide solution (50–100%)
▼ hyaluronidase 1500 units injection
▼ hydrocortisone 100 mg injection, and 1% cream
▼ sodium bicarbonate 8.4% injection*
▼ sodium chloride 0.9% injection
▼ sodium thiosulphate 50% injection*
▼ terfenadine 60 mg tablets
▼ water for injection (2 ml and 10 ml)
▼ selection of needles, syringes, alcohol wipes, cottonwool balls and sterile gauze
▼ directions to the nearest cold pack and heat pad.

* Overlabelled with directions for dilution.
Examples of the overlabels are shown below:

SODIUM BICARBONATE 8.4%
DO NOT USE UNDILUTED
5 ml of this solution should be added to 5 ml of water for injection and then 5 ml of this new solution added to a further 5 ml of water for injection. This will then give a 2.1% sodium bicarbonate solution.

SODIUM THIOSULPHATE 50%
DO NOT USE UNDILUTED
Dilute 1.2 ml of 50% sodium thiosulphate to 20 ml with water for injection. This will then give a 3% sodium thiosulphate solution.

APPENDIX 2

Contents of a 'simple' extravasation box:

▼ hyaluronidase 1500 units
▼ hydrocortisone 100 mg injection, and 1% cream
▼ sodium chloride 0.9% injection
▼ water for injections (2 ml)
▼ selection of needles, syringes, alcohol wipes, cottonwool balls and sterile gauze
▼ directions to the nearest cold pack and heat pad.

7

*Monitoring and treatment
of adverse effects in
cancer chemotherapy*

INTRODUCTION

Despite significant efforts over the last ten years to develop antineoplastic compounds with fewer adverse effects, the toxicity of cancer chemotherapy remains one of the main obstacles to its effective use. Most of the currently available drugs have been selected on the basis of their activity against proliferating cells. Unfortunately this cytotoxic activity is not highly selective and does not discriminate between malignant cells and normal cells undergoing rapid division. As a result, cytotoxic drugs probably have the narrowest therapeutic index of any class of drug in common use.

The adverse effects occurring most frequently with this group of drugs in the days and weeks immediately following treatment include suppression of bone marrow activity, anorexia, nausea and vomiting, mucositis and alopecia. Patients will require supportive care, both in the hospital and in the community, to help overcome these problems. Organ toxicities, such as pulmonary toxicity, neurotoxicity and cardiotoxicity, are more drug specific and, unlike most of the acute adverse effects, may not be reversible. Long-term effects may not be apparent until months or years following treatment. These problems include infertility due to suppression of ovarian or testicular function and occasionally the induction of a secondary malignancy in patients who have previously been successfully treated. In addition, cytotoxic drugs can give rise to a whole spectrum of rare, unpredictable or idiosyncratic reactions. The use of cytotoxic drugs in combination, in an attempt to increase their activity, adds to the toxicity of treatment, despite efforts being made to combine agents with different dose-limiting toxicities.

Reductions in dose or delays in treatment as a result of toxicity may compromise the success of potentially curative therapy, but, for the majority of patients, chemotherapy is given to palliate the disease and sometimes to prolong life. This has a considerable bearing on the degree of toxicity considered to be 'acceptable' to the patient.

Managing the toxicity of chemotherapy involves a number of approaches. Treatment must be individually tailored for each patient and appropriate measures taken to avoid or minimize predictable toxicity. Adverse effects which do arise in spite of these measures must be treated and accurately documented. To contribute effectively to patient care the pharmacist must have a detailed knowledge of the drugs prescribed and must be able to anticipate potential adverse effects, in order to monitor prescribing and to advise on appropriate supportive therapy.

INDIVIDUALIZING THERAPY

Although each cytotoxic drug varies in its particular spectrum of toxicity, some general precautions can be taken to minimize the risk of predictable adverse effects occurring. Appropriate investigations must be carried out before treatment commences to ensure that the patient is fit for chemotherapy; in particular their haematological, renal and hepatic functions should be investigated. In general, patients with a white cell count below 3000/mm³ or a platelet count below 100 000/mm³ should not be given myelosuppressive cytotoxics.

Unlike most classes of drug, where a standard dose range can be safely recommended for the majority of patients, the dose of cytotoxic drugs must be individually calculated for each patient on the basis of their weight or, more commonly, on body surface area (*see* page 106). Doses may then require further adjustment in the presence of renal or hepatic impairment to ensure that delayed excretion does not result in increased toxicity.

Methotrexate serum concentrations are measured following high-dose therapy to help determine the dose and duration of folinic acid necessary for adequate rescue. The concept of individualizing treatment based on serum drug concentrations is being explored with other agents, largely to optimize the efficacy of treatment.

MANAGEMENT OF ADVERSE EFFECTS

Significant progress has been made in reducing the mortality and morbidity of cancer chemotherapy through the improved management of adverse effects. Ondansetron and granisetron, the 5HT$_3$ receptor antagonists, have been significant additions to the armoury of available antiemetics. Reduced mortality in the febrile neutropenic patient has been achieved by the prompt use of combinations of antibiotics, usually an aminoglycoside and an anti-pseudomonal penicillin, to provide broad spectrum cover. The availability of new antifungal and antiviral agents has also been invaluable. Despite these advances, successful treatment of chemotherapy-related toxicity is expensive, involves prolonged hospitalization and a reduction in patients' quality of life. Thus, patient management must focus on the **prevention** of toxicity.

1 Extravasation

Extravasation of many cytotoxic drugs can have disastrous consequences. The long-term outcome may be permanent tissue damage, despite the best efforts made to rescue the situation. In the absence of adequate treatment, the approach to this problem relies heavily on safe techniques for administration of cytotoxic drugs (*see* Chapter 6).

2 Nausea and vomiting

Occasionally cytotoxic regimens or single agents such as vincristine or fluorouracil do not require antiemetic drugs to be given routinely, but, for any cytotoxic causing severe or moderate emesis, antiemetics should always be prescribed prophylactically and not used on an 'as required basis' after vomiting has begun. Although the availability of new, effective antiemetics and better use of existing agents has improved the control of acute nausea and vomiting, delayed emesis remains a significant problem, particularly for patients who have received cisplatin. Antiemetics should be taken regularly by all patients following treatment with cisplatin. Dexamethasone is probably the most effective available agent at the present time for delayed emesis and should be the basis of therapy, but further work is required in this area. More detailed information can be found by referring to the reference list on page 171.

3 Infection

A number of measures can be taken to minimize the risk of infection developing. Good oral hygiene is important as the mouth is a major source of infection, particularly in neutropenic patients. Patients should be instructed to brush their teeth regularly with a soft toothbrush and use regular antiseptic mouthwashes following tooth brushing and after every meal. Prophylactic antifungal therapy may also be appropriate.

Focal sepsis is a particular problem with IV catheter sites and is more prevalent with the increased use of central venous catheters. Ideally lines should only be handled by trained staff, using strict aseptic techniques and following agreed procedures for handling.

The haematopoietic growth factors G-CSF and GM-CSF shorten the duration of neutropenia following chemotherapy, thus reducing the incidence of infection. They are also being exploited to allow increased intensity of treatment where bone marrow suppression is the dose-limiting toxicity, in the hope of improving response rates and survival.

4 Alopecia

In an effort to avoid alopecia, scalp cooling techniques have been developed using ice caps and more sophisticated refrigeration systems. The procedure itself is unpleasant and can only be used with agents with a short elimination half-life such as doxorubicin with a half-life of 30 minutes. The results of studies carried out over the last 15 years remain equivocal. Hair loss may be avoided when single-agent doxorubicin is used, but is less effective when doxorubicin is used in combination with other drugs capable of causing alopecia, or is used at doses above 40 mg/m^2. In the absence of reliable methods of avoiding alopecia, patients should be prepared for hair loss and given practical advice on coping with this, for example when to expect loss of hair, how rapidly this will occur and advice on obtaining a wig.

MONITORING TOXICITY

Safe administration of chemotherapy relies on clear and accurate documentation of all treatment given. The total cumulative dose administered should be recorded for drugs such as doxorubicin where this is critical. Both the response to and the toxicity of therapy should be carefully documented. A detailed assessment of response is normally carried out after a pre-determined number of treatment cycles, and toxicity is generally assessed following every cycle. The occurrence of toxicity may result in a dose reduction, delay or some other modification to treatment on subsequent cycles. A number of international rating scales are available for rating predictable, acute reactions arising from chemotherapy, including that of the World Health Organization (WHO) and National Cancer Institute (NCI). Standardizing the assessment of treatment-related toxicity in this way allows comparison to be made between published reports of clinical trials. One example is shown in Table 7.1.

Table 7.1: *An example of the classification for patient toxicity and response used in a monitoring chart*

	Toxicity grade (based on WHO ratings)				
	0	1	2	3	4
Alopecia	No change	Minimal hair loss	Moderate, patchy alopecia	Complete alopecia but reversible	Non-reversible alopecia
Nausea/ vomiting	None	Nausea	Transient vomiting	Vomiting requiring treatment	Intractable vomiting
Diarrhoea	None	Transient <2 days	Tolerable but >2 days	Intolerable requiring therapy	Haemorrhagic dehydration
Oral	No change	Soreness Erythema	Erythema, ulcers: can eat solids	Ulcers: requires liquid diet	Alimentation not possible
Neurotoxicity	None	Paraesthesiae, and/or decreased tendon reflexes	Severe paraesthesiae and/or mild weakness	Intolerable paraesthesiae and/or marked motor loss	Paralysis
Skin	No change	Erythema	Dry desquamation, vesiculation, pruritus	Moist desquamation, ulceration	Exfoliative dermatitis: necrosis requiring surgical intervention
Performance status	Capable of normal activity No restrictions	Incapable of strenuous activity Capable of light work Ambulatory	Ambulatory Capable of all self-care Unable to work Up and about >50% waking hours	Limited self-care Confined to bed/chair >50% waking hours	Completely disabled No self-care Totally confined to bed/chair

Source: Birmingham Oncology Treatment Chart, St Chad's Unit, City Hospital, Dudley Road, Birmingham.

CLINICAL MONITORING

Prescriptions for cancer chemotherapy are often complex, involving combinations of both parenteral and oral cytotoxic drugs, intravenous fluids and other supportive therapies. To monitor and check prescribing effectively the pharmacist must recognize and anticipate a whole range of potential problems. Table 7.2 presents a framework for monitoring the prescribing of cytotoxic drugs to help ensure that the treatment received by patients is optimal.

Table 7.2: *A checklist for prescription monitoring in cancer chemotherapy*

Patient details
    diagnosis
    age
    weight, height, body surface area
    haematological function
    renal function
    liver function
    underlying disease
    allergy
    previous treatment
    previous reaction to treatment i.e. toxicity from previous cycles requiring dose
        modification of subsequent cycles
    total exposure to drugs with cumulative toxicity, e.g. doxorubicin

Protocol
    is treatment prescribed according to established regimen or clinical trial protocol?
    is drug name clear and unambiguous?
    dose
    timing, scheduling number of days therapy
    have all drugs in regimen been prescribed?
    recommended dose modifications for organ dysfunction or previous toxicity
    stop date indicated for oral therapy

Administration
    appropriate route of administration
    suitable venous access
    appropriate infusion fluid and dilution
    appropriate rate of administration
    appropriate scheduling, with regard to time of day, day of week

Interactions
    with other prescribed therapy
    pharmaceutical interactions with concurrent IV therapy, or infusion fluids

Supportive care
    ensure appropriate adjuvant therapy prescribed, e.g.:
        antiemetics
        mouth care
        eye care
        hydration
        allopurinol
        prophylactic antibiotics/antifungals/antivirals
        growth factors
        antidotes; folinic acid, mesna

The following drug tables highlight the main acute toxicities of specific cytotoxic drugs which can occur in the initial weeks following treatment. They do **not** include all documented adverse effects of the drugs but attempt to provide a guide to clinical monitoring of chemotherapy. For example, allergic or hypersensitivity reactions have occurred with many cytotoxic drugs. For more comprehensive information the reader should refer to original reference sources. A rating scale has been used to indicate the incidence and severity of adverse effects (Table 7.3), however, these effects may be dependent on the dose and method of administration and will also be influenced by patient factors such as the presence of any pre-existing disease. In addition, the toxicity of treatment will be compounded if these agents are used in combination.

Table 7.3: *Toxicity rating scale and abbreviations used in the following tables*

+	occasional or mild
++	common or moderately severe
+++	invariable or dose limiting
FBC	full blood count
ECG	electrocardiogram
LFT	liver function tests
WBC	white blood cell
SIADH	syndrome of inappropriate anti-diuretic hormone secretion
CNS	central nervous system

CHEMOTHERAPEUTIC AGENTS

Aclarubicin

	Toxicity grading	Comment	Clinical monitoring/ intervention
Gastrointestinal tract			
Nausea/vomiting	++	Severe at doses greater than 120 mg/m²	Prophylactic antiemetics
Other	+++	Mucositis Oral ulceration Diarrhoea	Good mouth care
Haematological			
Myelosuppression	+++	WBC nadir days 14–21, recovery days 21–28 Thrombocytopenia Nadir days 7–14, recovery days 14–28	Pre-treatment FBC
Cutaneous			
Alopecia	+	–	–
Tissue necrosis (on extravasation)	Group 1/2	–	–
Cardiovascular	++ +	Acute cardiotoxicity Congestive heart failure	ECG monitoring Caution in patients with impaired cardiac function or previously treated with anthracyclines
Pulmonary	–	–	–
CNS	–	–	–
Renal/bladder	–	–	–
Hepatic	++	–	Monitor liver function and consider dose reduction in presence of hepatic impairment

Amsacrine

	Toxicity grading	Comment	Clinical monitoring/ intervention
Gastrointestinal tract			
Nausea/vomiting	++	–	Prophylactic antiemetics
Other	++	Mucositis	Prophylactic mouth care
Haematological			
Myelosuppression	+++	Prolonged Nadir days 10–16 Recovery days 21–25	Pre-treatment FBC
Cutaneous			
Alopecia	++	–	–
Tissue necrosis (on extravasation)	Group 1	–	–
Other	–	Irritant to intact skin	–
Cardiovascular	++	Rare, but potentially serious, ventricular arrhythmias and congestive heart failure	Pre-treatment ECG Caution in patients previously treated with anthracyclines Avoid in hypokalaemia
Pulmonary	–	–	–
CNS	–	–	–
Renal/bladder	–	–	–
Hepatic	–	Cholestasis	Monitor liver function and consider reduction in presence of hepatic impairment

Asparaginase

	Toxicity grading	Comment	Clinical monitoring/ intervention
Gastrointestinal tract			
Nausea/vomiting	+	Usually acute in onset and short-lived	–
Haematological			
Myelosuppression	+	Nadir day 14 Recovery day 21	Pre-treatment FBC
Coagulation	+	Depressed clotting factors	Monitor prothrombin time
Cutaneous			
Alopecia	–	–	–
Tissue necrosis (on extravasation)	Group 3	–	–
Cardiovascular	–	–	–
CNS	++	Encephalopathy	Monitor renal status
Renal/bladder	+	Mild decrease in renal function	Monitor renal function
Hepatic	+++	Liver enzyme abnormalities common Severe hepatotoxicity rare	Consider dose reduction in hepatic impairment
Other		Hypersensitivity	Consider intradermal test dose of 50 IU in 0.1–0.2 ml Observe for 3 hours Facilities for management of anaphylaxis should be available
	+++	Pyrexia and rigors	
	+	Hyperglycaemia	Monitor urine glucose
	+	Pancreatitis	Monitor amylase

Bleomycin

	Toxicity grading	Comment	Clinical monitoring/ intervention
Gastrointestinal tract			
Nausea/vomiting	+	Onset 3–6 hours	–
	+	Mucositis	
Haematological			
Myelosuppression	–	Uncommon	–
Cutaneous			
Alopecia	–	–	–
Tissue necrosis (on extravasation)	Group 3	–	–
Other	++	Hyperpigmentation of mucous membranes, skin and nails	–
Cardiovascular	–	–	–
Pulmonary	+++	Pneumonitis Fibrosis Post-operative respiratory failure	Monitor pulmonary function Regular chest X-rays Avoid cumulative doses greater than 500 IU Treatment with corticosteroids may be considered
CNS	–	–	Caution in patients undergoing surgery following treatment with bleomycin
Renal/bladder	++	–	Monitor renal function Consider dose reduction in renal impairment
Hepatic	–	–	–
Other	++	Fever	Prophylactic paracetamol or concomitant hydrocortisone

Carboplatin

	Toxicity grading	Comment	Clinical monitoring/ intervention
Gastrointestinal tract			
Nausea/vomiting	++	Onset 2–6 hours Duration 6–12 hours	Prophylactic antiemetics
Haematological			
Myelosuppression	+++	Mainly thrombocytopenia Nadir days 10–21 Recovery days 28–35	Pre-treatment FBC
Cutaneous			
Alopecia	+	Rare	–
Tissue necrosis (on extravasation)	Group 2	–	–
Cardiovascular	–	–	–
Pulmonary	–	–	–
CNS	+	Peripheral neuropathies Ototoxicity	– –
Renal/bladder	++	Nephrotoxicity mainly at high doses	Hydration with high doses Monitor renal function Consider dose modification on basis of renal function
Hepatic	–	–	–
Other	+	Electrolyte disturbance	Monitor biochemistry Supplement as required

Carmustine (BCNU)

	Toxicity grading	Comment	Clinical monitoring/ intervention
Gastrointestinal tract			
Nausea/vomiting	++	Dose related Onset 2–4 hours Duration 4–6 hours	Prophylactic antiemetics
Haematological			
Myelosuppression	++ WBC +++ platelets	Delayed Nadir 4–6 weeks	Pre-treatment FBC Treatment interval >6 weeks
Cutaneous			
Alopecia	+	Rare	–
Tissue necrosis (on extravasation)	Group 1	–	–
Cardiovascular	–	–	–
Pulmonary	–	Acute pulmonary infiltrate and/or fibrosis Also delayed onset pulmonary toxicity	–
CNS	+	Rare	–
Renal/bladder	–	–	–
Hepatic	–	Reversible elevation of LFTs	–
Other	++	Pain on injection	Administer slowly by infusion

Cisplatin

	Toxicity grading	Comment	Clinical monitoring/ intervention
Gastrointestinal tract			
Nausea/vomiting	+++	Onset 1–2 hours Duration 12–48 hours	Prophylactic antiemetics
Other	++	Diarrhoea Sudden onset	Anti-diarrhoeal prophylaxis for future cycles
Haematological			
Myelosuppression	+	Nadir days 14–23 Recovery days 21–35	
Cutaneous			
Alopecia	–	–	–
Tissue necrosis (on extravasation)	Group 1	–	–
Cardiovascular	–	–	–
Pulmonary	–	–	–
CNS	+++	Peripheral neuropathy Ototoxicity	Regular neurological examinations Audiometry
Renal/bladder	+++	Renal toxicity	Adequate pre- and post-treatment hydration, to maintain diuresis mannitol may be given Monitor renal function prior to each cycle and adjust dose accordingly
Hepatic	–	–	–
Other	+++ ++ +	Electrolyte imbalance: hypomagnesaemia hypocalcaemia hypersensitivity	Rarely symptomatic Monitor and supplement as appropriate

Cladribine

	Toxicity grading	Comment	Clinical monitoring/ intervention
Gastrointestinal tract			
Nausea/vomiting	+	Mild to moderate duration	Prophylactic antiemetics
Haematological			
Myelosuppression	+++	WBC nadir days 7–14, Recovery days 28–30	Pre-treatment FBC
Cutaneous			
Alopecia	+	–	–
Tissue necrosis (on extravasation)	Group 3	–	–
Rash	++	Occurs in approximately 50% of patients	–
Cardiovascular	–	–	–
Pulmonary	–	–	–
CNS	–	–	–
Renal/bladder	+	Rare but not unreported	–
Hepatic	+	Rare but not unreported	–
Other			
Fever	++	Due to tumour lysis	–

Cyclophosphamide

	Toxicity grading	Comment	Clinical monitoring/ intervention
Gastrointestinal tract			
Nausea/vomiting	++	Onset 4–12 hours Duration 4–10 hours	Prophylactic antiemetics
Other	++	Mucositis	Prophylactic mouth care
Haematological			
Myelosuppression	+++	Nadir days 10–14 Recovery days 21–28	Pre-treatment FBC
Cutaneous			
Alopecia	+++	Complete with IV therapy Partial with oral therapy	–
Tissue necrosis (on extravasation)	Group 3	–	–
Cardiovascular	+	Cardiac toxicity reported with high doses	–
Pulmonary	+	Interstitial pneumonitis Pulmonary fibrosis	–
CNS	–	–	–
Renal/bladder	+++	Haemorrhagic cystitis Tubular damage	Less problematic than ifosfamide Ensure adequate hydration Consider mesna at doses greater than 1.5 g/m^2 Monitor renal function
Hepatic	–	–	–
Other	+	SIADH	

Cytarabine

	Toxicity grading	Comment	Clinical monitoring/intervention
Gastrointestinal tract			
Nausea/vomiting	++	Dose related Onset 6–12 hours Duration 3–8 hours	Prophylactic antiemetics
Other	++	Mucositis Diarrhoea	Prophylactic mouth care
Haematological			
Myelosuppression	+++	Nadir days 14–18 Recovery days 21–28 Thrombocytopenia Rapid recovery	Pre-treatment FBC
Cutaneous			
Alopecia	+	+	–
Tissue necrosis (on extravasation)	Group 3	–	–
Cardiovascular	–	–	–
Pulmonary	++	Respiratory distress Pulmonary oedema	–
CNS	++	Toxicity at high dose, including dysarthria, ataxia	May be alleviated by pyridoxine
Renal/bladder	–	–	Reduce dose in renal impairment
Hepatic	+	Rare hepatic dysfunction	Monitor liver function and modify dose as necessary
Other	++	Ocular toxicity: including conjunctivitis, and photophobia	Prophylactic steroid eye drops with high dose therapy
		'Cytarabine syndrome': fever, myalgia, bone pain, conjunctivitis, chest pain, malaise	Corticosteroids

Dacarbazine

	Toxicity grading	Comment	Clinical monitoring/ intervention
Gastrointestinal tract			
Nausea/vomiting	+++	Onset 1–3 hours Duration 1–12 hours	Prophylactic antiemetics
Haematological			
Myelosuppression	++	Nadir days 10–14 Recovery days 21–28	Pre-treatment FBC
Cutaneous			
Alopecia	+	Rare	–
Tissue necrosis (on extravasation)	Group 1	–	–
Cardiovascular	–	–	–
Pulmonary	–	–	–
CNS	–	–	–
Renal/bladder	–	–	–
Hepatic	+	Rare hepatotoxicity	–
Other	+	Rare 'flu-like syndrome, myalgia, fever, malaise starting within 7 days of treatment	–

Dactinomycin

	Toxicity grading	Comment	Clinical monitoring/ intervention
Gastrointestinal tract			
Nausea/vomiting	++	Onset 2–6 hours	Prophylactic antiemetics
Other	++	Mucositis	Prophylactic mouth care
Haematological			
Myelosuppression	++	Nadir days 10–14 Recovery days 21–28	Pre-treatment FBC
Cutaneous			
Alopecia	+	–	–
Tissue necrosis (on extravasation)	Group 1	–	–
Cardiovascular	–	–	–
Pulmonary	–	–	–
CNS	–	–	–
Renal/bladder	–	–	–
Hepatic	–	–	Monitor liver function Consider dose reduction in hepatic impairment

Daunorubicin

	Toxicity grading	Comment	Clinical monitoring/ intervention
Gastrointestinal tract			
Nausea/vomiting	++	Onset 2–6 hours	Prophylactic antiemetics
Other	++	Mucositis	Prophylactic mouth care
Haematological			
Myelosuppression	+++	Nadir days 9–14 Recovery days 21–28	Pre-treatment FBC
Cutaneous			
Alopecia	++	–	–
Tissue necrosis (on extravasation)	Group 1	–	–
Cardiovascular	+++	Cardiomyopathy	Monitor cardiac function Maximum cumulative dose 600 mg/m^2
Pulmonary	–	–	–
CNS	–	–	–
Renal/bladder	–	–	–
Hepatic	–	–	Monitor hepatic function Consider dose reduction for hepatic impairment

Daunorubicin liposomal

	Toxicity grading	Comment	Clinical monitoring/ intervention
Gastrointestinal tract			
Nausea/vomiting	+	–	Prophylactic antiemetics
Other	+	Mucositis is notably reduced	Prophylactic mouth care
Haematological			
Myelosuppression	+++	WBC nadir days 7–14 Recovery day 28	Pre-treatment FBC
Cutaneous			
Alopecia	+	–	–
Tissue necrosis (on extravasation)	Group 2/3	Potential for more severe injuries as liposomes break down	–
Cardiovascular	+	Markedly reduced compared to non-liposomal formation	–
Pulmonary	–	–	–
CNS	–	–	–
Renal/bladder	–	–	–
Hepatic	–	–	–
Other	++	Low-grade fever +/– fatigue	–

Docetaxel

	Toxicity grading	Comment	Clinical monitoring/ intervention
Gastrointestinal tract			
Nausea/vomiting	++	–	Prophylactic antiemetics
Other	++	Stomatitis and mucositis	Prophylactic mouth care
Haematological			
Myelosuppression	+++	Nadir days 7–9 Recovery days 14–16	Pre-treatment FBC
Thrombocytopenia	++	–	Pre-treatment platelet count
Cutaneous			
Alopecia	++	Completely reversible	–
Tissue necrosis (on extravasation)	Group 1/2	–	–
Skin erythema		Particularly of palms and soles, often associated with oedema leading to desquamation. Reversible, resolving within 21 days	
Cardiovascular	–	–	–
Pulmonary		Associated with hypersensitivity reactions and fluid retention	
CNS	+++	Paraesthesiae and dysaesthesiae are fairly common but rarely severe. Some loss of deep tendon reflex, irreversible	–
Renal/bladder	–	–	–
Hepatic	++	Increased alkaline phosphatase and transaminases	Monitor hepatic function
Other			
Hypersensitivity	+++	–	Reactions are dramatically reduced by the use of high-dose steroid (dexamethasone) 20 mg at 12 hours and 6 hours pre-infusion and immediately pre-treatment with H_1 and H_2 antihistamines

Docetaxel *Continued*

	Toxicity grading	Comment	Clinical monitoring/ intervention
Fluid retention	+++	Occurs in 61% of patients untreated and 43% of patients treated with hypersensitivity schedule, cumulative in incidence and severity	Pre-treatment according to hyper-sensitivity schedule, slowly reversible

Doxorubicin

	Toxicity grading	Comment	Clinical monitoring/ intervention
Gastrointestinal tract			
Nausea/vomiting	++	Onset 4–6 hours Duration 6 hours	Prophylactic antiemetics
Other	+++	Mucositis	Prophylactic mouth care
Haematological			
Myelosuppression	+++	Nadir days 10–14 Recovery days 21–28	Pre-treatment FBC
Cutaneous			
Alopecia	+++	–	–
Tissue necrosis (on extravasation)	Group 1	–	–
Cardiovascular	+++	Dose-limiting toxicity Cardiomyopathy arrhythmias	ECG monitoring Caution in patients with impaired cardiac function or previously treated with anthracyclines Maximum cumulative dose 450–550 mg/m^2
Pulmonary	–	–	–
CNS	–	–	–
Renal/bladder	–	–	–
Hepatic	++	Increased bilirubin Rare hepatocellular necrosis	Monitor hepatic function and modify dose as required
Other	–	Hyperpigmentation of skin, mucous membranes, nails	–

Epirubicin

	Toxicity grading	Comment	Clinical monitoring/ intervention
Gastrointestinal tract			
Nausea/vomiting	++	Onset 4–6 hours Duration 6 hours	Prophylactic antiemetics
Other	+++	Mucositis	Prophylactic mouth care
Haematological			
Myelosuppression	+++	Nadir days 10–14 Recovery days 21–28	Pre-treatment FBC
Cutaneous			
Alopecia	+++	–	–
Tissue necrosis (on extravasation)	Group 1	–	–
Cardiovascular	+++	Dose-limiting toxicity Cardiomyopathy arrhythmias	ECG monitoring Caution in patients with impaired cardiac function or previously treated with anthracyclines Maximum cumulative dose 950 mg/m^2
Pulmonary	–	–	–
CNS	–	–	–
Renal/bladder	–	–	–
Hepatic	++	Increased bilirubin Rare hepatocellular necrosis	Monitor hepatic function and modify dose as required
Other	–	Hyperpigmentation of skin, mucous membranes, nails	–

Etoposide

	Toxicity grading	Comment	Clinical monitoring/ intervention
Gastrointestinal tract			
Nausea/vomiting	++	Onset 3–8 hours Duration 12 hours	Prophylactic antiemetics
Other	++	Mucositis	Prophylactic mouth care
Haematological			
Myelosuppression	+++	Nadir days 14–16 Recovery days 21–28	Pre-treatment FBC
Cutaneous			
Alopecia	++	–	–
Tissue necrosis (on extravasation)	Group 2	–	–
Cardiovascular	+	Hypotension on rapid infusion	Administer over 1 hour
Pulmonary	–	–	–
CNS	–	–	–
Renal/bladder	–	–	Monitor renal function Consider dose modification in patients with renal impairment
Hepatic	–	–	Monitor liver function Consider dose modification in patients with hepatic impairment

Fludarabine

	Toxicity grading	Comment	Clinical monitoring/ intervention
Gastrointestinal tract			
Nausea/vomiting	+	Transient but occurring in up to 30% of patients	Prophylactic antiemetics
Other	+	Diarrhoea	Prophylactic diarrhoeals
Haematological			
Myelosuppression	+++	Nadir days 10–17 Recovery days 21–28	Pre-treatment FBC
Cutaneous			
Alopecia	–	–	–
Tissue necrosis (on extravasation)	Group 3	–	–
Cardiovascular	–	–	–
Pulmonary	+++	Interstitial pneumonitis due to cumulative dose	Steroids
CNS	+++	–	–
Renal/bladder	–	–	–
Hepatic	++	Elevation of hepatic transaminase and creatinine	Monitor hepatic function
Other	–	–	–

Fluorouracil

	Toxicity grading	Comment	Clinical monitoring/ intervention
Gastrointestinal tract			
Nausea/vomiting	+	Onset 3–6 hours Dose limiting	Prophylactic antiemetics
Other	+++	Diarrhoea	Treatment may need to be stopped, may need prophylactic anti-diarrhoeals
		Stomatitis	Possible benefit from sucralfate or prophylactic allopurinol suspension
Haematological			
Myelosuppression	+	Nadir day 14 Recovery days 21–25	Schedule dependent
Cutaneous			
Alopecia	+	–	–
Tissue necrosis (on extravasation)	Group 3	5FU 'burns' can cause problems with venous access	–
Cardiovascular	++	Rare vascular toxicity including angina/ cardiac spasm Myocardial infarction	Monitor cardiac function Caution in patients with cardiac disease
Pulmonary	–	–	–
CNS	+	Rare CNS dysfunction, ataxia, confusion, headaches	–
Renal/bladder	–	–	–
Hepatic	–	–	–

Gemcitabine

	Toxicity grading	Comment	Clinical monitoring/ intervention
Gastrointestinal tract			
Nausea/vomiting	+	Particularly schedule dependent	Prophylactic antiemetics
Haematological			
Myelosuppression	++	Dose limiting, but not cumulative WBC nadir days 8–12	Pre-treatment FBC
Thrombocytopenia	++	May be more problematic than neutropenia	–
Cutaneous			
Alopecia	+	–	–
Tissue necrosis (on extravasation)	Group 3	–	–
Rash	++	Generalized onset within 48–72 hours Presents an erythematous maculopapular rash of neck and extremities	Response to steroids
Cardiovascular	–	–	–
Pulmonary	–	–	–
CNS	–	–	–
Renal/bladder	–	–	–
Hepatic	–	–	–
Other	–	–	–

Idarubicin

	Toxicity grading	Comment	Clinical monitoring/ intervention
Gastrointestinal tract			
Nausea/vomiting	++	–	Prophylactic antiemetics
Other	++	Mucositis	Prophylactic mouth care
Haematological			
Myelosuppression	+++	–	Pre-treatment FBC
Cutaneous			
Alopecia	+++	–	–
Tissue necrosis (on extravasation)	Group 1	–	–
Cardiovascular	+++	Cardiomyopathy	Monitor cardiac function Caution in patients with cardiac disease or previously treated with anthracyclines
Pulmonary	–	–	–
CNS	–	–	–
Renal/bladder	–	–	Monitor renal function Consider dose reduction for renal impairment
Hepatic	–	–	Monitor hepatic function Consider dose reduction for hepatic impairment

Ifosfamide

	Toxicity grading	Comment	Clinical monitoring/ intervention
Gastrointestinal tract			
Nausea/vomiting	+++	Onset 1–2 hours Duration 12–24 hours	Prophylactic antiemetics
Haematological			
Myelosuppression	+++	Nadir days 5–10 Recovery days 14–21	Pre-treatment FBC
Cutaneous			
Alopecia	+++	Usually complete Onset 1–3 weeks	–
Tissue necrosis (on extravasation)	Group 3	–	–
Cardiovascular	–	–	–
Pulmonary	–	–	–
CNS	+++	Encephalopathy Neurotoxicity Confusion/lethargy	Assess risk factors: renal function, albumin, presence or absence of pelvic disease
Renal/bladder	+++	Haemorrhagic cystitis Urothelial toxicity Tubular damage	Prophylactic mesna required Ensure adequate hydration Monitor renal function Consider dose reduction in presence of renal impairment
Hepatic	–	–	–

Melphalan

	Toxicity grading	Comment	Clinical monitoring/ intervention
Gastrointestinal tract			
Nausea/vomiting	++	Onset 6–12 hours	Prophylactic antiemetics
Haematological			
Myelosuppression	++	Delayed Nadir days 10–18 Recovery 6–7 weeks	Pre-treatment FBC
Cutaneous			
Alopecia	–	Uncommon	–
Tissue necrosis (on extravasation)	Group 3	–	–
Cardiovascular	–	–	–
Pulmonary	+	Rare pulmonary fibrosis	–
CNS	–	–	–
Renal/bladder	–	–	Monitor renal function Consider dose reduction for renal impairment
Hepatic	–	–	–

Methotrexate

	Toxicity grading	Comment	Clinical monitoring/ intervention
Gastrointestinal tract			
Nausea/vomiting	++	Dose related	Prophylactic antiemetics with doses >100 mg/m²
Other	+++	Stomatitis	Ensure folinic acid rescue starts at 24 hours post-chemotherapy with doses >100 mg/m²
Haematological			
Myelosuppression	++	Dose related Nadir day 10 Recovery day 21	Pre-treatment FBC
Cutaneous			
Alopecia	–	–	–
Tissue necrosis (on extravasation)	Group 2	–	–
Cardiovascular	–	–	–
Pulmonary	–	–	–
CNS	–	–	–
Renal/bladder	+++	Electrolyte disturbance Tubular damage and destruction	Monitor renal function Maintain diuresis Maintain urinary pH at >7.5 with doses >1 g/m² monitor methotrexate plasma concentration and adjust folinic acid dose accordingly
Hepatic	–	–	–
Other	–	Conjunctivitis Sore, itching eyes	Symptomatic treatment with hypromellose 0.3% eye drops

Mitomycin

	Toxicity grading	Comment	Clinical monitoring/ intervention
Gastrointestinal tract			
Nausea/vomiting	+	Onset 1–4 hours	Prophylactic antiemetics
Haematological			
Myelosuppression	++	Nadir 3–4 weeks Recovery 6–8 weeks	Pre-treatment FBC
Cutaneous			
Alopecia	–	–	–
Tissue necrosis (on extravasation)	Group 1	–	–
Cardiovascular	–	–	–
Pulmonary	+	Pulmonary fibrosis	–
CNS	–	–	–
Renal/bladder	–	Renal toxicity	Monitor renal function
Hepatic	–	–	–

Mitozantrone

	Toxicity grading	Comment	Clinical monitoring/ intervention
Gastrointestinal tract			
Nausea/vomiting	+	–	Prophylactic antiemetics
	+	Mucositis	
Haematological			
Myelosuppression	+	Nadir day 14 Recovery day 21	Pre-treatment FBC
Cutaneous			
Alopecia	++	–	–
Tissue necrosis (on extravasation)	Group 2	–	–
Cardiovascular	++	Cardiomyopathy	Monitor cardiac function if cumulative dose >160 mg/m^2, in presence of cardiac disease or previous anthracycline therapy
Pulmonary	–	–	–
CNS	–	–	–
Renal/bladder	–	–	–
Hepatic	+	+	Particular problem in patients with bilirubins >35–40 Monitor hepatic function

Mustine

	Toxicity grading	Comment	Clinical monitoring/ intervention
Gastrointestinal tract			
Nausea/vomiting	+++	Onset 0.5–2 hours	Prophylactic antiemetics
Haematological			
Myelosuppression	+++	Nadir days 9–14 Recovery days 16–28	Pre-treatment FBC
Cutaneous			
Alopecia	++	–	–
Tissue necrosis (on extravasation)	Group 1	–	–
Cardiovascular	–	–	–
Pulmonary	–	Rarely pulmonary fibrosis	–
CNS	–	–	–
Renal/bladder	–	–	–
Hepatic	–	–	–

Paclitaxel

	Toxicity grading	Comment	Clinical monitoring/ intervention
Gastrointestinal tract			
Nausea/vomiting	++	Schedule-related onset 30 mins–3 hours	Prophylactic antiemetics
Other	+	Mucositis	Good mouth care
Haematological			
Myelosuppression	+++	Nadir days 9–11 Recovery day 15	Pre-treatment FBC
Cutaneous			
Alopecia	+++	Complete but reversible	–
Tissue necrosis (on extravasation)	Group 1/2	–	–
Cardiovascular	++	Commonly bradycardic, particularly problematic in patients with other risk factors	–
Pulmonary		Only in association with hypersensitivity reaction, burning sensation on soles of feet	–
CNS	+++	Peripheral neuropathies loss of deep tendon reflexes, fairly rapidly reversible	–
Renal/bladder	–	–	–
Hepatic	–	–	–
Other			
Hypersensitivity	+++	Probably due to the cremophor vehicle rather than paclitaxel	Reactions are dramatically reduced, if not eliminated, by the use of high-dose steroid dexamethasone 20 mg at 12 hours and 6 hours prior to infusion and immediate pre-treatment with H_1 and H_2 antihistamines

Pentostatin

	Toxicity grading	Comment	Clinical monitoring/ intervention
Gastrointestinal tract			
Nausea/vomiting	++	–	Prophylactic antiemetics
Haematological			
Myelosuppression	+++	Nadir days 12–17 Recovery days 21–28	Pre-treatment FBC
Cutaneous			
Alopecia	–	–	–
Tissue necrosis (on extravasation)	Group 3	–	–
Others			
Skin rash	+	Only in patients with hairy-cell leukaemia	Topical hydrocortisone
Dry skin	++	–	Emollient creams
Cardiovascular	–	–	–
Pulmonary	–	–	–
CNS	++	Dose-dependent lethargy and fatigue Rarely coma and seizures	–
Renal/bladder	+++	Tubular toxicity leading to increased tubular creatine and acute renal failure	Monitor renal function Dose reduced in mild to moderate failure
Hepatic	–	–	–
Other			
Eye (keratoconjunctivitis)	+	–	Responds to steroid eye drops

Plicamycin

	Toxicity grading	Comment	Clinical monitoring/ intervention
Gastrointestinal tract			
Nausea/vomiting	++	Onset 4–6 hours Duration 12–24 hours	Prophylactic antiemetics
Haematological			
Myelosuppression	++	Mainly thrombocytopenia Nadir day 14 Recovery day 21	Pre-treatment FBC
Other	+	Coagulopathy	Monitor coagulation
Cutaneous			
Alopecia	–	Uncommon	–
Tissue necrosis (on extravasation)	Group 1	–	–
Cardiovascular	–	–	–
Pulmonary	–	–	–
CNS	–	–	–
Renal/bladder	–	Nephrotoxic	Monitor renal function Consider dose reduction for renal impairment
Hepatic	–	Hepatotoxic	Monitor hepatic function Consider dose reduction for hepatic impairment
Other	–	Hypocalcaemia	Monitor calcium level

Raltitrexed

	Toxicity grading	Comment	Clinical monitoring/ intervention
Gastrointestinal tract			
Nausea/vomiting	+++	Often only of moderate intensity	Prophylactic antiemetics
Other			
Diarrhoea	+++	Mild to moderate	Prophylactic anti-diarrhoeals
Haematological			
Myelosuppression	++	–	Pre-treatment FBC
Anaemia	+++	–	Pre-treatment FBC as required transfusion
Cutaneous			
Alopecia	–	–	–
Tissue necrosis (on extravasation)	Group 3	–	–
Rash	++	Erythematous or pruritic	–
Cardiovascular	–	–	–
Pulmonary	–	–	–
CNS	–	–	–
Renal/bladder	–	–	–
Hepatic	+++	Elevation of lower transaminases	Monitor liver function
Other			
Constitutional	+++	Asthma, malaise and 'flu-like symptoms, may be dose limiting	–

Thiotepa

	Toxicity grading	Comment	Clinical monitoring/ intervention
Gastrointestinal tract			
Nausea/vomiting	+	–	Antiemetics as required
Haematological			
Myelosuppression	++WBC +++platelets	Nadir day 14 Recovery 4 weeks	Pre-treatment FBC
Cutaneous			
Alopecia	–	Rare	–
Tissue necrosis (on extravasation)	Group 3	–	–
Cardiovascular	–	–	–
Pulmonary	–	–	–
CNS	–	–	–
Renal/bladder	–	–	–
Hepatic	–	–	–

Treosulfan

	Toxicity grading	Comment	Clinical monitoring/ intervention
Gastrointestinal tract			
Nausea/vomiting	++	Onset 0–4 hours Duration 4–12 hours	Prophylactic antiemetics
Haematological			
Myelosuppression	+++	Onset days 12–14 Nadir days 14–16 Recovery day 28	Pre-treatment FBC
Cutaneous			
Alopecia	+++	–	–
Tissue necrosis (on extravasation)	Group 1	–	–
Rash	+	Erythema with some skin pigmentation	–
Cardiovascular	–	–	–
Pulmonary	–	–	–
CNS	–	–	–
Renal/bladder	–	–	–
Hepatic	–	–	–
Other	–	–	–

Vinblastine

	Toxicity grading	Comment	Clinical monitoring/ intervention
Gastrointestinal tract			
Nausea/vomiting	+	Onset 4–8 hours	Antiemetics as required
Other	++	Constipation	Consider prophylactic laxatives
	+	Stomatitis	Prophylactic mouth care
Haematological			
Myelosuppression	++	Nadir day 10 Recovery days 14–21	Pre-treatment FBC
Cutaneous			
Alopecia	+	–	–
Tissue necrosis (on extravasation)	Group 1	–	–
Cardiovascular	–	–	–
Pulmonary	–	–	–
CNS	++	Neuropathy	–
Renal/bladder	–	–	–
Hepatic	–	–	Monitor hepatic function Consider dose reduction for hepatic impairment
Other	+	SIADH	–

Vincristine

	Toxicity grading	Comment	Clinical monitoring/ intervention
Gastrointestinal tract			
Nausea/vomiting	+	Onset 4–8 hours	Antiemetics as required
Other	++	Constipation	Consider prophylactic laxatives
	+	Stomatitis	Prophylactic mouth care
Haematological			
Myelosuppression	+	Nadir day 10 Recovery day 21	Pre-treatment FBC
Cutaneous			
Alopecia	+	–	–
Tissue necrosis (on extravasation)	Group 1	–	–
Cardiovascular	–	–	–
Pulmonary	–	–	–
CNS	+++	Neuropathy	–
Renal/bladder	–	–	–
Hepatic	–	–	Monitor hepatic function Consider dose reduction for hepatic/biliary impairment
Other	–	SIADH	–

Vindesine

	Toxicity grading	Comment	Clinical monitoring/ intervention
Gastrointestinal tract			
Nausea/vomiting	+	Onset 4–8 hours	Antiemetics as required
Other	+	Constipation	Consider prophylactic laxatives
Haematological			
Myelosuppression	++	Nadir days 3–5 Recovery days 7–10	Pre-treatment FBC
Cutaneous			
Alopecia	++	–	–
Tissue necrosis (on extravasation)	Group 1	–	–
Cardiovascular	–	–	–
Pulmonary	–	–	–
CNS	++	Neuropathy	–
Renal/bladder	–	–	–
Hepatic	–	–	Monitor hepatic function Consider dose reduction for hepatic/biliary impairment
Other	–	–	–

CYTOKINES

α Interferon

	Toxicity grading	Comment	Clinical monitoring/ intervention
Gastrointestinal tract			
Nausea/vomiting	+	Usualy accompanied by diarrhoea	–
Other	++	Anorexia	Regular monitoring of patient's weight
Haematological			
Myelosuppression	++	Nadir day 14 Recovery day 21	Pre-treatment FBC Monitor with regular FBCs
Cutaneous			
Alopecia	+	Mild to moderate	–
Tissue necrosis (on extravasation)	Group 3	–	–
Cardiovascular	+	Dose-related transient hypotension, arrhythmias, palpitations	Monitor cardiac function in at-risk patients
Pulmonary	–	–	–
CNS	++	Depression, confusion, dizziness, vertigo At high does: convulsions, coma, paraesthesiae, neuropathy	–
Renal/bladder	–	–	–
Hepatic	–	–	–
Other	–	'Flu-like symptoms: fever, chills, headaches, malaise Pain/reaction at injection site Elevated serum glucose levels	Administer injection in the evening Prophylactic paracetamol Rotate site of injection

Aldesleukin (IL-2)

	Toxicity grading	Comment	Clinical monitoring/ intervention
Gastrointestinal tract			
Nausea/vomiting	++	–	Prophylactic antiemetics
Other	++	Diarrhoea Mucositis	Anti-diarrhoeals
Haematological			
Myelosuppression	+	Anaemia Thrombocytopenia	Pre-treatment FBC
Cutaneous			
Alopecia	–	–	–
Tissue necrosis (on extravasation)	Group 3	–	–
Other	++	Erythematous rash	Prophylactic antihistamine
		Skin desquamation	Water-based lotion
Cardiovascular	+++	Hypotension/ arrhythmias Peripheral and pulmonary oedema Weight gain/dyspnoea Capillary leak syndrome	Monitor throughout treatment
Pulmonary			
CNS	++	Confusion Disorientation	–
Renal/bladder	+++	Nephrotoxic transient increase in serum creatinine. Potentially fatal decreases in glomerular filtration rates	Monitor renal function
Hepatic	++	Liver enzymes disturbance	Monitor hepatic function
Other	++	'Flu-like symptoms: fever, chills, malaise, nasal congestion	Prophylactic paracetamol

SOURCES OF INFORMATION

ABPI Data Sheet Compendium 1991–1992 (1991) DataPharm Publications, London.

Borison HL, McCarthy LE (1983) Neuropharmacology of chemotherapy induced emesis. *Drugs* **25(Suppl.1)**, 8–17.

Cain M, Tenni P (1992) *Drug therapy in cancer: a practical guide for health professionals*. Society of Hospital Pharmacists of Australia.

Chabner BA, Myers CE (1989) Clinical pharmacology of cancer chemotherapy. In: (DeVita VT *et al*. eds), *Cancer: principles and practice of oncology*, 3rd edition. Lippincott, New York, p. 356.

Dollery C (ed.) (1991) *Therapeutic drugs*. Churchill Livingstone, Edinburgh.

Fahey M *et al*. (1984) Prescription monitoring and the oncology patient. *Pharm. J.* **233**, 483–5.

Middleton J *et al*. (1985) Failue of scalp hypothermia to prevent hair loss when cyclophosphamide is added to doxorubicin and vincristine. *Cancer Treat. Rep.* **69**, 373–5.

Perry MC, Yarbro JW (1984) *Toxicity of chemotherapy*. Grune & Stratton, Orlando.

Priestman TJ (1989) *Cancer chemotherapy: an introduction*, 3rd edition. Springer-Verlag.

Reynold JEF (ed.) (1982) *The extra pharmacopoeia*, 29th edition. Pharmaceutical Press, London.

Souhami R, Tobias J (1986) *Cancer and its management*. Blackwell Scientific, Oxford.

Staley AP (1992) Management of symptoms associated with cancer treatment. (I). *Pharm. J.* **249**, 50–3.

Stanley AP (1992) Management of symptoms associated with cancer treatment. (II). *Pharm. J.* **249**, 90–2.

Tierney AJ (1987) Preventing chemotherapy induced alopecia in cancer patients: Is scalp cooling worthwhile? *J. Adv. Nurs.* **12**, 303–10.

Triozzi A, Laszlo J (1987) Optimum management of nausea and vomiting in cancer chemotherapy. *Drugs* **34**, 136–49.

WHO handbook for reporting results of cancer treatment (1989) WHO, Geneva.

Storage of cytotoxic drugs after reconstitution or repackaging: a statement regarding extended shelf-life

Many parenteral cytotoxics require reconstitution. In a centralized service, cytotoxic injections will normally be drawn up into a syringe or into an infusion container ready for administration. Manufacturers are currently required by licensing authorities to indicate on the data sheet and package insert that reconstituted drugs, with or without preservative, should be stored in a refrigerator (unless dictated by the chemical nature of the drug) and must be used within a specified period, usually not more than 24 hours. This is to ensure that, although the drug may be stable, any microorganisms introduced during the reconstitution procedures (assumed to be on the ward) will have insufficient opportunity to multiply and reach hazardous numbers before the injection is administered.

This recommendation or directive, therefore, will not usually relate to considerations of chemical stability. Consequently, provided that any manipulations undertaken to prepare the drug for administration are carried out under aseptic conditions, ensuring that an adequate level of sterility assurance is maintained, the shelf-life of such reconstituted or repackaged injections can be extended at the discretion of the responsible hospital pharmacist.

It is essential that good aseptic techniques are employed and adequate quality assurance programmes maintained. The shelf-life of such injectables can then be governed by chemical stability considerations together with local practice and procedures. This allows far greater flexibility and opportunities for greater efficiency in operating centralized cytotoxic services.

Guidance in each monograph regarding storage after reconstitution assumes that subsequent manipulations are undertaken under appropriate aseptic conditions. The monographs have been prepared from reviews of the literature, guidance from the respective manufacturer and the author's own studies and experience. However, responsibility for the final preparation must rest with the pharmacist responsible for the cytotoxic services.

Introduction to drug monographs: compendium of intravenous drugs in cancer chemotherapy

These monographs describe injectable cytotoxics, biologicals and adjuvant drugs used in cancer chemotherapy. Information has, wherever possible, been referenced to specific sources. Data and information from the particular manufacturer may originate from a variety of sources, including UK data sheets, package inserts and personal communications held on file by the author of each monograph. Since the content of data sheets changes frequently, the reader is referred to the current product data sheet for the latest information.

Each monograph has a common structure for ease of reference and uniformity. The purpose of each section is described below. The major aim in producing the monographs is to provide the user with all the available information for each injection concerning stability, in the context of a cytotoxic service operated by a pharmacy department.

1 General details

Under the heading Approved names, the first name(s) refers to INNM titles, followed by alternatives in common use.

As well as nomenclature, this section includes manufacturers and suppliers in the UK.

2 Chemistry

A summary of the chemical properties of the drug relevant to the injection form (structure, solubility, etc.).

3 Stability profile

A summary of the chemical stability of each drug is given, including chemical and physical parameters that influence stability after reconstitution and repackaging. Degradation pathways, when known, are included as background information. Important practical aspects, including container compatibility, and reported incompatibilities with other drugs are noted. Although useful for reference purposes, much of the data relate to short-term physical compatibility of admixtures in the laboratory, and are not necessarily applicable to the clinical setting. A summary of the stability of the reconstituted injection follows.

In light of the increasing use of ambulatory administration of cytotoxic drugs, a separate sub-section has been included for these specialized devices.

4 Clinical use

A brief summary of dosage regimens commonly used is included for guidance purposes only.

5 Preparation of injection

Details of how the injection is prepared for bolus injection and infusion, as relevant, are included, together with handling precautions and details concerning treatment of extravasation. With regard to injections prepared for different routes of administration, the pharmacist responsible for these services should ensure that everything possible is done to distinguish **intrathecal** injections, in particular, from those intended for other routes.

6 Destruction of drug or contaminated articles

The recommended methods of inactivating each cytotoxic drug are summarized under the headings Incineration, Chemical, and Contact with skin. The incineration conditions indicate the minimum temperatures recommended, usually by the manufacturer. *See* Chapter 6 for more details concerning safe handling.

NOTE: While the authors of each monograph have taken every care to provide accurate and complete information, as far as it is possible to do so, the authors or publishers cannot accept any liability for the information therein.

ACLARUBICIN

1 General details

Approved names: Aclarubicin, Aclacinomycin A.

Proprietary name: Aclarubicin injection.

Manufacturer or supplier: Medac Gessellschaft für Klinische Spezialpräparate mbH, Fehlandsträße 3, 20354 Hamburg, Germany.

Presentation and formulation details: Sterile, pyrogen-free, yellow or orange-yellow, freeze-dried powder in vials containing aclarubicin hydrochloride equivalent to 20 mg aclarubicin.[1]

Storage and shelf-life of unopened container: Three years, protected from light. Store at room temperature.[1]

2 Chemistry

Type: Aclarubicin is a cytotoxic antibiotic of the anthracycline group (Class II). It is used as the hydrochloride salt.

Molecular structure: A trisaccharide (containing L-cinerulose A, 2-deoxy-1-fucose, and L-rhodosamine), linked through a glycosidic bond to the C7 of a tetracyclic aglycone, aklavinone.[2]

Molecular weight: 848.34.

Formula: $C_{42}H_{53}NO_{15}HCl$.

Solubility: Aclarubicin is freely soluble in water and sparingly soluble in benzene and toluene.[2] The solubility of aclarubicin is pH-dependent. In buffered solution at pH 6 solubility is approximately 400 mg/ml, whereas at pH 7.4 it is only 0.05 mg/ml.[3]

3 Stability profile

3.1 Physical and chemical stability

According to the manufacturer reconstituted aqueous and saline solutions stored below 4°C should be used within 24 hours of preparation, or within six hours at room temperature when protected from light.[1] A review of the literature suggests that aclarubicin may be stable for longer periods.[4,5] However, very few data have been published. In addition, Krämer and Wenchel[4] quote 'in-house data', the full details of which have not been published. For these reasons further studies are needed to assess the long-term stability of aclarubicin.

The stability of aclarubicin hydrochloride in aqueous solution depends on a number of factors, the most important of which are pH, temperature, and the type of solvent used for reconstitution. Aclarubicin is also light-sensitive and may adsorb on to glass and certain plastics, in the same way as other anthracyclines.

Effect of pH: Aclarubicin is most stable at pH 5–6. At pH values greater than 7 the hydrochloride is insoluble and/or very slightly soluble degradation products are formed.[6] Aclarubicin is not stable at pH values less than 4.[3]

Poochikian *et al.*[5] studied the stability of aclarubicin (128 µg/ml) in glass at ambient temperature (21°C) in 5% glucose (pH 4.5), 0.9% sodium chloride (pH 6.2), lactated Ringer solution (pH 6.3) and Normosol-R (pH 7.4). Results showed that aclarubicin was more stable in 0.9% sodium chloride ($t_{90\%} = 108$ hours) than in 5% glucose ($t_{90\%} = 88$ hours), lactated Ringer solution ($t_{90\%} = 72$ hours) or Normosol-R ($t_{90\%} = 32$ hours). These data indicate that the stability of aclarubicin is highly dependent on the pH of the medium.

In acidic solution, the rate of degradation of the anthracyclines is strongly dependent on structural modifications in the amino sugar moiety.[7] As aclarubicin contains a trisaccharide its rate of degradation is likely to be different to doxorubicin, daunorubicin and epirubicin which all contain monosaccharides. However, there are no published data available to confirm this hypothesis. Acidic hydrolysis of aclarubicin is expected to result in cleavage of the glycosidic bond to yield a water-insoluble aglycone, aklavinone, and water-soluble amino sugar residues.

In alkaline solution, the rate of degradation of the anthracyclines is affected by structural modifications in the aglycone portion of the molecule.[8] As aclarubicin possesses a unique aglycone, aklavinone, its stability in alkaline media cannot be predicted from existing data for other anthracylines. In addition, its poor solubility in alkaline solution may preclude stability determination under these conditions.

Effect of light: Data on the photodegradation of doxorubicin, daunorubicin and epirubicin have been published[9,10] but there are no data available for aclarubicin. The rates of photodegradation of doxorubicin, daunorubicin and epirubicin have been reported to be similar and may be substantial at concentrations less than 100 µg/ml if solutions are exposed to light for sufficient time.[10] Exposure of very dilute solutions of aclarubicin to light promotes degradation.[1] At higher concentrations, such as those used for cancer chemotherapy (at least 500 µg/ml), no special precautions are necessary to protect freshly prepared solutions of doxorubicin, daunorubicin and epirubicin from light.[10] According to the manufacturer of aclarubicin all reconstituted solutions should be protected from light.[1]

Effect of temperature: At ambient temperature (21°C) Poochikian *et al.*[5] observed that aclarubicin was chemically stable (less than 10% degradation) in 5% glucose, 0.9% sodium chloride, lactated Ringer solution and Normosol-R for at least 48 hours. At 5°C aclarubicin (2 mg/ml) has also been stated to be stable in 0.9% sodium chloride, water for injections and 5% glucose for at least 14 days when protected from light.[6]

Container compatibility: Aclarubicin appears to be compatible with polypropylene, PVC, EVA and glass.[4-6] Doxorubicin, daunorubicin and epirubicin adsorb on to glass but not on to siliconized glass or polypropylene.[11] Therefore, aclarubicin may behave in a similar manner. In clinical practice, when aclarubicin is used at concentrations of approximately 500 µg/ml, adsorptive losses during storage and delivery are expected to be negligible.

Compatibility with other drugs: The manufacturer recommends that no other drugs are mixed with aclarubicin.[1]

3.2 Stability in clinical practice

Aclarubicin hydrochloride (2 mg/ml) appears to be chemically stable for at least 14 days, in 0.9% sodium chloride, water for injections and 5% glucose at 5°C when protected from light.[6] However, the manufacturer recommends that reconstituted solutions should be used within 24 hours if stored at 4°C or within six hours if stored at room temperature and protected from light. If 5% glucose or 0.9% sodium chloride are used to dilute aclarubicin their pH should be between 5 and 6.[1]

3.3 Stability in specialized delivery systems

No data are available.

4 Clinical use

Main indications: Remission induction in patients with acute non-lymphocytic leukaemia (ANLL) who are resistant or refractory to first-line chemotherapy. Aclarubicin may be used in combination regimens with other cytotoxic agents but the dosage may need to be reduced.[1]

Dosage and administration: Dosage is usually calculated on the basis of body surface area. The manufacturer gives the following recommendations:

▼ In adults, including the elderly, the usual initial dosage is 175–300 mg/m² over three to seven consecutive days, for example, 80–100 mg/m² daily for three days or 25 mg/m² daily for seven days.[1] Maintenance dosage should be treatments of 25–100 mg/m² given as a single infusion every three to four weeks.[1]

▼ In children, experience suggests that aclarubicin is well tolerated at the standard dosage level.[1]

The dosage schedules should, however, take into account the haematological status of the patient and the dosages of other cytotoxic drugs when used in combination. Aclarubicin should be used with caution in patients with impaired hepatic, renal or cardiac function. The total cumulative dosage administered should be decided according to the cardiological status of the patient. Most patients have received a maximum of 400 mg/m², however, larger doses in some patients have been used without ill consequence.[1]

5 Preparation of injection

Reconstitution: The contents of the 20 mg vial should be reconstituted with 10 ml of water for injections or 0.9% sodium chloride. After addition of the diluent and gentle shaking the contents of the vial will dissolve to produce a solution of 2 mg/ml.[1] The pH of the reconstituted solution is 5.0–6.5.[3] To prepare an infusion solution the required volume of reconstituted solution should be diluted with 200–500 ml of 0.9% sodium chloride or, if necessary, 5% glucose (with a pH value between 5 and 6). The final concentration should be between 0.2 and 0.5 mg/ml.[1]

Bolus administration: In Phase I–II trials, aclarubicin has been administered by bolus injection.[12–14] However, the manufacturer recommends that aclarubicin is administered by intravenous infusion over 30–60 minutes.[1]

Intravenous infusion: In Phase I–II trials aclarubicin has been given by short-term infusion using various schedules; 20 mg daily for 7–14 days,[15] 0.33–0.70 mg/kg daily for 7–20 days[16] and 60 mg/m² daily for five days.[17] In another study, short-term infusion (10–30 mg/m² daily for 10–30 days) was compared with bolus injection, 15 mg/m² daily for ten days.[18]

Extravasation: Irritant. May cause inflammation and induration on extravasation, but is unlikely to cause tissue necrosis[19–22] (*see* Chapter 6).

6 Destruction of drug or contaminated articles

Incineration: 1000°C.[1]

Chemical: 10% sodium hypochlorite (1% available chlorine)/24 hours.[6]

Contact with skin: Wash well with water, or soap and water. If the eyes are contaminated, immediate irrigation with 0.9% sodium chloride should be carried out.[1]

References

1 *ABPI Data Sheet Compendium 1994–95* (1995). DataPharm Publications Ltd, London, pp. 843–4.
2 Mori S *et al.* (1980) Physicochemical properties and stability of aclacinomycin A hydrochloride. *Jpn. J. Antibiot.* **33**, 618–22.
3 Medac GmbH. Personal communication.
4 Krämer I, Wenchel HP (1991) Viability of micro-organisms in antineoplastic drug solutions. *Eur. J. Hosp. Pharm.* **1**, 14–19.
5 Poochikian GK *et al.* (1981) Stability of anthracycline antitumour agents in four infusion fluids. *Am J. Hosp. Pharm.* **38**, 483–6.
6 Chemical and pharmaceutical documentation, Medac GmbH. Unpublished information.
7 Beijnen JH *et al.* (1985) Aspects of the chemical stability of daunorubicin and seven other anthracyclines in acidic solution. *Pharm. Weekbl. Sci. Edn.* **7**, 109–16.

8 Beijnen JH *et al.* (1986) Aspects of the degradation kinetics of doxorubicin in aqueous solution. *Int. J. Pharm.* **32**, 123–31.

9 Tavoloni N *et al.* (1980) Photolytic degradation of adriamycin. Communications. *J. Pharm. Pharmacol.* **32**, 860–2.

10 Wood MJ *et al.* (1990) Photodegradation of doxorubicin, daunorubicin and epirubicin measured by high-performance liquid chromatography. *J. Clin. Pharm. Ther.* **15**, 291–300.

11 Bosanquet AG (1986) Stability of solutions of antineoplastic agents during preparation and storage for *in vitro* assays. II. Assay methods, adriamycin and the other antitumour antibiotics. *Cancer Chemother. Pharmacol.* **17**, 1–10.

12 Machover D *et al.* (1984) Phase I–II study of aclarubicin for treatment of acute myeloid leukaemia. *Cancer Treat. Rep.* **68**, 881–6.

13 Mitrou PS *et al.* (1985) Aclarubicin (aclacinomycin A) in the treatment of relapsing acute leukaemias. *Eur. J. Cancer Clin. Oncol.* **21**, 919–23.

14 Mitrou PS (1987) Aclarubicin in single agent and combined chemotherapy of acute myeloid leukaemias. *Eur. J. Haematol.* **38** (Suppl. 47), 59–65.

15 Takahashi I *et al.* (1980) Treatment of refractory acute leukaemia with aclacinomycin A. *Acta Med. Okayama* **34**, 349–54.

16 Suzuki H *et al.* (1980) Phase I and preliminary phase II studies on aclacinomycin A in patients with acute leukaemia. *Jpn. J. Clin. Oncol.* **10**, 111–17.

17 Rowe JM *et al.* (1988) Aclacinomycin A and etoposide (VP-16-213): An effective regimen in previously treated patients with refractory acute myelogenous leukaemia. *Blood* **71**, 992–6.

18 Maral C *et al.* (1983) Aclacinomycin A: Present status of experimental and clinical studies. *Drugs Exptl. Clin. Res.* **IX**, 375–82.

19 Warrell RP Jr *et al.* (1982) Phase I–II evaluation of a new anthracycline antibiotic, aclacinomycin A, in adults with refractory leukaemia. *Cancer Treat. Rep.* **66**, 1619–23.

20 Majima H (1980) Preliminary clinical study of aclacinomycin A. In: (Carter SK, Sakurai Y eds), *Recent Results in Cancer Research.* **70**, 75–81.

21 Spehn J *et al.* (1983) Aclacinomycin A in thyroid cancer. *Proc. 13th International Congress Chemotherapy*, Vienna, 211/63–211/66.

22 Bedikian AY *et al.* (1983) Phase II evaluation of Aclacinomycin A (ACM-A, NSC208734) in patients with metastatic colorectal cancer. *Am. J. Clin. Oncol.* **6**, 187–90.

Prepared by Jayne Wood

AMSACRINE

1 General details

Approved names: Amsacrine, AMSA, m-AMSA.

Proprietary name: Amsidine Concentrate for Infusion.

Manufacturer or supplier: Parke-Davis Research Laboratories Ltd.

Presentation and formulation details: Orange/red solution of amsacrine in 2 ml ampoules containing 1.5 ml injection, 50 mg/ml amsacrine (75 mg/vial). The diluent vial contains 13.5 ml of 0.0353 M/L lactic acid solution. Amsacrine is dissolved in anhydrous N,N-dimethylacetamide (DMA). The diluent vial contains lactic acid in order to form the lactate salt of amsacrine when the drug is added to the diluent, under the acid conditions prevailing. The presence of DMA also prevents the formation of gelatinous material normally seen in aqueous amsacrine lactate solutions.

Storage and shelf-life of unopened container: Three years at ambient temperature not exceeding 25°C, protected from light.

2 Chemistry

Type: Acridine-like DNA intercalating agent.

Molecular structure: 4'-(Acridine-9-ylamino)methanesulphon-*m*-anisidine.

Molecular weight: 393.5.

Solubility: in water = 0.3 mg/ml

in DMA = 100 mg/ml.

3 Stability profile

3.1 Physical and chemical stability

Amsacrine is relatively stable in an aqueuous vehicle, provided reconstitution takes place in the presence of lactate ions, and pH remains acidic. It is stable for 48 hours after dilution in 5% glucose.[1] As the drug is incompatible with chloride or sulphate ions, saline must be avoided as a diluent. The hydrochloride salt of amsacrine is poorly water soluble.

Degradation pathways: 9(10H)-acridone, 9-chloroacridine and 4-aminomethane-sulphon-*m*-amsidine are formed as degradation products.

Physical stability is not significantly affected by normal temperature ranges. The drug is light-sensitive. After dilution in 5% glucose at a final concentration of 150 µg/ml, amsacrine is stable during exposure to diffuse daylight or fluorescent light over a 48 hour period.[1] Since amsacrine solutions are relatively insoluble in water, DMA is included in the drug diluent to prevent precipitation when the drug is reconstituted.

It has been reported that DMA may increase extraction of components of rubber or certain plastic material.[2] Consequently, it is recommended that only glass syringes should be employed to transfer the drug concentrate to the diluent vial and from vial to infusion. However, this study examined only leaching from PVC infusion containers and administration sets. Most plastic syringes are composed of polypropylene barrels with rubber plungers so this study is not relevant. The company points out that studies using the amsacrine/DMA solution in polypropylene syringes were not conclusive in demonstrating elution of these substances; however, contamination with such chemicals may affect the stability and toxicity profile of amsacrine and glass syringes should be used for the initial steps in the preparation of the infusion. Once diluted in 500 ml 5% glucose, however, DMA is sufficiently dilute not to interact with plastic infusion containers, sets or lines.[3] One other problem that can arise is the effect of DMA on the physical performance characteristics of syringes. Experience indicates that amsacrine concentrate does not affect the physical performance of polypropylene syringes.

Compatibility information: No further information available.

3.2 Stability in clinical practice

The reconstituted drug is stable in the diluent provided for 48 hours at room temperature and ambient lighting. It should be protected from exposure to strong daylight. Amsacrine is also stable after dilution in 5% glucose for 8 hours,[4] although there is evidence to indicate that such solutions are stable for 48 hours.[5]

Amsacrine must not be diluted in saline infusions.[4] Amsacrine diluted in 5% glucose at a concentration of 150 µg/ml is not degraded during exposure to diffuse daylight or fluorescent light over a 48 hour period.[3] It was also reported that amsacrine was not absorbed by PVC or polybutadiene-containing administration sets.[3]

3.3 Stability in specialized delivery systems

No data available.

4 Clinical use

Type of cytotoxic: Inhibitor of DNA.

Main indications: Acute leukaemia.

Dosage: Induction of remission – 90 mg/m²/day for five days. In patients with impaired hepatic or renal function, reduce the dose by 20–30% (60–75 mg/m²/day). Maintenance – 150 mg/m² as a single dose or 50 mg/m²/day for three days, repeated every 3–4 weeks.[4]

5 Preparation of injection

Dilution: Transfer 1.5 ml of amsacrine solution in DMA (in the ampoule) to the diluent vial, preferably using a glass syringe. The resulting solution contains 5 mg/ml amsacrine.

Bolus administration: Not recommended.

Intravenous infusion: Add required volume of diluted amsacrine to 500 ml 5% glucose infusion. Infuse over 60–90 minutes. Problems of phlebitis are more likely with higher concentrations and the Data Sheet recommends dilution of 75 mg amsacrine in 500 ml 5% glucose solution.[4]

Extravasation: Very damaging; no known antidote. Apply ice-pack to affected area (*see* Chapter 6).

6 Destruction of drug or contaminated articles

Incineration: >260°C.

Chemical: 10% sodium hypochlorite/24 hours (not recommended by the manufacturer).

Contact with skin: wash with soap and water.

References

1 D'Arcy PF (1983) Reactions and interactions in handling anticancer drugs. *Drug Intell. Clin. Pharm.*, **17**, 532–8.
2 Vishnuvajjala RB, Cradock JC (1984) Compatibility of plastic infusion devices with diluted N-methyl-formamide and N,N-dimethylacetamide. *Am. J. Hosp. Pharm.* **41**, 1160–3.
3 Cartwright-Shamoon JM *et al.* (1988) Examination of sorption and photo-degradation of amsacrine in intravenous burette administration sets. *Int. J. Pharm.* **42**, 41–6.
4 *ABPI Data Sheet Compendium 1995–96* (1995) DataPharm Publications Ltd, London, pp. 1176–8.
5 Trissel LA (1994) *Handbook on injectable drugs*, 8th edn. American Society of Hospital Pharmacists, Bethesda, USA.

Prepared by Michael Allwood

ASPARAGINASE

1 General details

Approved names: Crisantaspase, Erwinia L-asparaginase.

Proprietary name: Erwinase.

Manufacturer or supplier: Speywood Pharmaceuticals Ltd.

Presentation and formulation details: White, freeze-dried powder in 2 ml rubber-capped vials containing 10 000 IU asparaginase. Each pack contains 20 vials.

Inactive ingredients: Glucose 5.0 mg, sodium chloride 0.6 mg. 1 IU crisantaspase releases 1 μmol ammonia/minute from L-asparagine.

Storage and shelf-life of unopened container: Three years at 2–8°C.[1]

2 Chemistry

Type: Bacterial enzyme protein from *Erwinia chrysanthemi*.

Molecular weight: 130 000.

Activity: 700 U/mg.

Solubility in water: Highly soluble.[2]

3 Stability profile

3.1 *Physical and chemical stability*

Stable in solution for at least 20 days at 37°C. Denaturation of the protein and loss of enzyme activity occur outside physiological pH range (6–7.5).[3]

Degradation pathways: No information available.

Physical: Polymerization of the reconstituted enzyme solution occurs after 15 minutes. Gelatinous fibres are produced. Enzyme activity is retained. Polymerization is accelerated by contact with the rubber closure of the vial.[3]

Container compatibility: Stable in glass containers and glass or polypropylene syringes.[4] Avoid contact with rubber. No data on stability in plastic syringes, but most syringes contain a rubber plunger.

Compatibility with other drugs: The manufacturer recommends that asparaginase should not be mixed with other drugs.

3.2 *Stability in clinical practice*

Solutions should be administered as soon as possible after reconstitution since gelatinous fibres form after 15 minutes. The effect, however, is not progressive and does not affect the potency of the solution. Sterile solutions transferred to glass syringes retain potency for at least 20 days at 37°C.[4]

3.3 *Stability in specialized delivery systems*

No data available.

4 Clinical use

Type of cytotoxic: Therapeutic enzyme – not a true cytotoxic agent.

Main indications: Used in combination with other agents in treatment of acute lymphatic leukaemia and some other neoplastic conditions.

Dosage: 200 IU/kg bodyweight (5000–6000 IU/m² body surface area) by intramuscular injection three times per week for nine doses.[3] Also refer to current MRC protocols.

5 Preparation of injection

Reconstitution: The contents of the vial should be reconstituted with 1–2 ml of 0.9% sodium chloride injection and dissolved with gentle mixing to avoid contact with the rubber stopper.

Administration: The intramuscular route is preferred as it is associated with less risk of anaphylaxis. The solution may also be given by subcutaneous injection. Intravenous injection or infusion is rarely indicated but may be used if necessary.

Intravenous infusion: Administration by infusion is not usually necessary. Asparaginase is stable for at least seven days in solution in 0.9% sodium chloride and 5% glucose.[2] Enzyme activity may be adversely affected if the pH of the solution is outside the normal physiological range.[3]

Extravasation: Administration is usually by intramuscular or subcutaneous injection. No harmful local effects will result from extravasation of solutions given intravenously.

6 Destruction of drug or contaminated articles

Incineration: 800°C.

Chemical: Strong acids or alkalis denature the protein.

Contact with skin: Wash with water.

References

1 *ABPI Data Sheet Compendium 1991–92* (1991) DataPharm Publications Ltd, London, p. 1164–6.
2 Wade HE (1986) *Development of Erwinase (Erwinia Asparaginase).* Lecture to symposium: Erwinia asparaginase in the treatment of leukaemia. Frankfurt, Germany, 21 November 1986.
3 Speywood Pharmaceuticals Ltd (1988) Data on file.
4 Speywood Pharmaceuticals Ltd (1991) Data on file.

Prepared by Jonathan Oakes

BLEOMYCIN

1 General details

Approved names: Bleomycin, bleomycin sulphate.

Proprietary name: Bleomycin Lundbeck Injection.

Manufacturer or supplier: Lundbeck Ltd.

Presentation and formulation details: Cream-coloured freeze-dried plug of bleomycin sulphate equivalent to 15 IU bleomycin in a clear glass ampoule. Contains no excipients.

Storage and shelf-life of unopened container: Store at room temperature and protect from light.[1] Shelf-life is three years.

2 Chemistry

Type: Anti-tumour antibiotic.

Molecular structure: Glycopeptide. The drug consists of at least ten components, the main ones being bleomycin A_2 and bleomycin B_2.[2]

Solubility in water: Very soluble.

3 Stability profile

3.1 Physical and chemical stability

Bleomycin is reported to be stable at room temperature in 0.9% sodium chloride, protected from light for 28 days (data on file at company). Equally stable at 2–8°C.[2,3] Less stable in 5% glucose.

Degradation pathways: No information available.

Physical: Stable in pH range 4–10.[4] Light may cause bleomycin to break down.[1]

Container compatibility: Early studies suggested that bleomycin binds to PVC containers.[5,6] Subsequent work indicated that sorption does not occur, but adducts are formed in 5% glucose.[7] The stability of bleomycin in the following systems has been investigated by the manufacturer:

▼ 0.9% saline in an infusion bag (bleomycin 15 IU/100 ml)
▼ 5% glucose in an infusion bag (bleomycin 15 IU/100 ml)
▼ 0.95 saline in polypropylene syringes (bleomycin 60 IU/100 ml).

The stabilities of bleomycin A_2 and B_2 were evaluated after 28 days storage at room temperature in the dark. Bleomycin was found to be relatively stable in 0.9% sodium chloride with only 4% loss in infusion bags and 6% loss in plastic syringes. In contrast, a 54% loss occurred from the glucose solution in the infusion bag. It can be concluded that bleomycin is relatively stable in PVC containers and plastic syringes provided that the diluent is 0.9% saline.

Compatibility with other drugs: Bleomycin is reported to be physically compatible with a range of other drugs in situations such as brief mixing in a syringe or in a simulated 'Y' site injection.[4,8–16] It has been found to be incompatible with a number of drugs, including aminophylline, ascorbic acid, dexamethasone, diazepam, hydrocortisone sodium succinate, penicillin G, terbutaline, and any agents containing sulphydryl groups.[4] Methotrexate and mitomycin, whilst appearing to be compatible in 'Y' site studies, are not compatible in any stored mixture.[8]

3.2 Stability in clinical practice

The solution, after reconstitution in 0.9% sodium chloride, is stable for at least seven days, protected from light and stored in the refrigerator. After further dilution in 0.9% sodium chloride, in PVC containers, it is similarly stable. Drug diluted in 5% glucose or glucose/saline appears to be unstable and such diluents should be avoided.

3.3 Stability in specialized delivery systems

No data available.

4 Clinical use

Type of cytotoxic: Anti-tumour antibiotic.

Main indications: Squamous cell carcinoma, Hodgkin's disease and lymphomas, testicular teratoma, and malignant effusions of serous cavities.

Dosage: As single agent 15–30 IU twice or three times weekly up to a total of 100–500 IU, dependent on age and condition of patient; lower doses in combination therapy. For malignant effusions, use 60 IU in 100 ml 0.9% sodium chloride.

5 Preparation of injection

Dilution: Dissolve dose in up to 5 ml water for injection or 0.9% sodium chloride. (1% lignocaine may be used if pain occurs at injection site. Intramuscular use only.)

Bolus administration: Inject slowly or via fast-running drip.

Intravenous infusion: Dilute in up to 200 ml 0.9% sodium chloride and administer slowly.

Extravasation: Non-irritant.

6 Destruction of drug or contaminated articles

Incineration: 1000°C.

Chemical: 10% hypochlorite/24 hours.

Contact with skin: Wash with soap and water.

References

1 *ABPI Data Sheet Compendium 1995–96* (1995) DataPharm Publications Ltd, London, pp. 915–17.
2 McEvoy GK (ed.) (1985) *American Hospital Formulary service drug information.* American Society of Hospital Pharmacists, Bethesda, Maryland, USA.
3 Anon. (1981) *Outline guide for the use of cancer chemotherapeutic agents.* MD Anderson Hospital and Tumor Institute, University of Texas Cancer Center, Houston, Texas.
4 Dorr RT *et al.* (1982) Bleomycin compatibility with selected intravenous medications. *J. Med.* **13**, 121–30.

5 Benvenuto JA *et al.* (1981) Stability and compatibility of antitumor agents in glass and plastic containers. *Am. J. Hosp. Pharm.* **38**, 1914–18.

6 Adams J *et al.* (1982) Instability of bleomycin in plastic containers. *Am. J. Hosp. Pharm.* **39**, 1636.

7 Koberda M *et al.* (1990) Stability of bleomycin sulphate reconstituted in 5% dextrose or 0.9% sodium chloride injection stored in glass vials or PVC containers. *Am. J. Hosp. Pharm.* **47**, 2528–9.

8 Cohen MH *et al.* (1985) Drug precipitation within IV tubing: A potential hazard of chemotherapy administration. *Cancer Treat. Rep.* **69**, 1325–6.

9 Trissel LA, Martinez JF (1994) Physical compatibility of allopurinol sodium with selected drugs during simulated Y-site administration. *Am. J. Hosp. Pharm.* **51**, 1792–9.

10 Trissel LA, Martinez JF (1994) Physical compatibility of filgrastim with selected drugs during simulated Y-site administration. *Am. J. Hosp. Pharm.* **51**, 1907–13.

11 Trissel LA *et al.* (1991) Visual compatibility of fludarabine phosphate with anti-neoplastic drugs, anti-infectives, and other selected drugs during simulated Y-site injection. *Am. J. Hosp. Pharm.* **48**, 2186–9.

12 Trissel LA, Martinez JF (1993) Melphalan physical compatibility with selected drugs during simulated Y-site administration. *Am. J. Hosp. Pharm.* **50**, 2359–63.

13 Trissel LA *et al.* (1991) Visual compatibility of ondansetron hydrochloride with other selected drugs during simulated Y-site injection. *Am. J. Hosp. Pharm.* **48**, 988–92.

14 Trissel LA, Bready BB (1992) Turbidimetric assessment of the compatibility of taxol with selected other drugs during simulated Y-site injection. *Am. J. Hosp. Pharm.* **49**, 1716–19.

15 Trissel LA, Martinez JF (1994) Physical compatibility of piperacillin sodium plus tazobactam sodium with selected drugs during simulated Y-site administration. *Am. J. Hosp. Pharm.* **51**, 672–8.

16 Trissel LA, Martinez JF (1994) Visual, turbidimetric, and particle-content assessment of compatibility of vinorelbine tartrate with selected drugs during simulated Y-site injection. *Am. J. Hosp. Pharm.* **51**, 495–9.

Prepared by Richard Needle

CARBOPLATIN

1 General details

Approved names: Carboplatin, JM8.

Proprietary names: Paraplatin.

Manufacturer or supplier: Bristol-Myers Squibb Pharmaceuticals Ltd, David Bull Laboratories Ltd (DBL).

Presentation and formulation details: Vials containing 50, 150 and 450 mg carboplatin, as a 10 mg/ml solution in water for injection.[1]

Storage and shelf-life of unopened container: 24 months at room termperature.

2 Chemistry

Type: Platinum-containing complex.

Molecular structure: Cis-diamine (1,1-cyclobutanedicarboxylato) platinum.

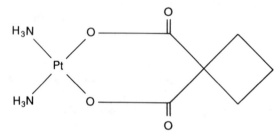

Molecular weight: 371.24.

Solubility in water: 18.6 mg/ml.[2]

3 Stability profile

3.1 Physical and chemical stability

Carboplatin is relatively stable in aqueous solutions. Degradation is accelerated by chloride and hydroxyl ions.[3] The $t_{95\%}$ values for carboplatin in 0.9% sodium chloride and water for injections at 25°C are 52.7 and 29.2 hours respectively.[3]

Degradation pathways: Carboplatin degrades by two simultaneous pathways summarized in Figure 1[3,4] and described as follows:

▼ hydrolytic reactions which give 'activated' platinum species, including cisplatin
▼ nucleophilic substitution with chloride or other nucleophiles resulting in the replacement of the cyclobutanecarboxylate ligands with chloride.

One degradation product is cisplatin.

Degradation obeys pseudo first-order kinetics.[3] The overall rate of reaction can be simplified in the following reaction:

$$K_{obs} = K_1 + K_2 (Cl^-)$$

where K_{obs} = observed degradation constant
K_1 = hydrolytic rate constant
K_2 = chloride-dependent nucleophilic substitution rate constant.

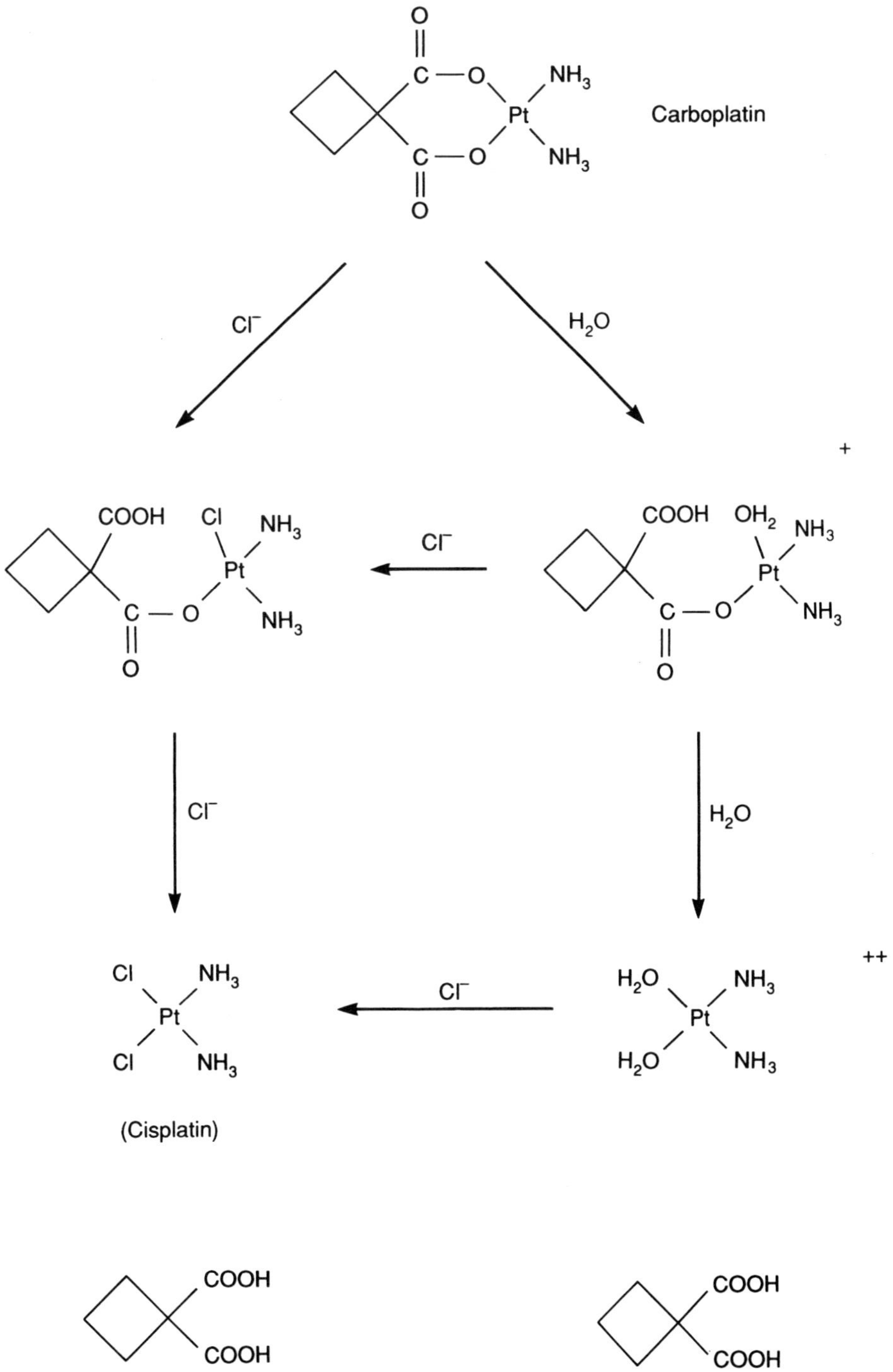

Figure 1: *Degradation pathways for carboplatin in chloride-containing solutions*

Values of K_1 and K_2 at 25°C were 9.74×10^{-4}/h and 3.14×10^{-3}/h, respectively.[3] Apparent first-order kinetics is obeyed.

The range of degradation products (some are intermediates) possibly include:

▼ monosubstitution with Cl^-
▼ disubstitution with Cl^- (cisplatin)
▼ monosubstitution with water
▼ substitution with water and chloride ions.

The aquated 'intermediates' are likely to be the most toxic (but also the species with most anti-tumour activity). They can form various dimers, trimers and other oligomers in their own right.

Effect of pH: Carboplatin is relatively stable within the range pH 4–6.5.[3] Degradation rate constants increase rapidly above pH 6.5.[3] The $t_{95\%}$ values for carboplatin at pH 7.0 stored at 4°C in the absence and presence of chloride ions (equivalent to 0.9% sodium chloride) are 737 and 559 hours respectively.[3]

Effect of temperature: The stability of carboplatin at various temperatures in different vehicles is summarized in Table 1.[3,5]

Table 1: *The effect of temperature on the stability of carboplatin in different infusions*

Temp. (°C)	Conc. (mg/ml)	$t_{95\%}$ (hours) in:		
		0.9% Sodium chloride	Water for injections	5% Glucose
4	3.7	24.0	32.0	40
21	3.7	22.0	32.0	44
25	1.0	29.2	52.7	–
37	3.7	9.0	14.0	16

Certain frozen solutions may also be stable.[6]

Effect of light: Carboplatin is not especially light-sensitive.

Container compatibility: Carboplatin is compatible with PVC infusion containers[4] and plastic syringes.[5,7]

Compatibility with other drugs: Mixing of carboplatin with any drug solution containing chloride ions (e.g. hydrochloride salts) leads to accelerated degradation. Physical compatibility of carboplatin with etoposide has been reported although no details are provided of concentration or conditions.[8] In the presence of a citrate buffer, a solution of carboplatin 0.1 mg/ml and 5-FU 1 mg/ml in glucose 5% showed <3% loss of carboplatin after 48 hours at room temperature.[9] Lokich and Anderson also report that a combination of carboplatin 1 mg/ml, etoposide 0.2 mg/ml and ifosfamide 2 mg/ml showed[10] <10% degradation over seven days at room temperature. Compatibility with a range of drugs is reported by Trissel.[11]

3.2 Stability in clinical practice

If diluted in water for injections or 5% glucose as directed, carboplatin is stable for at least eight hours at room temperature or 24 hours stored in the refrigerator.[1] Cheung *et al.*[4] have reported that carboplatin, 0.1 or 1 mg/ml, in 5% glucose, 0.9% sodium chloride or a range of other infusions, is stable for 24 hours at 25°C. It has also been reported that carboplatin, 1 mg/ml, in 0.9% sodium chloride, is stable for 24 hours at 5°C, with less than 1% degradation.[12] Carboplatin, 10 mg/ml, stored in plastic syringes is stable for at least five days at 4°C with no loss recorded over that period.[7] Benaji et al. reported that a solution of 2.4 mg/ml in 5% glucose showed no loss of carboplatin after storage for nine days at room temperature, in the dark, in a PVC bag.[13] Lokich and Anderson report that carboplatin solutions of unspecified concentration showed <10% degradation for up to seven days at room temperature.[10]

3.3 Stability in specialized delivery systems

The stability of carboplatin in ambulatory pumps has been reported. Sewell et al.[7] reported that carboplatin, 10 mg/ml, in plastic syringes showed 3.1% degradation after storage for 24 hours at 37°C. In a later study, carboplatin, 1 mg/ml, diluted in water for injections, stored in the reservoir of the Parker Micropump, was stable for 14 days at either 4°C or 37°C.[14]

4 Clinical use

Main indications: First and second line therapy of advanced ovarian carcinoma of epithelial origin and small cell carcinoma of the lung. Carboplatin is also used in treating testicular and bladder tumours in combination with other cytotoxic drugs.

Dosage and administration: Carboplatin is administered intravenously. Recommended dosage in previously untreated adult patients with normal kidney function is 400 mg/m^2 as a single IV dose administered by short-term (15–30 minutes) infusion.

The following formula may be used to calculate the dose of carboplatin:

$$Dose = AUC \times (GFR + 25)$$

where AUC = desired area under the plasma concentration curve, the value depending on individual chemotherapy protocols; it may vary from 2 to 12.[15] GFR = glomerular filtration rate. Therapy should not be repeated until four weeks after the previous carboplatin course. Reduction of initial dosage by 20–25% is recommended for those patients with risk factors, such as myelosuppressive treatment. Carboplatin should not be used in patients with severe pre-existing renal impairment (creatinine clearance at or below 20 ml/minute).

5 Preparation of injection

Bolus administration: Solution may be administered by slow intravenous injection (over 15–30 minutes) using an infusion pump.

Intravenous infusion: Dilute the injection (10 mg/ml) to as low as 500 µg/ml (1 : 20) in 5% glucose or 0.9% sodium chloride.[1]

Extravasation: Mildly irritant (*see* Chapter 6).

6 Destruction of drug or contaminated articles

Incineration: 1000°C.

Chemical: Dilute in large volumes of water; allow to stand for 48 hours.

Contact with skin: Wash with water.

References

1 *ABPI Data Sheet Compendium 1995–96* (1995) DataPharm Publications Ltd, London, pp. 263–5.

2 Harrap KR (1986) Paraplatin preclinical development. In *Abstracts of a symposium on paraplatin*, Imperial College, London, 1986, pp. 3–7. Bristol Myers Oncology.

3 Allsop MA *et al.* (1991) The degradation of carboplatin in aqueous solutions containing chloride or other selected nucleophiles. *Int. J. Pharm.* **69**, 197–210.

4 Cheung Y *et al.* (1987) Stability of cisplatin, iproplatin, carboplatin and tetraplatin in commonly used infusion solutions. *Am. J. Hosp. Pharm.* **44**, 124–30.

5 Institute of Cancer Research, London (1988) Personal communication.

6 Bosanquet AG (1989) Stability of solutions of antineoplastic agents during preparation and storage for *in vitro* assays. *Cancer Chemother. Pharmacol.* **23**, 197–207.

7 Sewell GJ *et al.* (1987) The stability of carboplatin in ambulatory continuous infusion regimens. *J. Clin. Pharm. Ther.* **12**, 427–32.

8 Salamone FR, Muller RJ (1990) Intravenous admixture compatibility of cancer chemotherapeutic agents. *Hosp. Pharm.* **25**, 567–70.

9 Sewell GJ *et al.* (1994) Stability studies on admixtures of 5-fluorouracil with carboplatin and 5-fluorouracil with heparin administration in continuous infusion regimens. *J. Clin. Pharm. Ther.* **19**, 127–33.

10 Lokich J, Anderson N (1995) Infusional cancer chemotherapy: Historical evolution and future development at the Cancer Center of Boston. *Cancer Invest.* **13**, 202–26.

11 Trissel LA (1994) *Handbook of Injectable Drugs*, 8th edn. American Society of Hospital Pharmacists, Bethesda, Maryland, USA.

12 Perrone RK *et al.* (1989) Extent of cisplatin formation in carboplatin admixtures. *Am. J. Hosp. Pharm.* **46**, 258–9.

13 Benaji B *et al.* (1994) Stability and compatibility of cisplatin and carboplatin with PVC bags. *J. Clin. Pharm. Ther.* **19**, 95–100.

14 Northcott M *et al.* (1991) The stability of carboplatin, diamorphine, 5-fluorouracil and mitozantrone infusions in an ambulatory pump under storage and prolonged in-use conditions *J. Clin. Pharm. Ther.* **16**, 123–9.

15 Calvert AH *et al.* (1989) Carboplatin dosage: prospective evaluation of a simple formulation based on renal function. *J. Clin. Oncol.* **7**, 1748–56.

Prepared by Tim Root

CARMUSTINE

1 General details

Approved name: Carmustine, BCNU.

Proprietary name: Bicnu.

Manufacturer or supplier: Bristol-Myers Pharmaceuticals Ltd.

Presentation and formulation details: White, freeze-dried flaky powder in 30 ml capacity vial, containing 100 mg carmustine, with diluent vial containing 3 ml absolute alcohol.

Storage and shelf-life of unopened container: Three years at 2–8°C, protect from light.

2 Chemistry

Type: Nitrosourea.

Molecular structure: N,N'-bis(2-chloroethyl)-1-nitrosourea.

$$\underset{\underset{ClCH_2CH_2N}{}}{\overset{\overset{NO}{|}}{}} - \underset{}{\overset{\overset{O}{||}}{C}} - NHCH_2CH_2Cl$$

Molecular weight: 214.04.

Melting point: 27°C (Merck Index quotes 30–32°C).

Solubility: 4 mg/ml in water; 150 mg/ml in 95% ethanol.

3 Stability profile

3.1 Physical and chemical stability

Carmustine is relatively unstable after reconstitution. Its stability depends on a number of factors. The most important chemical factor is pH.

Degradation pathways (in aqueous solution):[1] BCNU degrades to:

2-chloroethylamine hydrochloride + acetaldehyde + nitrogen + carbon dioxide.
($Cl.CH_2CH_2NH_3HCl + CH_3CHO + N_2 + CO_2$).

Carmustine has a very low melting point (27°C according to the manufacturer,[2] although another source quotes 30–32°C).[3] The drug, if melted, liquifies to become an oily film in the base of the vial. The physical change may also be associated with decomposition and such vials must be discarded. There is slow decomposition at room temperature. One report suggests 3% degradation in 36 days.[4]

The manufacturer indicates that the reconstituted injection decomposes by zero-order kinetics.[2] Thus, at ambient temperature, this report anticipated losses of 6% in three hours, whilst at 4°C losses of 4% in 24 hours are to be expected (the pH of the reconstituted injection is 5.6–6.0).

Studies[5,6] indicate that carmustine is most stable in aqueous buffered solutions between pH 3.5 and 5.0. In more acid conditions, there is a small increase in degradation rate whilst at pH above 4.8, degradation rates increase rapidly. For example at pH 5.0 (buffer) $t_{95\%}$ = 5 hours (24°C) or 60 hours (4°C), but at pH 7.3

(buffer) $t_{95\%}$ = 40 minutes (22°C) or 9 hours (4°C). Degradation may also be accelerated by buffering agents, especially phosphates.[1] The pH will rise during degradation in unbuffered medium, causing an acceleration in degradation rate with time. It has been suggested that because of the importance of pH, diluted solutions will be more stable in 5% glucose than in 0.9% sodium chloride.[6]

Effect of light: Fredriksson et al.[6] have shown that carmustine is relatively light-sensitive. Under artificial laboratory conditions using a light cabinet, the reaction rates at various light intensities were reported. Samples were placed in covered Petri dishes, not accurately reflecting degradation rates in practice. The authors reported a value for $t_{90\%}$ of 2.9 hours at an intensity of 1000 lux (a relatively high light intensity). The light-induced degradation rate is reduced in a bulk solution packed in a glass or plastic infusion container. Degradation may also occur during passage of the infusion through the administration set. Unfortunately the data from this report cannot be used to predict the outcome of light exposure in practice, but they do indicate the need to protect the drug from light exposure during storage after reconstitution and dilution into infusions. Information summarized from the manufacturer suggests, in contrast, that the drug is stable for 8 hours at 25°C exposed to fluorescent light.[2]

Effect of freezing: One report suggests that the drug is stable in infusions when in the frozen state,[6] but further studies are necessary to confirm this observation since evidence is somewhat conflicting.[7]

Container compatibility: Benvenuto et al.[8] indicated that infusions of carmustine in 5% glucose may be less stable in PVC than in glass containers. Some sorption to plastic containers (PVC Viaflex) was indicated. Losses of the order of 10% after 0.5–1 hour and 35% after 4 hours were evident (drug concentration = 1.25 mg/ml in 5% glucose at pH 4.4). However, these tests were carried out in 50 ml bags; in 500 ml bags, the surface area to volume ratio is lower so absorption rates may be reduced.

More recent studies[5] suggest that carmustine interacts with PVC, EVA and polyurethane administration sets, whilst no sorption to polyethylene was apparent. Tests under simulated infusion conditions from glass bottles suggest that if 500 ml of drug (0.20 mg/ml) are infused over one hour, about 4.6% (4.6 mg) of the dose is lost by sorption, but over two hours 6.5% (6.5 mg) will be lost.

However, all of these tests were conducted at a drug concentration of about 0.2 mg/ml. No studies on the effect of drug concentration were reported. It is likely that the losses may be substantially reduced (as a proportion of the total dose) at higher drug concentrations.

The evidence, therefore, indicates that carmustine binds to some plastics, especially PVC, but the full clinical implications regarding dose delivery from an infusion are yet to be fully quantified. In practice, it may be relatively unimportant.

Compatibility with other drugs: Carmustine (1.5 µg/ml) has been reported to be physically compatible with teniposide (100 µg/ml),[9] filgrastim (30 µg/ml)[10] and vinorelbine (1 µg/ml).[11]

3.2 Stability in clinical practice

After reconstitution in the vial the injection can be stored for up to two days in the refrigerator. After dilution in 0.9% sodium chloride or 5% glucose in glass or polyethylene containers, the resulting infusion may be stored for up to two days in the refrigerator.[2] If diluted in an infusion in a PVC container, it should not be stored, but used as soon as possible.

Carmustine is unstable after addition to any infusion containing sodium bicarbonate (due to alkaline pH).

3.3 Stability in specialized delivery systems

No data available.

4 Clinical use

Type of cytotoxic: Nitrosourea, alkylating agent.

Main indications: Brain tumours. In combination therapy for multiple myeloma, Hodgkin's disease and other lymphomas.

Dosage: 200 mg/m² every six weeks as a single agent, but adjusted if necessary according to haematological response. Lower doses are used in combination with other chemotherapeutic agents.

5 Preparation of injection

Dilution: To each vial add 3 ml diluent (absolute ethanol), dissolve contents and then dilute with 27 ml water for injections. Resulting solution contains 3.3 mg in 1 ml of 10% ethanol. Dissolution may be faster if vial and diluent are allowed to equilibrate at room temperature.

Bolus administration: Not recommended but if essential, inject very slowly via the bolus site of a fast-running drip infusion.

Intravenous infusion: Dilute in 5% glucose (up to 500 ml), preferably in a glass or polyethylene (e.g. Polyfusor) container and administer over one to two hours as a slow infusion. Protect the contents from light by covering the infusion with a light-protecting overwrap if infused over two hours, or exposed to sunlight. Do not store in a PVC container but use immediately after preparation. Non-PVC containing sets (e.g. Sureset, Avon Medical) are recommended.

Extravasation: Vesicant; damaging (*see* Chapter 6).

6 Destruction of drug or contaminated articles

Incineration: 1000°C.[2]

Chemical: 8.4% sodium bicarbonate solution/24–48 hours.

Contact with skin: Wash with copious amounts of water. In some cases of local irritancy apply sodium bicarbonate solution.

References

1 Montgomery JA *et al.* (1967) The modes of decomposition of 1,3-bis (2-chloroethyl)-1-nitrosourea and related compounds. *J. Med. Chem.* **10**, 668–74.

2 *ABPI Data Sheet Compendium 1995–96* (1995). DataPharm Publications Ltd, London, pp. 311–12.

3 Trissel LA (1994) *Handbook on injectable drugs*, 8th edn. American Society of Hospital Pharmacists, Bethesda, Maryland, USA.

4 Kleinman LM *et al.* (1976) Investigational drug information. *Drug Intell. Clin. Pharm.* **10**, 48–9.

5 Lasker PA, Ayres JW (1977) Degradation of carmustine in aqueous media. *J. Pharm. Sci.* **66**, 1073–6.

6 Fredriksson K *et al.* (1986) Stability of carmustine – kinetics and compatibility during administration. *Acta Pharm. Suec.* **23**, 115–24.

7 Bosanquet AG (1985) Stability of solutions of antineoplastic agents during preparation and storage for *in vitro* assays. General considerations and nitrosoureas and alkylating agents. *Cancer Chemother. Pharmacol.* **14**, 83–95.

8 Benvenuto JA *et al.* (1981) Stability and compatibility of antitumour agents in glass and plastic containers. *Am. J. Hosp. Pharm.* **38**, 1914–18.

9 Trissel LA, Martinez JF (1994) Screening for Y-site physical incompatibilities. *Hosp. Pharm.* **29**, 1010–17.

10 Trissel LA, Martinez JF (1994) Compatibility of filgrastim with selected drugs during simulated Y-site administration. *Am. J. Hosp. Pharm.* **51**, 1907–13.

11 Trissel LA, Martinez JF (1994) Visual, turbidimetric and particle-content of compatibility of vinorelbine tartrate with selected drugs during simulated Y-site injection. *Am. J. Hosp. Pharm.* **51**, 495–9.

Prepared by Michael Allwood

CISPLATIN

1 General details

Approved names: Cisplatin, cis-DDP.

Proprietary name: Cisplatin.

Manufacturer or supplier: David Bull Laboratories Ltd (DBL), Erba Ltd, Pharmacia Ltd.

Presentation and formulation details: Supplied (a) in 10, 50 and 100 ml vials, as a solution containing in each ml, 1 mg cisplatin, 9 mg sodium chloride, 1 mg mannitol in water for injections (DBL), or (b) as a yellowish-white lyophilized powder in vials containing 10 and 50 mg cisplatin, with sodium chloride and mannitol (DBL, Pharmacia). The solution, and the powder after reconstitution, are clear, practically colourless, with a pH usually between 3.5 and 5.5.

Storage and shelf-life of unopened container: Both the powder and the solution preparations should be stored at controlled room temperature (15–25°C) and protected from direct bright sunlight. Protection from normal room fluorescent light is also recommended. Unopened vials of the drug are stable for two to three years (dependent on the manufacturer).

2 Chemistry

Type: Platinum-containing complex.

Molecular structure: The platinum atom is surrounded in a plane by two chloride atoms and two ammonia molecules, in the *cis* position, platinum diammino dichloride.

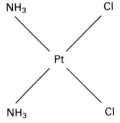

Molecular weight: 300.1.

Solubility: 1 mg/1 ml in water; 1 g in 42 ml of dimethyl formamide.

3 Stability profile

3.1 Physical and chemical stability

Cisplatin is unstable in an aqueous vehicle unless chloride ions are present. For example, losses of 30–35% in four hours, or 70–80% in 24 hours at 25°C have been reported.[1] The minimum concentration of sodium chloride providing an acceptable level of stability is about 0.3% w/v.[2]

Solutions of cisplatin in 0.9% sodium chloride are relatively stable for at least 24 hours at ambient temperatures. It should be noted that an equilibrium will be established between cisplatin and chloride ions in solution. In 0.9% sodium chloride, approximately 97% cisplatin will be present at equilibrium.[1,3] This level

Table 1: *Stability of cisplatin injection in 0.9% sodium chloride*

Time	Storage condition 20°C			
	Viaflex container/bag		Glass bottle	
	Exposed to light: % cisplatin	Protected from light: % cisplatin	Exposed to light: % cisplatin	Protected from light: % cisplatin
0 day	100.0 pH 4.60	100.0 pH 4.90	100.0 pH 4.90	100.0 pH 4.95
4 days	89.2 + 0.2* pH 5.90	100.0 + 0.1 pH 4.87	83.8 + 0.2 pH 6.76	99.5 + 0.1 pH 5.35
7 days	85.9 + 0.2 pH not recorded	100.5 + 0.3	79.0 + 0.1	100.2 + 0.1
14 days	77.2 + 0.2 pH 6.85	99.8 + 0.1 pH 4.70	70.1 + 0.2 pH 7.23	99.5 + 0.3 pH 4.86

* The figures represent the mean + standard deviation.

of degradation does not seriously compromise therapeutic efficacy or toxicity profiles. Other studies have indicated that dilutions of cisplatin injection in 0.9% sodium chloride are chemically stable (<5% degradation) for four days at 4°C, two days at 25°C or 30 days at –15°C.[4] The pH does not appear to be an important factor in cisplatin injection stability after dilution in recommended infusion fluids. Cisplatin is also stable in 0.9% sodium chloride in the presence of magnesium sulphate and potassium chloride for up to 24 hours.[5]

Degradation pathways: Cisplatin undergoes nucleophilic displacement of the chloride ligand by water in aqueous media[3] (*see* Figure 1). It is believed that the major route of decomposition involves the displacement of one chloride ion. The loss of the second chloride ion may not contribute substantially to the overall decomposition rate. The reaction is reversible. When enough liberated chloride ions accumulate in the medium, the reaction reaches an equilibrium. The equilibrium drug concentration depends on the concentration of chloride ions present. (Cisplatin can re-form in decomposed drug solutions with the addition of sufficient amounts of chloride.)

The reactions can be described by first-order kinetics, dependent principally on chloride ion concentration. Only the first reaction is of practical significance.[1,3]

Effect of light: Cisplatin is relatively sensitive to daylight, but reports confirm that the drug is not adversely affected by normal room lighting after dilution in 0.9% sodium chloride[1,5] (*see* Table 1). The solutions at the concentration of 150 mg cisplatin per 1000 ml 0.9% sodium chloride injection remained clear, colourless and free from particulate matter during the testing period.

Effect of temperature: Temperature appears to have little influence on the stability of cisplatin after dilution. However, because of limited solubility of cisplatin, especially in chloride-containing solutions, the cooling of diluted solutions can lead to precipitation. Studies have also shown that precipitates of cisplatin may be redissolved without further degradation by placing in a water bath heated to 70°C for four hours.[5] Concentrations of 1 mg/ml remain in solution at ambient temperature, while refrigeration can lead to precipitation within one hour.[4,6] Solutions

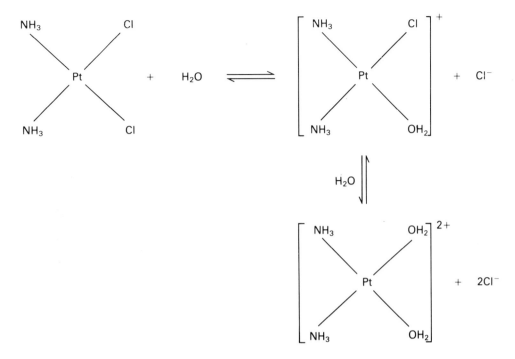

Figure 2: *Degradation pathways proposed for cisplatin*

stored in a refrigerator should contain NMT 0.6 mg/ml if stored for 24 hours, or NMT 0.5 mg/ml if stored for 24–72 hours.[7] Further studies have shown that solutions containing 0.05–0.2 mg/ml remain potent for four days at 4°C.[4]

Container compatibility: Cisplatin diluted in 0.9% sodium chloride is stable in glass or PVC containers.[2,4] Cisplatin reacts with aluminium and care should be taken to avoid contact of injections with metal items containing aluminium. Stainless steel is compatible.[8]

Compatibility with other drugs: Cisplatin injection is compatible with mannitol and magnesium sulphate injection.[4] However, it has been suggested that mannitol–cisplatin complexes may form if diluted mixtures are stored for several days.[9] Mannitol should therefore be added immediately before administration if 'diuresis' doses are required. Cisplatin has been reported to be physically compatible with fluorouracil,[10,11] etoposide,[10,12] cytarabine,[10] ifosfamide, cyclophosphamide and floxuridine,[13] and a range of other drugs.[9]

3.2 Stability in clinical practice

Reconstituted or diluted cisplatin injections are stable, if diluted in 0.9% sodium chloride, for 20 hours at 25°C but will precipitate on refrigeration.[7] In practice, the appropriate dose should be diluted in 2 l 0.9% sodium chloride infusion, giving concentrations in the range 0.1–0.2 mg/ml. At such concentrations precipitation will not occur on refrigeration. Such dilute infusions are stable for four days at 4°C in PVC containers.[4] If precipitation is seen as a result of refrigeration the solution should be discarded. Infusions may, however, be frozen at –15°C for up to 30 days and thawed at room temperature for 48 hours before use.[9]

The stability of cisplatin solutions (1 and 1.6 mg/ml) in plastic infusion bags was studied for up to 14 days at 25, 37 and 60°C. No evidence of any decomposition product was seen. Some precipitation was seen in the 1.6 mg/ml solution at temperatures below 37°C.[14] Cisplatin solutions 0.6 mg/ml in 0.9% sodium chloride and in 5% glucose showed <4% loss after storage for nine days at room temperature, in the dark, in PVC.[13] Lokich and Anderson report that solutions of unspecified concentration showed <10% degradation after 14 days storage at room temperature.[15]

3.3 Stability in specialized delivery systems

Cisplatin 1 mg/ml in 0.9% sodium chloride in the medication cassette (CADD-1 pump, Deltec, Pharmacia) stored at 25°C has been reported to be stable for seven days, although 10% loss was recorded after 14 days.[16]

4 Clinical use

Type of cytotoxic: Platinum-containing complex. The exact mechanism of action has not been determined conclusively but the drug has biochemical properties similar to those of alkylating agents.

Main indications: Cisplatin is used for many indications and in varying doses, commonly 20–100 mg/m^2.

5 Preparation of injection

Reconstitution: Cisplatin powder should be dissolved in water for injection to give a 1 mg/ml solution. The manufacturer recommends cisplatin solution to be added to 2 l of 0.9% sodium chloride solution or 4%/0.18% glucose/sodium chloride solution. At The Royal Marsden Hospital, doses of up to 100 mg/m^2 cisplatin are added to as little as 250 ml of 0.9% sodium chloride solution. Larger doses are added to 500–1000 ml. The resulting infusion bag should be protected from light and stored at room temperature.

Bolus administration: Must not be used.

Intravenous infusion: The manufacturers recommend that cisplatin solution be infused over six to eight hours, although at The Royal Marsden Hospital a dose of less than 100 mg in 250 ml 0.9% sodium chloride is infused over 30 minutes. Larger doses are often given over one to two hours or longer if renal function is particularly poor. Pre- and post-hydration are essential to induce diuresis during and after the cisplatin infusion. This is to ensure adequate renal clearance of cisplatin and varies according to the dose.

   Below are The Royal Marsden Hospital procedures for pre-and post-hydration, for doses of cisplatin between 20–100 mg/m^2.

▼ Pre-hydrate with 1 l 0.9% sodium chloride + 20 mmol KCl over 12 hours, followed by 200 ml 20% mannitol over 30 minutes.
▼ Post-hydration regimen: 2 l 0.9% sodium chloride + 20 mmol KCl + 1 g magnesium sulphate over 12 hours.

Extravasation: Irritant (*see* Chapter 6).

6 Destruction of drug or contaminated articles

Incineration: 800°C.

Chemical: Dilute in large volume of water, allow to stand for 48 hours.

Contact with skin: Wash with copious amounts of water. Apply a cream if transient stinging is experienced. (NB: Some individuals are sensitive to platinum and a skin reaction may occur.)

References

1 Hincal AA *et al.* (1979) Cisplatin stability in aqueous parenteral vehicles. *J. Parenteral Drug. Assoc.* **33**, 107–16.

2 Cheung YH *et al.* (1987) Stability of cisplatin, iproplatin, carboplatin and tetraplatin in commonly used intravenous solutions. *Am . J. Hosp. Pharm.* **44**, 124–30.

3 Le Rey RH (1970) Some quantitative data on cis-dichlorodiammineplatinum (II) species in solution. *Cancer Treat. Rep.* **63**, 231–3.

4 La Follette JM *et al.* (1985) Stability of cisplatin admixtures in polyvinyl chloride bags. *Am. J. Hosp. Pharm.* **42**, 2652.

5 DBL Ltd. Personal communication. Unpublished data.

6 Green RF *et al.* (1979) Stability of cisplatin in aqueous solution. *Am. J. Hosp. Pharm.* **36**, 38–43.

7 *ABPI Data Sheet Compendium 1995–96* (1995) DataPharm Publications Ltd, London, pp. 1251–3.

8 Bohart RD, Ogawa G (1979) An observation on the stability of cis-dichlorodiammineplatinum (II): A caution regarding its administration. *Cancer Treat. Rep.* **63**, 2117–18.

9 Trissel LA (1994) *Handbook on injectable drugs,* 8th edn. American Society of Hospital Pharmacists, Bethesda, Maryland, USA.

10 Salamone FR, Muller RJ (1990) Intravenous admixture compatibility of cancer chemotherapeutic agents. *Hosp. Pharm.* **25**, 567–70.

11 Stewart CF, Fleming RA (1990) Compatibility of cisplatin and fluorouracil on 0.9% sodium chloride injection. *Am. J. Hosp. Pharm.* **47**, 1373–7.

12 Stewart CF, Hampton EM (1989) Stability of cisplatin and etoposide in intravenous admixtures. *Am. J. Hosp. Pharm.* **46**, 1400–4.

13 Benaji B *et al.* (1994) Stability and compatibility of cisplatin and carboplatin with PVC bags. *J. Clin. Pharm. Ther.* **19**, 95–100.

14 Hrubisko M *et al.* (1992) Suitability of cisplatin solutions for 14-day continuous infusion by ambulatory pump. *Cancer Chemother. Pharmacol.* **29**, 252–5.

15 Lokich J, Anderson N (1995) Infusional cancer chemotherapy: Historical evolution and future development at the Cancer Center of Boston. *Cancer Invest.* **13**, 202–26.

16 Pharmacia Deltec Inc. (1991) Personal communication. *Am. J. Hosp. Pharm.* **46**, 1400–4.

Prepared by Tim Root

CLADRIBINE

1 General details

Approved name: Cladribine.

Proprietary name: Leustat.

Manufacturer or supplier: Janssen-Cilag Ltd.

Presentation and formulation details: 20 ml flint glass vials containing 10 ml solution. Each ml contains 1.0 mg cladribine and 9 mg (0.15 mEq) sodium chloride. The solution has a pH of 5.5–8.0. Phosphoric acid and/or dibasic sodium phosphate may be added to adjust pH.[1]

Storage and shelf-life of unopened containers: Store at 2–8°C,[1] protected from light. Freezing does not adversely affect stability. If freezing occurs, thaw naturally to room temperature. Do not use heat or microwave.

2 Chemistry

Type: Purine nucleoside antineoplastic.

Molecular structure: 72-Chloro-6-amino-9-(2-deoxy-β-D erythropentofuranosyl) purine.

Molecular formula:

Molecular weight: 285.7.

3 Stability profile

3.1 Physical and chemical stability

Cladribine injection (1.0 mg/ml) stored at 2–8°C, is stable for at least 18 months.[1] The drug solution has been found to lose less than 5% of activity in seven days at 37°C. When diluted to a concentration of 0.15–0.3 mg/ml in 0.9% sodium chloride containing 0.9% benzyl alcohol as the preservative, the solution is chemically stable for at least 14 days.

Solubility: A stable white, to off-white, crystalline powder sparingly soluble in water. Dissolves more easily in 0.9% sodium chloride at 60–65°C. The pH of the injection is 5.5–8.0.[1]

3.2 Stability in clinical practice

Infusions of cladribine are chemically and physically stable for at least 24 hours at room temperature under normal room fluorescent light in PVC (Viaflex) infusion containers.[1]

3.3 Stability in specialized delivery systems

Cladribine infusions have demonstrated acceptable chemical and physical stability for at least seven days in Deltec (Pharmacia) medication cassettes.[2]

4 Clinical use

Type of cytotoxic: Antimetabolite.

Main indications: Active hairy cell leukaemia. It also has activity in other haematologic malignancies, especially advanced refractory chronic lymphocytic leukaemia and low-grade lymphocytic lymphoma.

The safety and efficacy of cladribine has not been established in children. In early clinical trials, doses of 6.2–7.5 mg/m²/day for five days via continuous infusion have been used.

5 Preparation of injection

Reconstitution: Cladribine must be diluted in 0.9% sodium chloride prior to administration. The dose required is added to 500 ml 0.9% sodium chloride. The use of 5% glucose as a diluent is not recommended because of poor stability of cladribine.[1]

Bolus administration: Must not be used.

Intravenous infusion: Continuous infusion over 24 hours. This procedure is repeated daily for seven days.

Extravasation: Non-irritant.

6 Destruction of drug or contaminated articles

Incineration: No specific information available.

Chemical: No specific information available.

Contact with skin: No specific information available.

References

1 *ABPI Data Sheet Compendium 1995–1996* (1995) DataPharm Publications Ltd, pp. 426–8.
2 Micromedex (1995) *Drug Evaluation Monograph.* Vol. 84.

Prepared by Yaacov Cass

CYCLOPHOSPHAMIDE

1 General details

Approved names: Cyclophosphamide, cyclophospham.

Proprietary names: Endoxana, cyclophosphamide.

Manufacturer or supplier: ASTA Medica Ltd, Pharmacia Ltd.

Presentation and formulation details: Sterile, white powder in vials containing: 107 mg, 214 mg, 535 mg or 1069 mg of cyclophosphamide BP, equivalent to 100 mg, 200 mg, 500 mg or 1000 mg respectively, of anhydrous cyclophosphamide. Sodium chloride is also present to render the solution isotonic after reconstitution with the recommended amount of water for injections.[1,2]

Storage and shelf-life of unopened container: Five years, below 25°C, protected from light.[1,2]

2 Chemistry

Type: A cytotoxic which is converted in the body to an active alkylating agent with properties similar to those of mustine.[3]

2.1 Cyclophosphamide (Pharmacia)

Molecular structure: Contains 2-[bis (2-chloroethyl) amino]-perhydro-1,3,2 oxazaphosphorine-2-oxide monohydrate.

Formula: $C_7H_{15}Cl_2N_2O_2P.\ H_2O$.

Molecular weight: 279.1.

Melting point: 49.5–53°C.[3]

2.2 Endoxana (Asta Medica Ltd)

Molecular structure: Contains the anhydrous salt 2-[bis (2-chloroethyl)amino]-tetrahydro-2H-1,3,2 oxazaphosphorine-2-oxide.

Formula: $C_7H_{15}N_2O_2PCl_2$.

Molecular weight: 261.08.

Melting point: 41– 45°C.[4]

Solubility: Cyclophosphamide is soluble 1 in 25 parts of water and 0.9% sodium chloride and 1 in 1 of alcohol.[3,5]

3 Stability profile

3.1 Physical and chemical stability

The manufacturer states that when mixed with glucose saline infusion solution, cyclophosphamide is chemically stable for 24 hours at room temperature (25°C) or for six days when stored under refrigeration. However, as there is no preservative contained in the formulation the above solution should be used within eight hours unless prepared under strict aseptic conditions.[1] A review of the literature reveals that cyclophosphamide may be chemically stable for longer periods if stored at 4°C.

The loss of cyclophosphamide monohydrate from aqueous solution results from hydrolysis, loss of a chloride ion, or both.[6-9] Degradation follows first-order kinetics and is accompanied by a slight downward shift in pH which does not appear to affect the kinetics of drug loss. During degradation the solution remains colourless. Increase in temperature accelerates the rate of breakdown, as can the presence of benzyl alcohol.[10]

Effect of pH: Hirata *et al.*[6] showed that the rate constant for drug loss at 75°C was independent of pH (pH 2–10). Outside these limits acidic and basic catalysis was observed. In solutions between pH 2 and pH 14 cyclophosphamide degrades via a bicyclic compound, and a number of secondary intermediates, to give N-(2-hydroxyethyl)-N'-(3-hydroxypropyl) ethylenediamine.[7,11,12] The mechanism for hydrolysis of cyclophosphamide proposed by Chakrabarti and Friedman[11] is shown in Figure 1. Under more acidic conditions (pH ≤ 1) cyclophosphamide degrades via a different mechanism to yield bis (2-chloroethyl) amine and 3-aminopropan-1-ol.[6,12]

Effect of light: There are no published data which have systematically compared photodegradation of cyclophosphamide with degradation in identical solutions stored in the dark. Two studies have examined degradation in solutions of cyclophosphamide which were not protected from light. Gallelli[13] observed that cyclophosphamide, 4 mg/ml in 0.9% sodium chloride, stored in glass vials, exhibited 3.5% decomposition over a period of 24 hours at room temperature. Benvenuto *et al.*[14] observed that solutions of cyclophosphamide, 6.6 mg/ml in 5% glucose in both PVC and glass, were stable for 24 hours at room temperature. From these data it is difficult to draw conclusions about the effect of light on the stability of cyclophosphamide.

Effect of temperature: If heated above 32°C cyclophosphamide may decompose to a damp-looking gel which should not be used.[1] The effect of briefly heating cyclophosphamide has been studied. Heating a solution containing 21 mg/ml of cyclophosphamide to 50 or 60°C for 15 minutes resulted in a negligible loss of potency.[15] However heating to 70 or 80°C for 15 minutes resulted in approximately 10 and 23% decomposition respectively.[15] For this reason, the use of heat to speed up dissolution of cyclophosphamide is not recommended since decomposition may result.[15]

Brooke *et al.*[10] observed a 2% loss in potency in a solution of cyclophosphamide, 20 mg/ml, in glass vials, after four days storage at room temperature (24–27°C) and an 8% loss after 17 weeks at 4°C. The rate constants for drug loss recorded in that study were not significantly different for solutions reconstituted with water for injections, 5% glucose or glucose/saline admixtures.

Kirk *et al.*[16] studied the stability of cyclophosphamide in glass ampoules, polypropylene syringes and PVC infusion containers. In PVC infusion bags (Viaflex, Baxter), polypropylene syringes (Becton Dickinson, Plastipak), and glass ampoules, cyclophosphamide showed no appreciable degradation after four weeks at 4°C. After 19 weeks at 4°C, 5.7% and 8% degradation was observed in solutions stored in syringes and minibags respectively.

The effect of freezing cyclophosphamide was also investigated by Kirk *et al.*[16] Results showed that in syringes, PVC minibags or glass ampoules, no appreciable

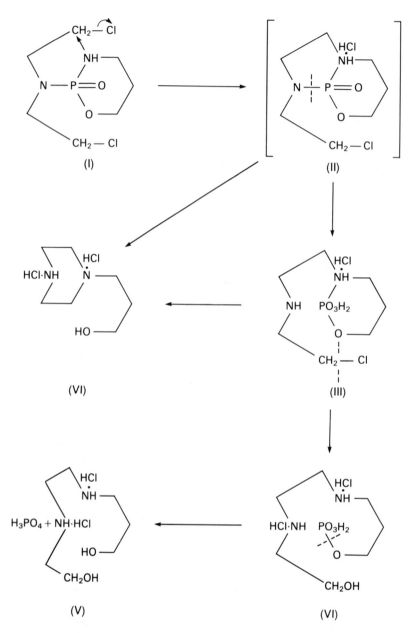

Figure 1: *Degradation of cyclophosphamide*[11]

degradation occurred after four weeks storage at −20°C. After 19 weeks, 4% and 8% degradation was observed in syringes and infusion bags respectively. However, two problems were encountered with freezing cyclophosphamide. First, at higher concentrations (20 mg/ml) precipitation occurred during thawing. Although dissolution occurred after vigorous shaking the possibility of injecting particles into the patient arises. Second, during freezing the integrity of polypropylene syringes was compromised by a marked contraction of the plungers allowing seepage of fluid past the plunger and on to the inner surface of the barrel. Although this probably represents a negligible drug loss, the potential risk of microbial contamination is unacceptable. Therefore, freezing of cyclophosphamide in plastic syringes is not recommended.

The effect of thawing cyclophosphamide in a microwave has also been investigated.[16] Results indicated that during microwave thawing uneven distribution of energy may occur and lead to overheating and consequent degradation. For this reason, thawing solutions in a microwave is not recommended.

Container compatibility: Cyclophosphamide is compatible with glass, PVC and polypropylene.[16] It is not adsorbed on to either PVC or polypropylene. Adsorption on to glass has not been documented. In clinical practice, when cyclophosphamide is used at concentrations of approximately 20 mg/ml, adsorptive losses during storage are likely to be negligible.[16]

Compatibility with other drugs: Cyclophosphamide is compatible with, and may be infused in 5% glucose, 0.9% sodium chloride or mixtures of glucose and saline.[17] The manufacturers recommend that no other drugs are mixed with cyclophosphamide.

3.2 Stability in clinical practice

Cyclophosphamide is compatible with glass, PVC and polypropylene containers and appears to be chemically stable for at least 28 days at 4°C. Solutions of cyclophosphamide should not be frozen.[16]

3.3 Stability in specialized delivery systems

Cyclophosphamide (2 to 20 mg/ml) is stable for 15 days in 0.9% sodium chloride at 4°C in the Baxter infusor. At a concentration of 20 mg/ml in water for injections it is also stable in the CADD pump for 14 days at 4°C and 24 hours at 35°C.[18]

4 Clinical use

Main indications: As a single agent, and in combination chemotherapy, cyclophosphamide has been used successfully to induce and maintain regressions in a wide range of neoplastic diseases including leukaemias, lymphomas, soft tissue and osteogenic sarcomas, paediatric malignancies and adult solid tumours; in particular breast and lung carcinoma.[2]

Dosage and administration. The dose, route and frequency of administration should be determined by the tumour type, tumour stage, the general condition of the patient and whether other chemotherapy or radiation is to be administered concurrently. The following sample regimens may serve as guides:

▼ low dose: 80–240 mg/m² (2–6 mg/kg) as a single dose intravenously each week, or in divided doses orally
▼ medium dose: 400–600 mg/m² (10–15 mg/kg) as a single dose intravenously, each week
▼ high dose: 800–1600 mg/m² (20–40 mg/kg) as a single dose, intravenously at 10–20 day intervals
▼ higher doses should be used only at the discretion of a physician experienced in cytotoxic chemotherapy.

It is recommended that the dose of cyclophosphamide is reduced when it is given in combination with other antineoplastic agents or radiotherapy, and in patients with bone marrow depression. Cyclophosphamide should also be used with caution in patients with renal and/or hepatic failure.[2]

Cyclophosphamide is metabolized to a compound (acrolein) which is toxic to the bladder. During treatment, a large urine output (a minimum of 100 ml/hr) should be maintained to avoid haemorrhagic cystitis.[1] In addition, intravenous or oral mesna may be given concurrently.[2]

5 Preparation of injection

Reconstitution: The contents of a vial are reconstituted with water for injections (5 ml per 100 mg of anhydrous cyclophosphamide). After addition of the diluent and vigorous shaking, the contents of the vial will dissolve to produce a solution of 20 mg/ml. Formation of a solution may be delayed because of the slow dissolution rate of cyclophosphamide in aqueous media. The pH of an aqueous solution is between 4.0 and 6.0.[2] Water for injections preserved with benzyl alcohol should not be used for preparation.[10,19]

Bolus administration: Cyclophosphamide is usually given directly into a vein, over two or three minutes, or directly into the tubing of a fast-running intravenous infusion. Cyclophosphamide injection may also be given intraperitoneally or intrapleurally but these routes offer no therapeutic advantage over the intravenous route.[1] Cyclophosphamide has been given intraarterially and by local perfusion.

Intravenous infusion: High doses of cyclophosphamide may be added to an infusion of 5% glucose, 0.9% sodium chloride or glucose/saline and infused over one to two hours. Both prolonged intermittent and continuous infusion of cyclophosphamide have been studied.[20–24] In a phase I study of a 72 hour continuous infusion patients received 300 mg/m²/day to 750 mg/m²/day.[22] Another study employed a five-day continuous infusion at a rate of 400 mg/m²/day.[20] Protracted infusion of cyclophosphamide has been reported by Lokich *et al.*[24] at doses of 50 to 100 mg/m²/day for periods of 28 days or more.

Extravasation: Non-irritant (*see* Chapter 6).

6 Destruction of drug or contaminated articles

Incineration: 900°C.[4,25]

Chemical: 0.2 M potasssium hydroxide in methanol solution/one hour or 5% sodium hypochlorite solution/24 hours.[4,25]

Contact with skin: Wash well with water, or soap and water. If the eyes are contaminated immediate irrigation with 0.9% sodium chloride should be carried out.[1,2]

References

1 *ABPI Data Sheet Compendium 1995–96* (1995) DataPharm Publications Ltd, London, pp. 100–1.

2 *ABPI Data Sheet Compendium 1995–96* (1995) DataPharm Publications Ltd, London, pp. 1254–5.

3 Anon. (1993) *The Extra Pharmacopoeia.* 30th edn. (JEF Reynolds ed.), Pharmaceutical Press, London, pp. 465–7.

4 ASTA Medica Ltd. Personal communication.

5 Dorr RT, Fritz WL (1980) *Cancer Chemotherapy Handbook*, Elsevier, Amsterdam, p. 342.

6 Hirata M *et al.* (1967) Studies on cyclophosphamide. Part 1. Chemical determination and degradation kinetics in aqueous media. *Shionogi Kenkyusho Nempo* **17**, 107–13.

7 Friedman OM (1967) Recent biologic and chemical studies of cyclophosphamide (NSC 26271). *Cancer Chemother. Reports* **51**, 327–33.

8 Arnold H, Klose H (1961) Die hydrolyse hexacyclisher N-lostphosphamidester in gepufferten system. *Arzneimittel-Forsch.* **11**, 159–63.

9 Friedman OM (1965) Studies on the hydrolysis of cyclophosphamide. I. Identification of N-(2-hydroxyethyl)-N′-(3-hydroxypropyl) ethylenediamine as the main product. *J. Am. Chem. Soc.* **87**, 4978–9.

10 Brooke D *et al.* (1973) Chemical stability of cyclophosphamide in parenteral solutions. *Am. J. Hosp. Pharm.* **30**, 134–7.

11 Chakrabarti JK, Friedman OM (1973) Studies on the hydrolysis of cyclophosphamide II. Isolation and characterization of intermediate hydrolytic products. (I). *J. Heterocyclic Chem.* **10**, 55–8.

12 Zon G *et al.* (1977) High resolution nuclear magnetic resonance investigations of the chemical stability of cyclophosphamide and related phosphoramidic compounds. *J. Am. Chem. Soc.* **99**, 5785–95.

13 Gallelli JF (1967) Stability studies of drugs used in intravenous solutions; Part one. *Am. J. Hosp. Pharm.* **24**, 425–33.

14 Benvenuto JA *et al.* (1981) Stability and compatibility of antitumour agents in glass and plastic containers. *Am. J. Hosp. Pharm.* **38**, 1914–18.

15 Brooke D *et al.* (1975) Effect of briefly heating cyclophosphamide solutions. *Am. J. Hosp. Pharm.* **32**, 44–5.

16 Kirk B *et al.* (1984) Chemical stability of cyclophosphamide injection. The effect of low temperature storage and microwave thawing. *Br. J. Parenter. Ther.* **1**, 90–7.

17 Trissel LA (1994) *Handbook of Injectable Drugs*, 8th edn. American Society of Hospital Pharmacists, Bethesda, USA.

18 Baxter Healthcare Ltd. Personal communication.

19 D'Arcy PF (1983) Handling anticancer drugs. *Drug Intell. Clin. Pharm.* **17**, 532–8.

20 Tchekmedyian NS *et al.* (1986) Phase I clinical and pharmacokinetic study of cyclophosphamide administered by 5-day continuous intravenous infusion. *Cancer Chemother. Rep.* **18**, 33–8.

21 Solidoro A *et al.* (1981) Intermittent continuous IV infusion of high dose cyclophosphamide for remission induction in acute lymphocytic leukaemia. *Cancer Treat. Rep.* **65**, 213–18.

22 Bedikian AY, Bodey GP (1983) Phase I study of cyclophosphamide (NSC 26271) by 72-hour continuous intravenous infusion. *Am. J. Clin. Oncol.* **6**, 365–8.

23 Smith DB *et al.* (1986) A phase II study of cyclophosphamide as a 24 hour infusion in advanced non small cell lung cancer. *Eur. J. Cancer Clin. Oncol.* **22**, 435–7.

24 Lokich JJ, Botha A (1984) Phase I study of continuous infusion cyclophosphamide for protracted duration: A preliminary report. *Cancer Drug Deliv.* **1**, 329–32.

25 Pharmacia Ltd. Personal communication.

Prepared by Jayne Wood

CYTARABINE

1 General details

Approved names: Cytarabine, arabinosylcytosine, ara-C, cytosine arabinoside.

Proprietary names: Alexan, Alexan 100, Cytosar, Cytarabine.

Manufacturer or supplier: Pfizer Ltd, Upjohn Ltd, David Bull Laboratories Ltd (DBL).

Presentation and formulation details:

▼ Alexan: 2 ml and 5 ml ampoules of an isotonic solution of cytarabine 20 mg/ml. Inactive excipients include sodium chloride, sodium lactate and sodium hydroxide.

▼ Alexan 100: 1 ml and 10 ml ampoules of a hypertonic solution of cytarabine 100 mg/ml. Inactive excipients include sodium lactate and lactic acid.

All solutions of Alexan and Alexan 100 are preservative free.[1]

▼ Cytosar: An off-white, sterile, freeze-dried cake of 100 mg or 500 mg cytarabine in a vial. Cytosar is supplied as a single vial with diluent (water for injections) or as ten vials without diluent.[2]

▼ Cytarabine: Vials containing 100 mg, 500 mg and 1000 mg with preserved diluent supplied.[3]

Storage and shelf-life of unopened container: Alexan solution in unopened ampoules is stable for three years when stored below 15°C.[1,4] Vials of Cytosar and Cytarabine (DBL) are stable for three and two years respectively when stored at room temperature.[3,5]

2 Chemistry

Type: A pyrimidine nucleoside analogue that kills cells undergoing DNA synthesis. Its actions are specific for the S phase of the cell cycle.[6]

Molecular structure: 4-amino-1-β-D arabinofuranosylpyrimidin-2-(1H)-one.

Molecular weight: 243.2.

Formula: $H_9H_{13}N_3O_5$.

Solubility: Cytarabine is soluble 1 in 10 parts of water and is very slightly soluble in alcohol.[6]

3 Stability profile

3.1 *Physical and chemical stability*

The manufacturer states that ampoules of Alexan should be discarded within 24 hours of opening. Alexan and Alexan 100 are stable for at least 24 hours following dilution with 0.9% sodium chloride or 5% glucose infusion.[1] After reconstitution the manufacturers recommend that Cytosar should be discarded immediately and not stored.[2] A review of the literature reveals that cytarabine may be chemically stable for longer periods.

Effect of pH: In aqueous buffered solution, cytarabine is broken down by hydrolytic deamination to uracil arabinoside.[7] Cytarabine is most stable in the neutral pH region and has been calculated to retain 90% potency for six and a half months in 0.06 M phosphate buffer, pH 6.9, at 25°C. The rate of degradation of cytarabine in alkaline solution is approximately ten times as great as in acidic solution.[8]

In aqueous buffered solutions cytarabine (I) has been shown to undergo hydrolytic deamination to form the inactive nucleoside arabinosyluracil (II). In the acid to neutral region, pH 0–7.8, I undergoes deamination to yield II via an intermediate, which is formed in maximum yield at pH 2–3, and is not formed in detectable yields at pH 5.5–7.8. The observed rate constant for the loss of I in the absence of buffer catalysis was found to pass through a maximum value at approximately pH 2.8. The proposed mechanism for the acid-catalysed degradation of cytarabine in aqueous solution, from Notari *et al.*[8] is shown in Figure 1.

The loss of I in alkaline solution is not accompanied by a corresponding increase in the concentration of II. Instead the degradation of I in alkaline solution is characterized by a complete loss of UV absorption spectra. This suggests that the pyrimidine ring is hydrolysed. Figure 2 illustrates the probable reaction pathways for loss of I in alkaline solution proposed by Notari *et al.*[8] based on the work of Fox *et al.*[9]

Effect of light: At a concentration of 5 mg/ml in Elliots B and lactated Ringer's solution, cytarabine exhibited no change in concentration over seven days, under fluorescent light, at room temperature and at 30°C. In 0.9% sodium chloride no decomposition occurred after 24 hours, but a 3% loss at room temperature and a 6% loss at 30°C, was observed over seven days.[10] Benvenuto *et al.*[11] studied the stability of cytarabine (2 mg/ml) in glass and PVC bags (Viaflex, Baxter) in 5% glucose, stored at room temperature and exposed to normal daylight. Results showed that cytarabine was stable for 24 hours. These data indicate that photodegradation of cytarabine does not appear to be significant.

Effect of temperature: At a concentration of 800 mg/l one group suggest that cytarabine, in 0.9% sodium chloride, and 5% glucose, showed no significant loss of activity over a period of 13 days,[4] whereas at a concentration of 500 mg/l, in the same solvents another group indicate that cytarabine is stable for up to 48 hours.[5]

Gannon and Sesin[12] studied the stability of cytarabine in glass and polypropylene syringes at 25 and 5°C. Results showed that cytarabine (20 mg/ml) was more stable at 5°C in glass than plastic. The maximum decrease in potency over the seven day period of study in any of the containers was 2.9%. However, in that study cytarabine concentration was measured using ultraviolet spectrophotometric assay. High-performance liquid chromatographic (HPLC) assay is a more accurate, specific and reliable method of quantitation of drug concentration. Those authors indicated that further study was warranted using HPLC assay to confirm the overall stability of cytarabine.

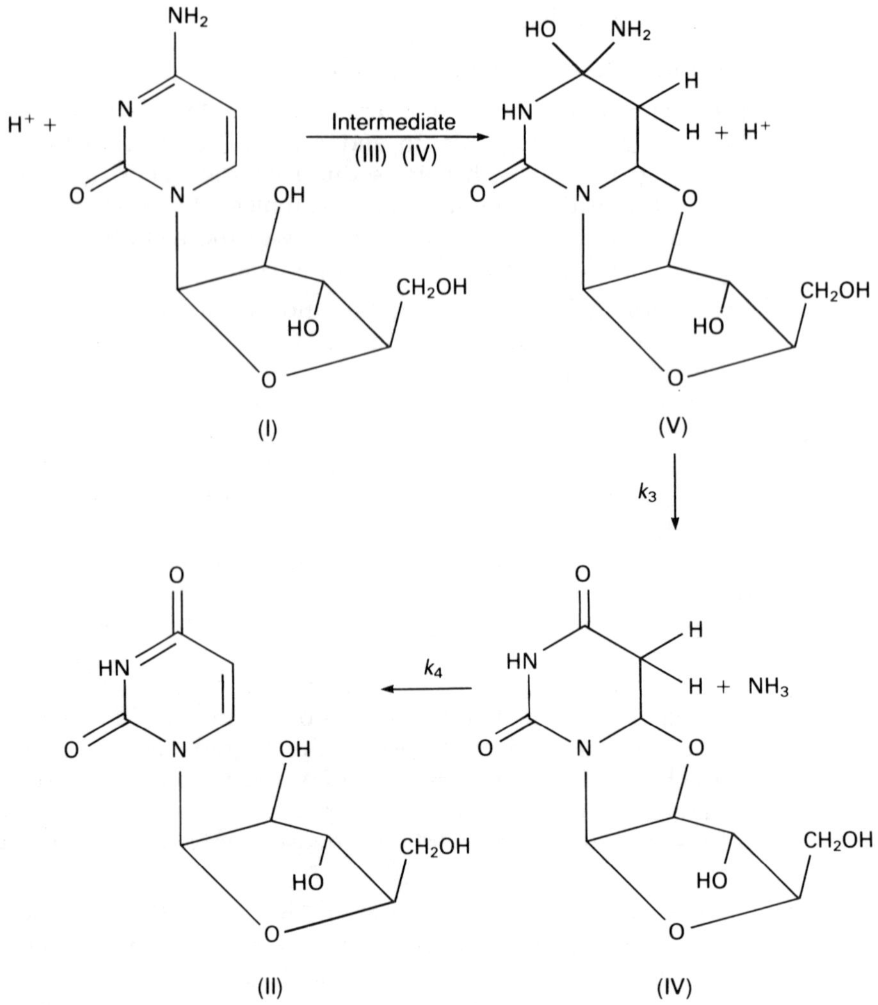

Figure 1: *Proposed mechanism for the acid-catalysed degradation of cytarabine*[8]

Munson *et al.*[13] studied the stability of cytarabine in 5% glucose and glucose/saline in glass and PVC containers, with added sodium bicarbonate, at 22 and 8°C. Stability in water for injections in plastic syringes (Pharmaseal) was also studied at 22, 8 and –10°C. Results showed that in plastic syringes cytarabine, 20 mg/ml and 50 mg/ml, was chemically stable for one week at all temperatures studied. Addition of sodium bicarbonate, 50 mEq/l, to solutions had no effect on the chemical stability of cytarabine for at least one week either at 22 or 8°C.[13] Weir and Ireland[14] observed that cytarabine (100 mg in 5 ml, 500 mg in 10 ml and 1 g in 20 ml) in polypropylene syringes was chemically stable for at least 30 days at 4 and 21°C.

In another study, cytarabine, 40 mg/ml and 80 mg/ml, reconstituted with water for injections, was shown to be stable in 5 ml (Becton-Dickinson, Plastipak) syringes for at least 15 days when stored at 4 and 25°C and for seven days at 37°C, however storage at –20°C resulted in precipitation.[5] Kirk *et al.*[15] noted that freezing cyclophosphamide in polypropylene syringes resulted in contraction of

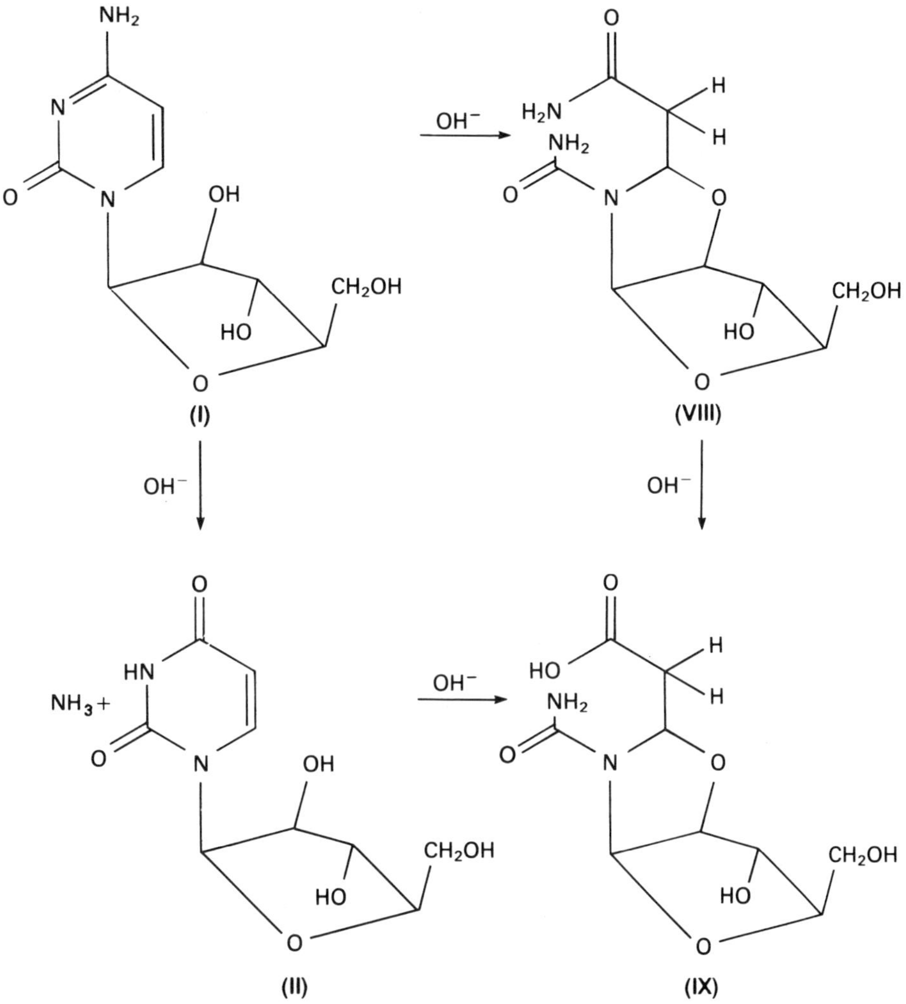

Figure 2: *Proposed mechanism for the degradation of cytarabine in alkaline solution*[8]

the plunger and seepage of the drugs past the barrel. Although this probably represents a negligible drug loss, the potential risk of microbial contamination is unacceptable. For this reason freezing of cytarabine in polypropylene syringes is not recommended.

Container compatibility: Cytarabine is compatible with glass, PVC and polypropylene.[12,13] Adsorption of cytarabine on to glass has not been documented. Adsorption on to PVC is negligible at concentrations greater than or equal to 0.5 mg/ml.[5] In clinical practice, when cytarabine is used at concentrations between 0.5 mg/ml and 20 mg/ml, adsorptive losses during storage and delivery are likely to be negligible.

Compatibility with other drugs: Cytarabine appears to be physically incompatible with methotrexate sodium,[4] 5-fluorouracil and heparin sodium.[16] The manufacturers recommend that no other drugs are mixed with cytarabine.

3.2 Stability in clinical practice

Cytarabine is compatible with glass, PVC and polypropylene.[12,13] Cytarabine appears to be chemically stable for at least one week, and possibly one month, when reconstituted with water for injections, 5% glucose and/or sodium chloride when stored at 4°C.[5,13] It is important to note that bacterially contaminated intrathecal injections could pose very grave risks and consequently such solutions should be administered as soon as possible after reconstitution.[17]

3.3 Stability in specialized delivery systems

Cytarabine (20 mg/ml) is stable in 0.9% sodium chloride in the CADD pump for 14 days at 4°C.[18] Cytarabine (25 and 1.25 mg/ml in 0.9% sodium chloride and 5% glucose) is stable in 80 ml EVA reservoirs (RES80 A, Celsa Laboratories, Chasseneuil, France) for 28 days at 4 and 22°C and for seven days at 35°C.[19] Cytarabine (1 mg/ml in Elliots B solution) showed no appreciable drug decomposition when stored for up to 15 days in an Infusaid Model 400 implantable pump at 37°C.[20]

4 Clinical use

Main indications: Induction of clinical remission and/or maintenance therapy in patients with acute myeloid leukaemia, acute non-lymphoblastic leukaemias, acute lymphoblastic leukaemias, blast crises of chronic myeloid leukaemia and diffuse histiocytic lymphomas (non-Hodgkin's lymphomas of high malignancy).[1]

Dosage for Alexan: For remission induction, the dose is 100–200 mg/m²/day or 3–6 mg/kg/day. When rapid IV injection is used administer 100 mg/m² twice daily. However, when continuous infusion is employed 100 mg/m² is given daily as a starting dose. For remission maintenance the following doses are recommended:

▼ leukaemias: 75–100 mg/m²/day or 1.5–3 mg/kg/day for five consecutive days once a month, or for one day each week
▼ CNS leukaemias: 10–30 mg/m² three times weekly, intrathecally.

Dosage for Alexan 100: Evidence suggests that the maximum tolerated dose is 3 g/m² every 12 hours for six days. High-dose Alexan is reserved for the treatment of resistant or refractory cases of leukaemia.[1]

Dosage for Cytosar: For continuous treatment a dose of 2 mg/kg/day for ten days, as a starting dose is given by bolus injection. If no antileukaemic effect and no toxicity is observed the dose may be increased to 4 mg/kg/day until a therapeutic response or toxicity occurs. Alternatively, 0.5–1.0 mg/kg/day may be given as an infusion of up to 24 hours duration. After ten days the dose may be increased to 2 mg/kg/day subject to toxicity. Treatment is continued until remission or toxicity occurs.[2]

For intermittent treatment an intravenous dosage of 3–5 mg/kg/day is administered on each of five consecutive days. After a two to nine day rest period a further course is given. Treatment is continued until a response or toxicity occurs.[2] Remissions which have been induced by cytarabine may be maintained by intravenous or subcutaneous injection of 1 mg/kg once or twice weekly.[2]

5 Preparation of injection

Reconstitution: The contents of the vial (Cytosar) may be reconstituted with water for injections, 0.9% sodium chloride or 5% glucose. When reconstituted with the accompanying diluent (water for injections) gentle shaking of the vial will produce a solution containing 20 mg/ml (100 mg vial) or 50 mg/ml (500 mg vial) of cytarabine.[2]

Bolus administration: Alexan is administered by intravenous, intrathecal, intramuscular and subcutaneous injection. For intrathecal injection it is recommended that 5–8 ml of cerebrospinal fluid (CSF) is drawn up, mixed with the injection solution in the syringe and slowly re-injected. Intramuscular and subcutaneous injections are usually used only in maintenance therapy.[1]

Subcutaneous injection of Alexan 100 is not recommended, at present, due to a lack of clinical data. Intrathecal or intramuscular use of Alexan 100 is contra-indicated due to slight hypertonicity of the formulation.[1] Cytarabine (Cytosar) may be administered by intravenous infusion or injection or by subcutaneous injection.[2]

Intravenous infusion: In high-dose schedules Alexan 100 should be administered by continuous intravenous infusion in either 0.9% sodium chloride or 5% glucose solution. To reduce toxicity the duration of the infusion should not be less than one hour.[1] Continuous infusions of cytarabine have ranged from eight to 12 hours to 120 to 168 hours.[1,21] Kreis *et al.*[22] investigated a low-dose infusion given over 21 days. Slevin *et al.*[23] compared intravenous and subcutaneous infusions. Results in that study showed that subcutaneous infusion was well tolerated without any local discomfort or excoriation. Continuous infusions (compared to bolus doses) show more pronounced gastrointestinal side-effects.[1]

Extravasation: Mildly irritant (*see* Chapter 6).

6 Destruction of drug or contaminated articles

Incineration: 1000°C.[1,3,5]

Chemical: Hydrochloric acid/24 hours.[1,3,5]

Contact with skin: Wash well with water, or soap and water. If the eyes are contaminated immediate irrigation with 0.9% sodium chloride should be carried out.[1,2,5]

References

1 *ABPI Data Sheet Compendium 1995–96* (1995) DataPharm Publications Ltd, London, pp. 1218–20.
2 *ABPI Data Sheet Compendium 1995–96* (1995) DataPharm Publications Ltd, London, pp. 1863–4.
3 David Bull Laboratories. Personal communication.
4 Pfizer Ltd. Personal communication.
5 Upjohn Ltd. Personal communication.
6 Anon. (1993) *The Extra Pharmacopoeia.* 30th edn. (JEF Reynolds ed.), Pharmaceutical Press, London, pp. 471–3.
7 Notari RE (1967) A mechanism for the hydrolytic deamination of cytosine arabinoside in aqueous buffer. *J. Pharm. Sci.* **56**, 804–9.
8 Notari RE *et al.* (1972) Arabinosylcytosine stability in aqueous solutions: pH profile and shelflife predictions. *J. Pharm. Sci.* **61**, 1189–96.
9 Fox JJ *et al.* (1966) Nucleosides XXXVI. Transformation of arabinopyrimidine nucleosides (1). *Tetrahedron Lett.* **40**, 4927–34.

10 Cradock JC *et al.* (1978) Evaluation of some pharmaceutical aspects of intrathecal methotrexate sodium, cytarabine and hydrocortisone sodium succinate. *Am. J. Hosp. Pharm.* **35**, 402–6.

11 Benvenuto JA *et al.* (1981) Stability and compatibility of antitumour agents in glass and plastic containers. *Am. J. Hosp. Pharm.* **38**, 1914–18.

12 Gannon PM, Sesin GP (1983) Stability of cytarabine following repackaging in plastic syringes and glass containers. *Am. J. Int. Ther. Clin. Nutr.* **10**, 11–16.

13 Munson JW *et al.* (1982) Cytosine arabinoside stability in intravenous admixtures with sodium bicarbonate and in plastic syringes. *Drug Intell. Clin. Pharm.* **16**, 765–7.

14 Weir PJ, Ireland DS (1990) Chemical stability of cytarabine and vinblastine injection. *Br. J. Phar. Pract.* **12**, 53–6.

15 Kirk B *et al.* (1984) Chemical stability of cyclophosphamide injection: The effect of low temperature storage and microwave thawing. *Br. J. Parenter. Ther.* **1**, 90–7.

16 Trissel LA (1994) *Handbook of Injectable Drugs.* 8th edn. American Society of Hospital Pharmacists, Bethesda, USA.

17 Sarubbi FA *et al.* (1978) Nosocomial meningitis and bacteraemia due to contaminated Amphotericin B. *J. Am. Med. Assoc.* **35**, 402–6.

18 Baxter Healthcare Ltd. Personal communication.

19 Rochard EB *et al.* (1992) Stability of fluorouracil, cytarabine, or doxorubicin hydrochloride in ethylene vinylacetate portable infusion-pump reservoirs. *Am. J. Hosp. Pharm.* **49**, 619–23.

20 Keller JH, Ensminger WD (1982) Stability of cancer chemotherapy agents in a totally implanted pump drug delivery system. *Am. J. Hosp. Pharm.* **39**, 1321–3.

21 Spriggs DR *et al.* (1985) Continuous infusion of high dose cytarabine a phase I and pharmacological study. *Cancer Res.* **45**, 3932–6.

22 Kreis W *et al.* (1985) Pharmacokinetics of low dose 1-β-D arabinofuranosylcytosine given by continuous IV infusion over 21 days. *Cancer Res.* **45**, 4698–501.

23 Slevin ML *et al.* (1983) Subcutaneous infusion of cytosine arabinoside – A practical alternative to intravenous infusion. *Cancer Chemother. Pharmacol.* **10**, 112–14.

Prepared by Jayne Wood

DACARBAZINE

1 General details

Approved name: Dacarbazine.

Proprietary name: DTIC-Dome.

Manufacturer or supplier: Bayer (UK) Ltd.

Presentation and formulation details: A colourless or ivory-coloured powder in amber glass vials containing 100 mg or 200 mg dacarbazine as the citrate salt. The 100 mg vial contains 100 mg citric acid and 50 mg mannitol. The 200 mg vial contains 100 mg citric acid and 37.5 mg mannitol. The vials do not contain any preservatives.

Storage and shelf-life of unopened container: Three years stored at 2–8°C and protected from light.

2 Chemistry

Type: Triazene, alkylating agent.

Molecular structure: 5-(3,3-dimethyl-1-1-triazeno) imidazole-4-carboxamide.

Molecular weight: 182.2.

Solubility: 1 mg/ml in water and 60 mg/ml in 10% citric acid.

3 Stability profile

3.1 Physical and chemical stability

Dacarbazine is relatively stable after reconstitution and further dilution, the reconstituted drug being stable for at least 72 hours if stored at 2 to 8°C.[1] After further dilution in 0.9% sodium chloride or 5% glucose, there is less than 1% degradation after 24 hours storage at 4°C, if protected from light.[1,2]

Dacarbazine is very sensitive to daylight.[3-6] Exposure to sunlight causes rapid degradation.[4] However, exposure to artificial (fluorescent) light or diffuse daylight is far less detrimental. Kirk,[4] in a detailed study, has shown that approximately 4–6% losses were recorded during administration under conditions of 'normal' room lighting (diffuse daylight and fluorescent light), whilst solutions exposed to strong daylight showed losses of the order of 12% in 90 minutes. Photodegradation is indicated by a colour change from yellow to pink.

Degradation pathways: The mechanisms described by Kirk[4] have been elucidated by Horton and Stevens.[7] The degradation route of dacarbazine (DTIC) in solutions of different pH either exposed to daylight or maintained in the dark are shown in Figure 1; the principal degradation products are 5-diazoimidazole-4-carboxamide (DIAZO-IC: II), 2-azahypoxanthine (III), a metastable intermediate carbene moiety (IV) and 4-carbamoylimidazolium-5-olate (V).

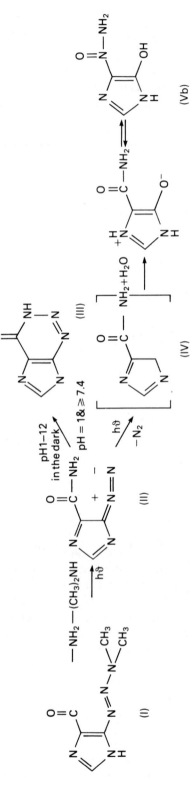

Figure 1: *The degradation route of dacarbazine (DTIC) in solutions of different pH, either exposed to daylight or maintained in the dark*

The primary degradation product of photolysis is 5-diazoimidazole-4-carboxamide (DIAZO-IC). Further degradation then occurs to conjugated polymers, which gives rise to the pink coloration. It has been suggested that these polymers are responsible for localized side-effects at the site of injection.[3] This has not been confirmed.

Container compatibility: Dacarbazine is compatible with PVC containers and administration sets[4,5,8] and with Amberset (Avon Medical Ltd).[4] There is no further information on the compatibility of dacarbazine with other delivery systems, such as plastic syringes.[5]

Compatibility with other drugs: Dacarbazine forms an immediate precipitate with hydrocortisone sodium succinate, but not with hydrocortisone sodium phosphate, nor with lignocaine 1 to 2%.[9] Dacarbazine is physically compatible with heparin in 5% glucose.[9] A white precipitate has been observed when tubing containing dacarbazine (25 mg/ml) was flushed with heparin (100 units/ml).[10] Physical compatibility of dacarbazine with the following drugs has been documented: bleomycin, carmustine, cyclophosphamide, cytarabine, dactinomycin, doxorubicin, methotrexate, 5-fluorouracil,[11] paclitaxel,[2,12] melphalan, fludarabine and vinorelbine.[2] No details of concentrations or conditions are, however, available.[11]

3.2 Stability in clinical practice

After reconstitution with water for injections, the resulting 10 mg/ml solution is stable in the vial for 72 hours at 4°C, protected from light, or eight hours at normal temperature.[1,2,5]

This solution can be diluted further in 5% glucose or 0.9% sodium chloride infusions and the resulting solution is stable for 24 hours at 2–8°C. Dacarbazine is very sensitive to UV light and all unnecessary exposure to daylight should be avoided. During administration, the infusion container should be protected from exposure to daylight. The use of a UV light-protecting administration set should be recommended for administration in daylight conditions.[4]

3.3 Stability in specialized delivery systems

No data available.

4 Clinical use

Type of cytotoxic: Alkylating agent.

Main indications: As a single agent in metastatic malignant melanoma, sarcoma, Hodgkin's disease. In combination with other drugs for carcinoma of colon, ovary, breast, lung, testicular teratoma and some solid tumours in children.

Dosage and administration: 2–4.5 mg/kg/day for ten days repeated every 28 days. 650–1450 mg/m² repeated every four to six weeks. 750–1200 mg/m² repeated every 21 days. 250 mg/m²/day for five days repeated every 21 days. Paediatric dosage is 200–250 mg/m²/day for five days, repeated every 28 days. (These are the regimens used at The Royal Marsden Hospital.)

5 Preparation of injection

Reconstitution: The 100 mg vial is reconstituted with 9.9 ml water for injections and the 200 mg vial with 19.7 ml water for injections, both giving a final concentration of 10 mg/ml and a pH of 3.0 and 4.0.

Bolus administration: Inject IV slowly over one to two minutes.

Intravenous infusion: Dilute in 125–250 ml 0.9% sodium chloride or 5% glucose. Infuse over 15–30 minutes.

Extravasation: Moderately damaging. No specific antidote.

6 Destruction of drug or contaminated articles

Incineration: 500°C.

Chemical: 10% sulphuric acid for 24 hours.

Contact with skin: Wash with water.

References

1 *ABPI Data Sheet Compendium 1995–96* (1995) DataPharm Publications Ltd, London, pp. 191–2.
2 Trissel LA (1994) *Handbook on Injectable Drugs,* 8th edn. American Society of Hospital Pharmacists, Bethesda, Maryland, USA.
3 Baird SM, Willoughby MLN (1978) Photodegradation of dacarbazine. *Lancet* **ii**, 681.
4 Kirk B (1987) The evaluation of a light-protecting giving set. *Intensive Ther. & Clin. Monitor.* **8,** 78–86.
5 Bayer (UK) Ltd. Personal communication. Unpublished data.
6 Institute of Cancer Research, London (1988) Personal communication. Unpublished data.
7 Horton JK, Stevens MFG (1981) A new light on the photodecomposition of the antitumour drug DTIC. *J. Pharm. Pharmacol.* **33**, 808–11.
8 Benvenuto JA *et al.* (1981) Stability and compatibility of antitumour agents in glass and plastic containers. *Am. J. Hosp. Pharm.* **38**, 1914–18.
9 Dorr RT (1979) Incompatibilities with parenteral anticancer drugs. *Am. J. Intravenous Ther.* **6**, 42–52.
10 Nelson RW *et al.* (1987) Visual incompatibility of decarbazine and heparin. *Am. J. Hosp. Pharm.* **44**, 2028.
11 Salamone FR, Muller RJ (1990) Intravenous admixture compatibility of cancer chemotherapeutic agents. *Hosp. Pharm.* **25**, 567–70.
12 Goldspiel BR (1994) Pharmaceutical issues: Preparation, administration, stability and compatibility with other medications. *Ann. Pharmacother.* **28**, S23–S26.

Prepared by Tim Root

DACTINOMYCIN

1 General details

Approved names: Dactinomycin, actinomycin D.

Proprietary name: Cosmegen Lyovac.

Manufacturer or supplier: Merck, Sharpe & Dohme Ltd.

Presentation and formulation details: Yellow lyophilized powder in vial, containing 500 μg dactinomycin. Each vial contains 20 mg mannitol.

Storage and shelf-life of unopened container: Five years when stored in cool, dry place protected from light.

2 Chemistry

Type: Antibiotic.

Molecular structure: Actinomycin (thr-val-pro-sar-meval).

Molecular weight: 1255.5.

Solubility: Soluble in water.

3 Stability profile

3.1 Physical and chemical stability

Degradation in aqueous solution is pH dependent. The pH of reconstituted drug is 5.5–7.0 and it is most stable between pH 5 and 7. One report indicates approximately 2–3% degradation in six days at 25°C at these pH values (30 μg/ml).[1] At pH 9.0, 80% loss was noted under the same conditions.[1]

Degradation pathways: Alkaline conditions – ring opening of the acridine-like centre.[2]

Physical: Degradation is reduced at lower temperatures. In aqueous solution, degradation at 2–6°C is negligible over a six day period.[1]

Container compatibility: Syringes – no information available. Dactinomycin is reported to be compatible with glass and PVC containers for infusions.[3]

No information is available on the compatibility of administration sets, but it should be noted that dactinomycin is compatible with PVC.[2]

There is evidence of dactinomycin binding to certain types of in-line filters.[4] For example, when 500 µg was diluted in 500 ml infusion fluid a total of 67 µg (approximately 13%) was subsequently bound to the in-line cellulose acetate membrane filter. Binding to polycarbonate filters has also been reported.[4] When dactinomycin, 500 µg/ml,[5] was injected through a 0.2 µm nylon filter (Utipor, Pall) 87% of the drug was delivered.[6]

Compatibility with other drugs and excipients: No further information available. Incompatible with benzyl alcohol and other preservatives; avoid preserved diluents for reconstitution.

3.2 Stability in clinical practice

The drug is relatively stable after reconstitution in water for injections and may be stored at 2–6°C for seven days. The drug is also reasonably stable after further dilution in 0.9% sodium chloride or 5% glucose showing less than 10% degradation after 24 hours at ambient temperature.[3] It should be protected from daylight during storage. The reconstituted drug is also stable when frozen.[7]

3.3 Stability in specialized delivery systems

No data available.

4 Clinical use

Type of cytotoxic: Cytotoxic antibiotic.

Main indications: Wilms' tumour; rhabdomyosarcoma; carcinoma of testis or uterus.

Dosage: Adults, up to 400–600 µg/m²/day, for up to five days; children, 15 µg/kg, for up to five days.

5 Preparation of injection

Reconstitution: Add 1.1 ml water for injections and shake to dissolve. The injection may be stored for up to seven days at 2–6°C.

Bolus administration: Inject into the tubing of a fast-running infusion of 5% glucose or 0.9% sodium chloride.

Intravenous infusion: Add to up to 500 ml 0.9% sodium chloride or 5% glucose. The infusion may be stored for 24 hours at 2–6°C.

Stability in plastic syringes: No information available.

Extravasation: Very damaging (*see* Chapter 6).

6 Destruction of drug or contaminated articles

Incineration: 1000°C.

Chemical: 5% trisodium phosphate, or 20% sodium hydroxide/24 hours.

Contact with skin: Wash in water or sodium phosphate solution.

References

1 Crevar GE, Slotnick IJ (1964) A note on the stability of actinomycin D. *J. Pharm. Pharmacol.* **16**, 429.

2 Johnson AW (1960) The chemistry of antinomycin D and related compounds. *Ann. New York Acad. Sci.* **89**, 336–41.

3 Benvenuto JA *et al.* (1981) Stability and compatibility of antitumor agents in glass and plastic containers. *Am. J. Hosp. Pharm.* **38**, 1914–18.

4 Rusmin S *et al.* (1977) Effect of inline filtration on the potency of drugs administered intravenously. *Am. J. Hosp. Pharm.* **34**, 1071–4.

5 *ABPI Data Sheet Compendium 1995–96* (1995) DataPharm Publications Ltd, London, pp. 991–3.

6 Ennis CE *et al.* (1983) *In vitro* study of inline filtration of medication commonly administered to paediatric patients. *J. Parenter. Enteral Nutr.* **7**, 156–8.

7 Bosanquet AG (1986) Stability of solutions of antineoplastic agents during preparation and storage for *in vitro* assays II. Assay methods, adriamycin and other antitumour antibiotics. *Cancer Chemother. Pharmacol.* **17**, 1–10.

Prepared by Michael Allwood

DAUNORUBICIN

1 General details

Approved name: Daunorubicin.

Proprietary name: Cerubidin.

Manufacturer or supplier: Rhône-Poulenc Rorer UK Ltd.

Presentation and formulation details: Sterile, pyrogen-free, orange-red, microcrystalline powder in vials of 20 mg of daunorubicin as the hydrochloride, with mannitol as a stabilizing agent.[1]

Storage and shelf-life of unopened container: Three years, stored at room temperature protected from sunlight.[1]

2 Chemistry

Type: A cytotoxic antibiotic consisting of an amino sugar moiety linked through a glycosidic bond to the C7 of a tetracyclic aglycone, daunosamine. It forms a stable complex with DNA and interferes with the synthesis of nucleic acids. The cytotoxic effects of daunorubicin are most marked on cells in the S phase.[2]

Molecular structure: (1S, 3S)-3-acetyl-1,2,3,4,6,11-hexahydro-3,5,12-trihydroxy-10-methoxy-6,11-dioxonaphthacen-1-yl-3-amino-2,3,6-trideoxy-α-L-lyxopyranoside hydrochloride.

Molecular weight: 564.00.

Formula: $C_{27}H_{29}NO_{10}HCl$.

Solubility: Daunorubicin is soluble in water for injections, 5% glucose and 0.9% sodium chloride.[2]

3 Stability profile

3.1 Physical and chemical stability

The manufacturer states that the reconstitution solution is stable for up to 24 hours, at 2–8°C, when protected from strong daylight. The literature reveals that daunorubicin may be chemically stable for longer periods although few data have been published.[3–5]

The stability of daunorubicin depends on a number of factors. Degradation in aqueous solution is pH-dependent. Daunorubicin is also light-sensitive and adsorbs on to glass and certain plastics.

Effect of pH: Daunorubicin becomes progressively more stable as the pH of the drug fluid admixture becomes more acidic (pH 7.4–4.5).[4] Maximum stability is observed at approximately pH 5.[6] Decomposition of daunorubicin has been studied by Beijnen *et al.*[7,8] Acidic hydrolysis of daunorubicin (pH below 3.5), which is shown in Figure 1, yields a red-coloured, water-insoluble aglycone, daunorúbicinone and a water-soluble amino sugar, daunosamine.

At pH values above 3.5, two major degradation products are formed, both of which are aglycones; 7,8-dehydro-9,10-desacetyldaunorubicinone and 7,8-9,10-bisanhydrodaunorubicinone.[6,8] The proposed mechanism for this degradation is shown in Figure 2.

On addition to strongly alkaline solution, a colour change from red to a deep blue-purple is observed and rapid degradation of daunorubicin occurs. Analysis of the decomposition of daunorubicin at pH 8.0 showed formation of seven possible degradation products, the three major ones were: 7,8–9,10 bisanhydro-daunorubicinone (I), 7-deoxydaunorubicinone (II) and 7,8,-dehydro-9,10-desacetyl-daunorubicinone (III). The structures of these products are shown in Figure 3. Low yields of the remaining four compounds prevented full characterization and structure elucidation.[9]

Effect of light: Results from a study in which the rates of photodegradation of doxorubicin, daunorubicin and epirubicin were compared, indicated that the rate of photodegradation of all three analogues was similar.[10] This suggests that the rate of photodegradation of daunorubicin may be significant at concentrations less than 100 µg/ml if solutions are exposed to light for sufficient time. However, at higher concentrations, such as those used for cancer chemotherapy, (at least 500 µg/ml) no special precautions appear to be necessary to protect freshly prepared solutions of daunorubicin from light.[10]

Effect of temperature: Poochikian *et al.*[4] observed that daunorubicin (20 µg/ml) was stable for 72 hours in 5% glucose and 0.9% sodium chloride in glass containers at 21°C. In that study solutions were not protected from light and, at the low concentrations used, photodegradation may represent a considerable proportion of the overall degradation. Conversely, in a well-controlled study, where the solutions were protected from light, Beijnen *et al.*[5] reported that daunorubicin was stable, in polypropylene tubes, for 28 days in 5% glucose (pH 4.7), 3.3% glucose with 0.3% sodium chloride (pH 4.4) and 0.9% sodium chloride (pH 7.0) at 25°C.[5] Daunorubicin has also been reported to be stable for seven days at room temperature.[3] Wood *et al.*[11] observed that daunorubicin was stable in 5% glucose (pH 4.36) and 0.9% sodium chloride (pH 5.20 and 6.47) in PVC minibags for at least 43 days at 25, 4 and –20°C. Repeated freezing and thawing of solutions stored at –20°C did not cause degradation. In the same study daunorubicin was also reported to be stable for at least 43 days when reconstituted with water for injections and stored in polypropylene syringes at 4°C. Dine *et al.*[12] reported that daunorubicin (16 µg/ml in 5% glucose and 0.9% sodium chloride) was stable in PVC infusion bags (Macopharma Laboratories) for seven days at 4°C when protected from light.

Container compatibility: Daunorubicin is compatible with polypropylene, PVC and glass.[11,13] Daunorubicin adsorbs on to glass but not on to siliconized glass or polypropylene.[14] In clinical practice, when daunorubicin is used at concentrations of at least 500 µg/ml, adsorptive losses during storage and delivery are negligible.[11,13]

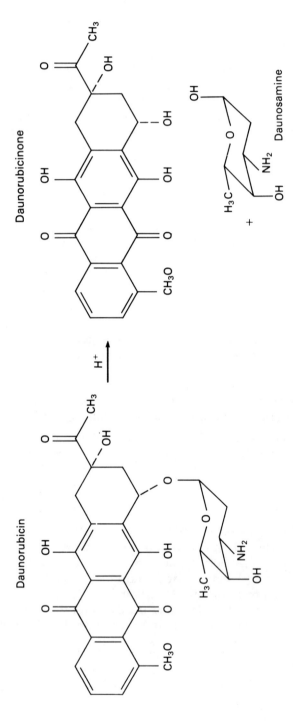

Figure 1: *Degradation pathway of daunorubicin in acidic solution*

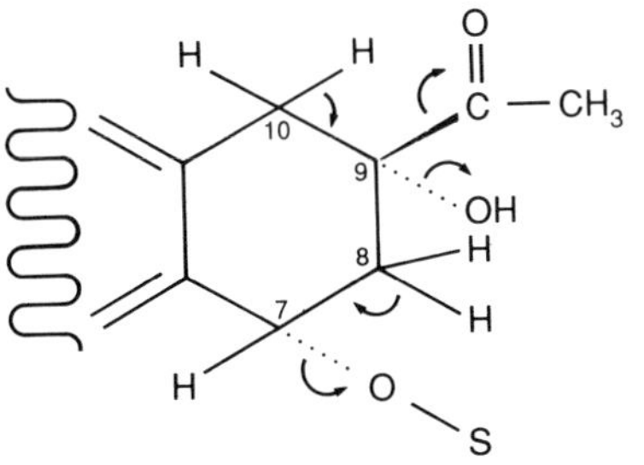

Figure 2: *Degradation scheme of daunorubicin (pH above 4). S refers to the daunosamine sugar moiety*[6]

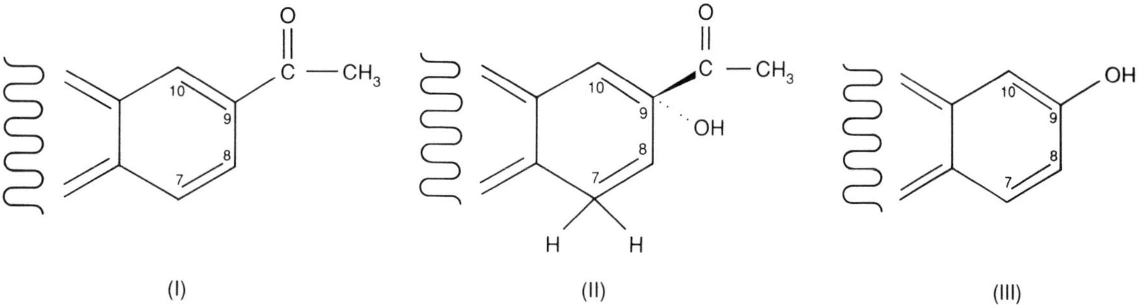

(I)   (II)   (III)

Figure 3: *Structure of the major degradation products of daunorubicin at pH 8*[9]

Compatibility with other drugs: Daunorubicin is incompatible with dexamethasone sodium phosphate and heparin sodium.[1] The manufacturer recommends that no other drugs are mixed with daunorubicin.

3.2 Stability in clinical practice

Daunorubicin is compatible with polypropylene, PVC and glass.[11,13] Daunorubicin appears to be chemically stable for at least 28 days in PVC minibags (100 µg/ml) in 5% glucose and 0.9% sodium chloride at 4°C and –20°C and for at least 28 days in polypropylene syringes (2 mg/ml) at 4°C.[11]

3.3 Stability in specialized delivery systems

No data available.

4 Clinical use

Main indications: In the treatment of acute leukaemia daunorubicin is particularly effective in inducing remissions in acute myelogenous and lymphocytic leukaemias.[1] Daunorubicin should not be used in patients recently exposed to, or with existing chicken pox or herpes zoster.[1]

Dosage and administration:

▼ remission induction (adults): For remission induction a dose of 40–60 mg/m² on alternate days is given for a course of up to three injections
▼ acute myelogenous leukaemia (adults): The recommended dose is 45 mg/m²/day

▼ acute lymphoblastic leukaemia (adults): The recommended dose is 45 mg/m²/day
▼ children: In children over two years the dose is the same as for adults. In children under two years, or less than 0.5 m² surface area, the dose is 1 mg/kg/day
▼ elderly: Daunorubicin should be used with care in patients with inadequate bone marrow reserves due to old age. A reduction of up to 50% of the dosage is recommended.

The number of injections required varies from patient to patient and must be determined in each case by response and tolerance. Dosage should be reduced in patients with impaired hepatic or renal function. A 25% reduction is recommended in patients with serum bilirubin concentrations between 1.2 and 3 mg/100 ml and a 50% reduction in patients with serum bilirubin levels above 3 mg/100 ml, or creatinine levels above 265 μmol/l.

When administered with other cytotoxic agents, with overlapping toxicity, dosage should be suitably reduced. A cumulative dose of 600 mg/m² in adults, 300 mg/m² in children over two years or 10 mg/kg in children under two years should not be exceeded as above this level the risk of irreversible congestive cardiac failure increases greatly.[1] The cumulative dose should be limited to 400 mg/m² when radiation to the mediastinum has been administered previously.[1] Cardiotoxicity may be more frequent in children and the elderly.

5 Preparation of injection

Reconstitution: The contents of the 20 mg vial are reconstituted with 4 ml of water for injections. After addition of the diluent and gentle shaking the contents of the vial will dissolve to produce a solution of 5 mg/ml.[1]

Bolus administration: Administration is only by the intravenous route. The manufacturer recommends that the calculated dose is further diluted with 0.9% sodium chloride to give a final concentration of 1 mg/ml. This solution should be injected, over a period of 20 minutes, into the side arm of a freely-running intravenous infusion of 0.9% sodium chloride. This technique minimizes the risk of thrombosis or perivenous extravasation, which can lead to severe cellulitis or vesication.[1]

Intravenous infusion: Although daunorubicin has been used as a continuous infusion in a phase I trial in previously treated patients with leukaemia, no phase II evaluation was conducted because of somewhat limited antileukaemic activity in patients who had previously received other anthracycline therapy.[15] In a study where fractionated daunorubicin was given to 16 patients with acute myeloid leukaemia a good response rate was obtained, coupled with a low incidence of side-effects. In addition, no significant cardiotoxicity was observed despite total doses of up to 1363 mg/m² of daunorubicin.[16]

Extravasation: Potent vesicant (*see* Chapter 6).

6 Destruction of drug or contaminated articles

Incineration: 700°C.[17]

Chemical: 10% sodium hypochlorite (1% available chlorine)/24 hours.[1]

Contact with skin: Wash well with water, soap and water, or sodium bicarbonate solution. If the eyes are contaminated immediate irrigation with 0.9% sodium chloride should be carried out.[1]

References

1 Daunorubicin: *Package Insert 1994* (1995) Rhône-Poulenc Rorer UK Ltd.

2 Anon. (1994) *The Extra Pharmacopoeia.* 30th edn. (JEF Reynolds ed.), Pharmaceutical Press, London, 474–5.

3 Trissel LA (1994) *Handbook of Injectable Drugs*, 8th edn, American Society of Hospital Pharmacists, Bethesda, USA.

4 Poochikian GK *et al.* (1981) Stability of anthracycline antitumour agents in four infusion fluids. *Am. J. Hosp. Pharm.* **38**, 483–6.

5 Beijnen JH *et al.* (1985) Stability of anthracycline antitumour agents in infusion fluids. *J. Parenter. Sci. Technol.* **39**, 220–2.

6 Beijnen JH *et al.* (1986) Aspects of the degradation kinetics of daunorubicin in aqueous solution. *Int. J. Pharm.* **31**, 75–82.

7 Beijnen JH *et al.* (1985) Aspects of the chemical stability of daunorubicin and seven other anthracyclines in acidic solution. *Pharm. Weekbl. (Sci. Edn),* **7**, 109–16.

8 Beijnen JH *et al.* (1986) Aspects of the degradation kinetics of doxorubicin in aqueous solution. *Int. J. Pharm.* **32**, 123–31.

9 Beijnen JH *et al.* (1987) Structure elucidation and characterization of daunorubicin degradation products. *Int. J. Pharm.* **34**, 247–57.

10 Wood MJ *et al.* (1990) Photodegradation of doxorubicin, daunorubicin and epirubicin measured by high-performance liquid chromatography. *J. Clin. Pharm. Ther.* **15**, 291–300.

11 Wood MJ *et al.* (1990) Stability of doxorubicin, daunorubicin and epirubicin in plastic syringes and minibags. *J. Clin. Pharm. Ther.* **15**, 279–89.

12 Dine T *et al.* (1992) Stability and compatibility of four anthracyclines: doxorubicin, daunorubicin, epirubicin and pirarubicin with PVC infusion bags. *Pharm.Weekbl. (Sci. Edn)* **14**, 365–9.

13 Wood MJ (1989) MPhil Thesis, University of Aston, Birmingham, UK.

14 Bosanquet AG (1986) Stability of solutions of antineoplastic agents during preparation and storage for *in vitro* assays. II. Assay methods, adriamycin and the other antitumour antibiotics. *Cancer Chemother. Pharmacol.* **17**, 1–10.

15 Legha SS *et al.* (1987) Anthracyclines: In: (JJ Lokich ed.), *Cancer Chemotherapy by Infusion*, MTP Press Ltd, Lancaster.

16 Donohue SM, Boughton BJ (1989) Fractionated anthracycline therapy in acute myeloblastic leukaemia in adults. *Cancer Chemother. Pharmacol.* **23**, 401–2.

17 Rhône-Poulenc Rorer UK Ltd. Personal communication.

Prepared by Jayne Wood

DAUNORUBICIN LIPOSOMAL

1 General details

Approved name: Liposomal daunorubicin.

Proprietary/other names: Daunoxome.

Manufacturer or supplier: Nexstar Ltd.

Presentation and formulation details: Daunoxome is a translucent, red emulsion in single dose vials. Each vial contains 50 mg of daunorubicin encapsulated in liposomes composed of cholesterol (180 mg) and the phospholipid distearoyl-phosphatidylcholine (DSPC) (15 mg). The average diameter of the liposomes is 45 nm. The lipid to drug ratio is 18 : 1 (total lipid : daunorubicin base), equivalent to a 10 : 5 : 1 molar composition of DSPC : cholesterol : daunorubicin. The liposomes encapsulating daunorubicin are suspended as a medium of 2.125 mg sucrose, 94 mg glycine with 7 mg calcium chloride dehydrate.[1] The liposome emulsion is red and clear to slightly opalescent in appearance.

Storage and shelf-life of unopened container: Store at 2–8°C. Do not freeze. Protect from light.

2 Chemistry

Type: Cytotoxic anthracycline antibiotic.

Molecular structure: As for daunorubicin, but enclosed in a carrier system consisting of a unilamellar liposome.

Molecular formula: See monograph for daunorubicin.

Molecular weight: A particle suspension.

pH of suspension: 4.5–6.5.

3 Stability profile

3.1 Physical and chemical stability

Undiluted liposomal daunorubicin stability studies are ongoing. Solutions diluted in 5% glucose are physically stable for up to six hours.[1]

Compatibility with other drugs: No interaction with other drugs has been recorded. Daunorubicin liposomal has been safely administered with zidovudine, dideoxy-cytidine and GCSF. The product is reported to be incompatible with heparin or docamethasome.[1]

3.2 Stability in clinical practice

The manufacturer indicates that the diluted injection should be administered within six hours of preparation.[1] Daunoxome must not be diluted using 0.9% sodium chloride or any other electrolyte solution.[1]

3.3 Stability in specialized delivery systems.

No data available.

4 Clinical use

Daunoxome is a liposomal preparation formulated to maximize the selectivity of daunorubicin for solid tumours *in situ*.

While in the circulation the daunoxome formulation helps to protect the entrapped daunorubicin from chemical and enzymatic degradation, minimizes protein binding and generally decreases uptake by normal (non-reticuloendothelial system) tissues. The specific mechanism by which daunoxome is able to deliver daunorubicin in solid tumours *in situ* is not known. However, it is believed to be a function of increased permeability of the tumour neovasculature to particulates in the size range of daunoxome. Thus, by decreasing non-specific binding to normal tissues and plasma proteins, selective binding to normal tissues and plasma proteins and selective extravasation in the tumour; neovasculature pharmacokinetics are favourably shifted towards an accumulation of daunoxome in tumour tissue. Once within the tumour environment, daunoxome vesicles enter the tumour cells intact. Daunorubicin is then released over time directly into the cells, where it is able to exert its antineoplastic activity.

Main indications: Advanced HIV-associated Kaposi's, failed on conventional chemotherapy – clinical trials phase IV are currently underway.

Dosage and administration: The recommended dose is 40 mg/m^2 every two weeks.[1] Dilute in 5% glucose to a concentration in the range of 0.2–1 mg daunorubicin/ml and administer intravenously over 30–60 minutes.

Paediatrics and use in the elderly: Safe use in these two groups has not been established.

5 Preparation of injection

Reconstitution: Should be diluted in 5% glucose to a concentration of 0.2 per mg daunorubicin/ml.

Intravenous infusion: Administer by intravenous injection or infusion for 30–60 minutes. Do not use 0.9% sodium chloride or any other infusion. An in-line filter is not recommended for the intravenous infusion of daunoxome. However, if such a filter is used, the mean pore diameter of the filter should not be less than 5 μm.[2]

Extravasation: In contrast to conventional daunorubicin, no local tissue necrosis has been observed with daunoxome.[1]

6 Destruction of drug or contaminated articles

Incineration: No specific information available.

Chemical: No specific information available.

Contact with skin: No specific information available.

Reference

1 *Daunoxome Data Sheet* (1995) Nexstar Limited, Cambridge, 24 August.
2 Personal communication (1995), Vestar Ltd.

Prepared by Yaacov Cass

DOCETAXEL

1 General details

Approved name: Taxotere.

Proprietary name: Docetaxel.

Synonyms: RP 56976, NSC 628503.

Marketing authorization holder: Rhône-Poulenc Rorer SA, 20 Avenue Raymond Aron, 92165, Antony Cedex, France.

Manufacturer or supplier: Rhône-Poulenc Rorer UK Ltd.

Presentation and formulation details: Taxotere concentrate for infusion is a clear viscous, yellow to brown-yellow solution, containing 40 mg/ml docetaxel (anhydrous) and 1040 mg polysorbate 80. The solvent for docetaxel is a 13% w/w solution of ethanol in water.[1] Taxotere is also supplied as single-dose vials containing 20 or 80 mg docetaxel anhydrous. Each box contains one taxotere concentrate vial (20 mg: green cap, or 80 mg: red cap) and one corresponding 'solvent for taxotere' vial (transparent cap), in a blister pack.[1]

Storage and shelf-life of unopened container: Docetaxel vials should be stored in the refrigerator and protected from bright light. The shelf-life under these conditions is 15 months for docetaxel 80 mg and 12 months for docetaxel 20 mg.[1]

2 Chemistry

Type: Taxoid obtained by semisynthesis from a non-cytotoxic precursor, 10-deacetyl-baccatin III extracted from the needles of the European Yew tree, *Taxus baccata*.

Mechanism of action: Promotes assembly of microtubules (necessary for mitosis) and prevents their disassembly, 'freezing' the cell skeleton leading to inhibition of mitosis and cell death.

Molecular structure: (2R,3S)-N-carboxy-3-phenylisoserine, N-tert-butylester, 13-ester with 5β, 20 epoxy-1,2α,4,7β,10β,13α-hexahydroxytax-11-en-9-one 4-acetate 2 benzoate, tihydrate. The molecular structure of docetaxel differs from paclitaxel in two ways: a hydroxy group replaces an acetyl group on the 10-position of the baccatin III and an $OC(CH_3)_3$ moiety replaces a benzamide phenyl group in the 3' position on the C13 side chain.

Molecular weight: 807.9.

Solubility: Limited in water, but soluble in polysorbate 80.

3 Stability profile

3.1 Physical and chemical stability

Unopened docetaxel concentrate is stable for 15 months (80 mg presentation) or 12 months (20 mg presentation) when refrigerated. Docetaxel premix solution is stable for eight hours refrigerated, or at room temperature. Docetaxel infusion solution should be used as soon as possible.[1,2]

Incompatibilities: None known.

3.2 Stability in clinical practice

No data available.

3.3 Stability in specialized delivery systems

No data available.

4 Clinical use

Main indications: Monotherapy of advanced or metastatic breast cancer. Patients who are resistant to, or have recurrent disease after, a cytotoxic therapy or who have relapsed during an adjuvant cytotoxic therapy. The cytotoxic therapy should have included an anthracycline.

Recommended dose: 100 mg/m² as a one hour intravenous infusion every three weeks.

Dosage reductions: Reduce to 75 mg/m² in cases of mild liver impairment, febrile neutropenia, neutrophils less than 500/mm³ for more than one week, severe or cumulative cutaneous reactions or severe peripheral neuropathy. If symptoms persist, reduce to 55 mg/m², or discontinue.

Contraindications: Increased serum bilirubin and/or ALT and AST values >3.5 times the ULN with alkaline phosphatase >6 times ULN.

Other tumour types: Clinical trials are ongoing in NSCLC, ovarian, head and neck and other tumour types, where docetaxel has shown promising activity in pre-clinical and Phase I trials.

Availability: Docetaxel was the first anticancer drug to be approved under the new EMEA concertation procedure and is licensed for breast cancer in 12 European countries, and in breast cancer and NSCLC in Australia, Mexico, Canada, South Africa and Uruguay with approvals pending in the US and Japan.

5 Preparation of injection

Docetaxel 80 mg: The labelled strength is 80 mg docetaxel per vial and the labelled volume is 2 ml. Practically, docetaxel 80 mg vials contain 2.3 ml of the 40 mg/ml solution, equivalent to 94.4 mg docetaxel. The solvent vial has a labelled volume of 6 ml but has been correspondingly overfilled to contain 7.33 ml ± 5%. These overfill volumes have been established and validated during the development of docetaxel to compensate for liquid loss during preparation of the premix solution due to foaming, adhesion to the walls of the vial and 'dead volumes'. This overfill ensures that there is a minimum extractable premix volume of 8 ml containing 10 mg/ml docetaxel.

Docetaxel 20 mg: The labelled strength is 20 mg docetaxel per vial and the labelled volume is 0.5 ml. Practically, docetaxel 20 mg vials contain 0.59 ml of the 40 mg/ml solution, equivalent to 23.6 mg docetaxel. The solvent vial has a labelled volume of 1.5 ml but has been correspondingly overfilled to contain 1.83 ml ± 5%. This overfill ensures that there is a minimum extractable premix volume of 2 ml containing 10 mg/ml docetaxel.[1,2]

Preparation of premix solution: Remove the required number of boxes containing docetaxel concentrate vials and their corresponding solvent vials from the refrigerator and allow to stand for five minutes at room temperature. Using a syringe fitted with a needle, aseptically withdraw the entire contents of the solvent vial and inject it into the corresponding docetaxel concentrate vial. Remove the syringe and needle and shake the mixture manually for 15 seconds. Allow to stand for five minutes at room temperature, and then check that the solution is homogeneous and clear. Foaming is common due to the polysorbate 80 and may persist for up to five minutes. The premix solution is stable for eight hours in the refrigerator or at room temperature.[2]

Preparation of infusion solution: More than one premix vial may be necessary to obtain the required dose for the patient. Based on the required dose expressed in mg; use graduated syringes fitted with a needle to withdraw the necessary premix volume containing 10 mg/ml docetaxel (e.g. a dose of 140 mg would require 14 ml premix solution). Inject the premix solution into a standard PVC infusion bag containing 250 ml of 5% glucose or 0.9% sodium chloride solution. If a dose greater than 240 mg of docetaxel is required, use a larger volume of the infusion vehicle so that a concentration of 0.9% mg/ml docetaxel is not exceeded.[2]

Administration: The docetaxel infusion solution should be administered intravenously as soon as possible after preparation by a one-hour infusion at room temperature and normal lighting conditions. There is no need for special giving sets bottles or in-line filters.

Premedication: The premedication regimen is simple; 8 mg oral corticosteroid given twice-daily starting the day before docetaxel infusion for a total of five days.

Extravasation: Vesicant (*see* Chapter 6).

6 Destruction of drug or contaminated articles

Incineration: 1000°C.

Chemical: None recommended. All other waste, including contaminated packaging or cleaning materials and protective gloves must be placed with clinical waste for incineration.

Contact with skin: Wash with copious amounts of water.

Contact with eyes: Irrigate eye with copious amounts of water or saline, seek ophthalmic opinion.

References

1 Summary of Product Characteristics, July 1995.
2 Docetaxel Data Sheet – Rhône-Poulenc Rorer. 1995.

Prepared by Andrew Stanley and Yaacov Cass

DOXORUBICIN

1 General details

Approved name: Doxorubicin.

Proprietary names: Doxorubicin rapid dissolution, doxorubicin solution for injection.

Manufacturer or supplier: Pharmacia and Upjohn Ltd.

Presentation and formulation details:

▼ doxorubicin rapid dissolution: sterile, pyrogen-free, orange-red, freeze-dried powder in vials containing 10 mg and 50 mg doxorubicin hydrochloride with lactose and hydroxybenzoate. The inclusion of hydroxybenzoate 0.02% (which is a sub-preservative concentration) is to prevent gel formation, which used to occur occasionally on reconstitution of adriamycin. Adriamycin has been replaced by doxorubicin rapid dissolution.[1]
▼ doxorubicin solution for injection: sterile, red, mobile solution in vials of 10 mg and 50 mg, each containing doxorubicin hydrochloride as a 2 mg/ml solution in 0.9% sodium chloride injection.[2] The solution is adjusted to pH 3 with 0.5 M hydrochloric acid.[2]

Storage and shelf-life of unopened container:

▼ doxorubicin rapid dissolution: four years, at room temperature protected from light.[3]
▼ doxorubicin solution for injection: stored in the refrigerator (2–8°C). Two years at 2–8°C. Once removed from the refrigerator the shelf-life is 48 hours.[3]

2 Chemistry

Type: A cytotoxic antibiotic consisting of an amino sugar, daunosamine, linked through a glycosidic bond to the C7 of a tetracyclic aglycone, doxorubicinone. Doxorubicin may act by forming a stable complex with DNA and interfering with the synthesis of nucleic acids. It is most active against cells in the S phase.[4]

Molecular weight: 580.0.

Formula: $C_{27}H_{29}NO_{11}HCl$.

Solubility: Doxorubicin is soluble in water for injections, 5% glucose and 0.9% sodium chloride.[4]

3 Stability profile

3.1 Physical and chemical stability

The manufacturer states that reconstituted solutions of doxorubicin rapid dissolution are chemically stable for up to 48 hours at room temperature in normal artificial light.[1] Doxorubicin solution for injection, which has a pH of 3, is stable for 18 months at 2–8°C and for one month at room temperature.[3] A review of the literature reveals that doxorubicin appears to be chemically stable for longer periods[5–12] but data are limited and contradictory and require critical assessment.

Molecular structure: (1S,3S)-3-glycoloyl-1,2,3,4,6,11-hexahydro-3,5,12-trihydroxy-10-methoxy-6,11-dioxonaphthacen-1-yl 3-amino-2,3,6-trideoxy-α-L-lyxopyranoside hydrochloride.

The stability of doxorubicin depends on a number of factors, the most important of which are temperature, pH and the type of solvent used for reconstitution.[13,14] Doxorubicin is also light-sensitive and adsorbs on to glass and certain plastics.

Effect of pH: Doxorubicin becomes more stable as the pH of the drug infusion fluid admixture becomes more acidic (pH 7.4–4.5).[6] Maximum stability is observed at about pH 4.[15]

Decomposition in acidic solution has been studied by several authors.[16,17] Acidic hydrolysis of doxorubicin (pH below 4), which is shown in Figure 1, yields a red-coloured, water-insoluble aglycone, doxorubicinone and a water-soluble amino sugar, daunosamine.

On addition of doxorubicin to strongly alkaline solution, a colour change from red to deep blue-purple is observed and rapid degradation of doxorubicin occurs. Abdeen *et al.*[18] acidified and extracted a solution of doxorubicin in 2 M sodium hydroxide and isolated at least five components which were not identified. Analysis of degradation mixtures at pH 8.0 by Beijnen *et al.*[15] showed one major degradation product, 7,8-dehydro-9,10-desacetyldaunorubicinone. The proposed scheme for this conversion is shown in Figure 2.

Effect of light: The large differences in stability which have been reported by different groups for virtually identical experiments[6,19] may be partially explained by poor control of photodegradation. Photodegradation of doxorubicin may be substantial at concentrations below 100 μg/ml, if solutions are exposed to light for sufficient time.[19,20] However, at higher concentrations, such as those used for cancer chemotherapy (at least 500 μg/ml), no special precautions appear to be necessary to protect freshly prepared solutions of doxorubicin from light.[19,20]

Effect of temperature: In a well-controlled study Beijnen *et al.*[9] reported that doxorubicin was stable in 5% glucose (pH 4.7) and 3.3% glucose with 0.3% sodium chloride (pH 4.4), in polypropylene tubes, for 28 days at 25°C in the dark. However, in 0.9% sodium chloride (pH 7.0) significant degradation occurred after six days at the same temperature.

Wood *et al.*[21] reported that doxorubicin was stable in 0.9% sodium chloride (pH 6.47) in PVC minibags stored in the dark for 20 days at 25°C. In 5% glucose (pH 4.36) and 0.9% sodium chloride (pH 5.20 and pH 6.47) doxorubicin was stable in PVC minibags for at least 43 days at 4°C. In the same study, doxorubicin was also observed to be stable when reconstituted with water for injections and stored in polypropylene syringes at 4°C.[21]

Dine *et al.*[22] reported that doxorubicin (16 μg/ml in 5% glucose and 0.9% sodium chloride) was stable in PVC infusion bags (Macopharma Laboratories)

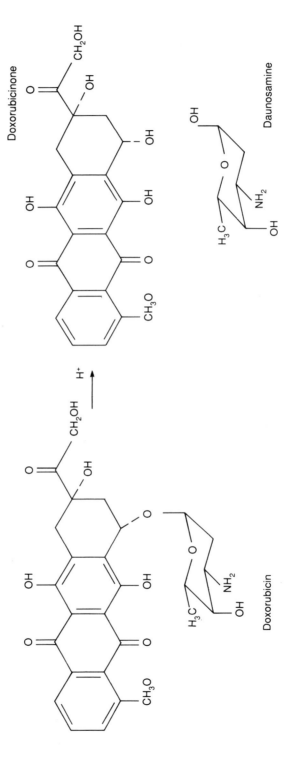

Figure 1: *Degradation pathway of doxorubicin in acidic solution*

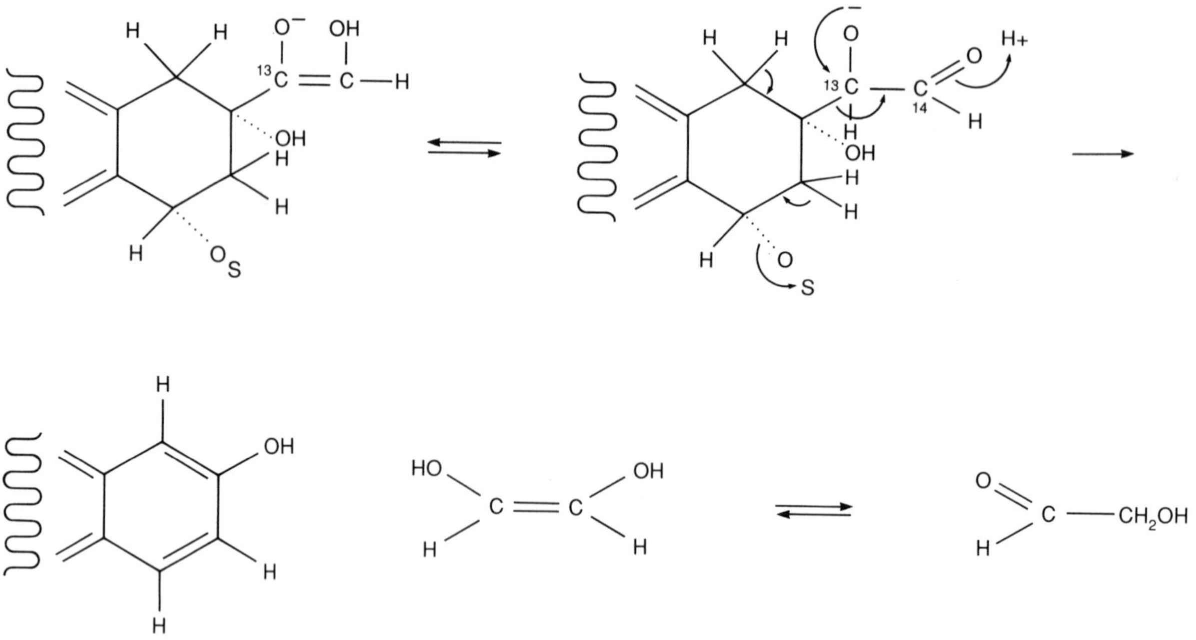

Figure 2: *Proposed degradation scheme for the conversion of doxorubicin to 7,8-dehydro-9,10-desacetyldaunorubicinone.[15] S refers to the daunosamine moiety*

for seven days at 4°C when protected from light. Walker *et al.*[23] reported that doxorubicin 2 mg/ml in 0.9% sodium chloride in glass vials and plastic syringes (Monoject and Terumo) and also 1 mg/ml in 0.9% sodium chloride in plastic syringes (Monoject) was stable when stored at 4 and 23°C while exposed to light for 124 days. Leaching of plasticizers from the syringes was not detected during the study period. Finally, Hoffman *et al.*[5] observed that solutions of doxorubicin (2 mg/ml) in water for injections, were stable for six months at 4°C. Those authors indicated that filtration through a 0.22 μm filter would ensure sterility without loss of drug.

Several authors have published data on the effects of freezing doxorubicin. Hoffman *et al.*[5] observed that aqueous solutions of doxorubicin (2 mg/ml) could be frozen and stored for one month at –20°C without significant degradation but indicated that doxorubicin reconstituted with sodium chloride should not be frozen. Conversely, doxorubicin has been reported to be stable in 0.9% sodium chloride, for 30 days[8] and two weeks,[12] respectively, at –20°C. Wood *et al.*[21] reported that doxorubicin was stable in 5% glucose (pH 4.36), 0.9% sodium chloride (pH 5.20 and pH 6.47) in PVC minibags for at least 43 days at –20°C.

The effects of thawing doxorubicin by microwave radiation have also been investigated.[8,12] Karlsen *et al.*[8] observed that the concentration of doxorubicin in PVC minibags declined significantly after four re-thawings in a microwave. Keusters *et al.*[12] compared the effects of freezing and thawing doxorubicin at room temperature with thawing in the microwave. Results showed that doxorubicin was stable for two weeks at –20°C when thawed by either method. After re-freezing and subsequent re-thawing a small, but significant, decrease in concentration was observed in solutions thawed by both methods. Alternatively, Hoffman *et al.*[5] observed that aqueous solutions of doxorubicin could be frozen and thawed at room temperature, seven times, without significant loss of potency.

Wood *et al.*[21] also observed that repeated freezing and thawing of solutions of doxorubicin in PVC minibags at room temperature did not lead to significant degradation.

Uneven distribution of energy can occur during microwave thawing which may overheat solutions and lead to degradation.[24] For this reason, thawing in a microwave is not recommended. If frozen, doxorubicin should be thawed at room temperature.

Container compatibility: Doxorubicin is compatible with polypropylene, PVC and glass.[21,25] It has been reported to be more stable in plastic (PVC) than glass.[7] Doxorubicin adsorbs on to glass and polyethylene but not on to siliconized glass or polypropylene.[10,25] Solutions which contain concentrations of 2 mg/ml do not adsorb to membrane filters but with more dilute solutions, especially when associated with small volumes, greater than 95% of doxorubicin adsorbs to cellulose ester membranes and about 40% binds to polytetrafluoroethylene (PTFE) membranes.[26,27] In clinical practice, when doxorubicin is used at concentrations of at least 500 μg/ml, adsorption during storage and delivery is negligible.[21,25]

Compatibility with other drugs: Doxorubicin is incompatible with heparin, dexamethasone sodium phosphate, hydrocortisone sodium succinate and diazepam as precipitation occurs. The manufacturers recommend that no other drugs are mixed with doxorubicin. Combinations of doxorubicin and fluorouracil or aminophylline result in a colour change from red to blue-purple which indicates the onset of rapid degradation of doxorubicin.[28]

A combination of doxorubicin and vincristine in 0.9% sodium chloride, and in a mixture of 2.5% glucose with 0.45% sodium chloride, appears to be stable for at least seven days.[29] A mixture of doxorubicin and vinblastine in 0.9% sodium chloride appears to be relatively stable for at least five days.[30]

3.2 Stability in clinical practice

Doxorubicin is compatible with polypropylene, PVC and glass.[21,25] Doxorubicin appears to be chemically stable in PVC minibags (100 μg/ml) for at least 28 days in 5% glucose or 0.9% sodium chloride when stored at 4°C and −20°C, and in polypropylene syringes (2 mg/ml) for at least 28 days at 4°C.[21]

Stability in specialized delivery systems: Both the commercially available preparations of doxorubicin (2 mg/ml in 0.9% sodium chloride) are stable in portable pump reservoirs (Pharmacia Deltec Medication Cassette 602100A) for up to 14 days at 3 and 23°C and for an additional 28 days at 30°C.[31] Doxorubicin (500 μg/ml and 1.25 mg/ml) is stable in 0.9% sodium chloride or 5% glucose solution in EVA reservoirs (RES80 A, Celsa Laboratories, Chasseneuil, France) for 14 days at 4 and 22°C and for seven days at 35°C.[32] Doxorubicin (200 μg/ml to 5 mg/ml) is stable in 0.9% sodium chloride for at least 15 days in the Baxter Infusor at 4°C.[33] At a concentration of 2 mg/ml doxorubicin is also stable in the CADD pump for 14 days at 4°C.[33] Doxorubicin (1.5 mg/ml) and vinblastine (150 μg/ml) and doxorubicin (500 μg/ml) and vinblastine (75 μg/ml) is stable for ten days in a Cormed ML6–46 reservoir pump.[34] Doxorubicin (concentration range 400 to 600 μg/ml) admixed with cyclophosphamide (concentration range 6 to 8 mg/ml) is stable for seven days in a Cormed ML6-46 reservoir pump.[34] Doxorubicin (3 mg/ml and 5 mg/ml in 0.9% sodium chloride) is stable for two weeks in the reservoir of a Medtronic DAD implantable infusion pump at 37°C.[35]

4 Clinical use

Main indications: Successfully used to produce regression in acute leukaemia, lymphomas, soft tissue and osteogenic sarcomas, paediatric malignancies and adult solid tumours, in particular breast and lung carcinomas. Doxorubicin is frequently used in combination regimens with other cytotoxics.[1]

Dosage: Dosage is usually calculated on the basis of body surface area. For single agent therapy, 60–75 mg/m^2 is given every three weeks. When administered in combination with other anti-tumour agents which possess overlapping toxicity, dosage may need to be reduced to 30–40 mg/m^2 every three weeks. The total dose for the cycle may be divided over three successive days (20–25 mg/m^2 on each day). Administration of doxorubicin on a weekly regimen (20 mg/m^2) has also been shown to be as effective as the three-weekly regimen and also leads to a reduction in cardiotoxicity. Dosage may need to be reduced in patients who have had prior treatment with other cytotoxics, in children and the elderly. If hepatic function is impaired, doxorubicin dosage should be reduced to 50% if serum bilirubin concentrations are between 1.2 and 3 mg/100 ml and to 25% if serum bilirubin concentrations are greater than 3 mg/100 ml. A cumulative dose of 450 mg to 550 mg/m^2 should only be exceeded with extreme caution, as above this level the risk of irreversible congestive cardiac failure increases greatly.[1,2]

5 Preparation of injection

Doxorubicin rapid dissolution: The contents of the 10 mg vial are reconstituted with 5 ml of water for injections or 0.9% sodium chloride, and the 50 mg vial with 25 ml of the same solvent. After addition of the diluent and gentle shaking without inversion the contents of the vial will dissolve within 30 seconds to produce a solution of 2 mg/ml.[1]

Bolus administration: Administration is most frequently by the intravenous route. The manufacturer recommends that the reconstituted solution is given over two to three minutes, via the tubing of a freely-running intravenous infusion of 0.9% sodium chloride, 5% glucose or sodium chloride with glucose. This technique minimizes the risk of thrombosis or perivenous extravasation, which can lead to severe cellulitis or vesication. Doxorubicin may also be administered by the intra-arterial or intravesical route. Intra-arterial administration is potentially extremely hazardous and should only be attempted by those fully conversant with the technique.[1,2]

Intravenous infusion: Although the optimum schedule of continuous infusion of doxorubicin has not been established, most current investigations can be grouped into two broad categories. Most experience has been acquired with a schedule of short-term infusions given over one to four days, with cycles repeated every three to four weeks. The most thoroughly investigated short-term infusion has been the 96-hour cycle which generally takes five days to complete. In more recent studies, patients have received infusions for several months or longer.

Based on the marked decrease in the cardiotoxicity seen with short-term infusions of doxorubicin, a number of investigators have recently initiated studies with low dose doxorubicin given as a continuous infusion on a more protracted basis.[36–39] With a daily dose of 1 to 2 mg/m^2 the maximum total daily dose has varied between 3 and 5 mg/m^2 for periods of several weeks to several months in responding patients. Some investigators have used higher daily doses for two-week cycles of therapy, followed by two weeks without chemotherapy to allow for recovery from side-effects.[40]

Extravasation: Potent vesicant (*see* Chapter 6).

6 Destruction of drug or contaminated articles

Incineration: 700°C.[3]

Chemical: 10% sodium hypochlorite (1% available chlorine)/24 hours.[1]

Contact with skin: Wash well with water, soap and water, or sodium bicarbonate solution. If the eyes are contaminated, immediate irrigation with saline should be carried out.[1]

References

1 *ABPI Data Sheet Compendium 1995–96* (1995) DataPharm Publications Ltd, London, pp. 1261–3.
2 *ABPI Data Sheet Compendium 1995–96* (1995) DataPharm Publications Ltd, London, pp. 1263–5.
3 Pharmacia Ltd. Personal communication.
4 Anon. (1993) *The Extra Pharmacopoeia*, 30th edn. (JEF Reynolds ed.), Pharmaceutical Press, London, pp. 475–7.
5 Hoffman DM *et al.* (1979) Stability of refrigerated and frozen solutions of doxorubicin hydrochloride. *Am. J. Hosp. Pharm.* **36**, 1536–8.
6 Poochikian GK *et al.* (1981) Stability of anthracycline antitumour agents in four infusion fluids. *Am. J. Hosp. Pharm.* **38**, 483–6.
7 Benvenuto JA *et al.* (1981) Stability and compatibility of antitumour agents in glass and plastic containers. *Am. J. Hosp. Pharm.* **38**, 1914–18.
8 Karlsen J *et al.* (1983) Stability of cytotoxic intravenous solutions subjected to freeze-thaw treatment. *Nor. Pharm. Acta* **45**, 61–7.
9 Beijnen JH *et al.* (1985) Stability of anthracycline antitumour agents in infusion fluids. *J. Parenter. Sci. Technol.* **39**, 220–2.
10 Bosanquet AG (1986) Stability of solutions of antineoplastic agents during preparation and storage for *in vitro* assays: II. Assay methods, adriamycin and the other antitumour antibiotics. *Cancer Chemother. Pharmacol.* **17**, 1–10.
11 Bouma J *et al.* (1986) Anthracycline antitumour agents: A review of physicochemical, analytical and stability properties. *Pharm. Weekbl. (Sci. Edn.)* **8**, 109–35.
12 Keusters L *et al.* (1986) Stability of solutions of doxorubicin and epirubicin in plastic minibags for intravesical use after storage at −20°C and thawing by microwave radiation. *Pharm. Weekbl. (Sci. Edn.)* **8**, 194–7.
13 Gupta PK *et al.* (1988) Investigation of the stability of doxorubicin hydrochloride using factorial design. *Drug Dev. Indust. Pharm.* **14**, 1657–71.
14 Janssen MJH *et al.* (1985) Doxorubicin decomposition on storage: Effect of pH, type of buffer and liposome encapsulation. *Int. J. Pharm.* **23**, 1–11.
15 Beijnen JH *et al.* (1986) Aspects of the degradation kinetics of doxorubicin in aqueous solution. *Int. J. Pharm.* **32**, 123–31.
16 Wasserman K, Bundgaard H (1983) Kinetics of the acid catalysed hydrolysis of doxorubicin. *Int. J. Pharm.* **14**, 73–8.
17 Beijnen JH *et al.* (1985) Aspects of the stability of doxorubicin and seven other anthracyclines in acidic solution. *Pharm. Weekbl. (Sci.)* **7**, 109–16.
18 Abdeen Z *et al.* (1985) Degradation of adriamycin in aqueous sodium hydroxide: Formation of a ring-A oxabicyclononenone. *J. Chem. Res. (S)*, 254–5.

19 Tavoloni N *et al.* (1980) Photolytic degradation of adriamycin. *J. Pharm. Pharmacol.* **32**, 860–2.

20 Wood MJ *et al.* (1990) Photodegradation of doxorubicin, daunorubicin and epirubicin measured by high-performance liquid chromatography. *J. Clin. Pharm. Ther.* **15**, 291–300.

21 Wood MJ *et al.* (1990) Stability of doxorubicin, daunorubicin and epirubicin in plastic syringes and minibags. *J. Clin. Pharm. Ther.* **15**, 279–89.

22 Dine T *et al.* (1992) Stability and compatibility of four anthracyclines: doxorubicin, daunorubicin, epirubicin and pirarubicin with PVC infusion bags. *Pharm. Weekbl. (Sci. Edn)* **14**(6), 365–9.

23 Walker S *et al.* (1991) Doxorubicin stability in syringes and glass vials and evaluation of chemical contamination. *Can. J. Hosp. Pharm.* **44**, 71–8, 88.

24 Williamson M, Luce JK (1987) Microwave thawing of doxorubicin hydrochloride admixtures not recommended. *Am. J. Hosp. Pharm.* **44**, 505, 510.

25 Wood MJ (1989) MPhil. Thesis, University of Aston, Birmingham, UK.

26 Pavlik EJ *et al.* (1982) Sensitivity of anticancer agents *in vitro*, standardising the cytotoxic response and characterizing the sensitivities of a reference cell line. *Gynecol. Oncol.* **14**, 243–61.

27 Pavlik EJ *et al.* (1984) Stability of doxorubicin in relation to chemosensitivity determinations: loss of lethality and retention of antiproliferative activity. *Cancer Invest.* **2**, 449–58.

28 Trissel LA (1994) *Handbook of Injectable Drugs*, 8th edn, American Society of Hospital Pharmacists, Bethesda, USA.

29 Beijnen JH *et al.* (1986) Stability of intravenous admixtures of doxorubicin and vincristine. *Am. J. Hosp. Pharm.* **43**, 3022–7.

30 Gaj E, Sesin P (1984) Compatibility of doxorubicin hydrochloride and vinblastine sulphate. The stability of a solution stored in Cormed reservoir bags or monoject plastic syringes. *Am. J. Int. Ther. Clin. Nutr.* **11**, 8–20.

31 Stiles ML, Allen LV (1991) Stability of doxorubicin hydrochloride in portable pump reservoirs. *Am. J. Hosp. Pharm.* **48**, 1976–7.

32 Rochard EB *et al.* (1992) Stability of fluorouracil, cytarabine, or doxorubicin hydrochloride in ethylene vinylacetate portable infusion-pump reservoirs. *Am. J. Hosp. Pharm.* **49**, 619–23.

33 Baxter Healthcare Ltd. Personal communication.

34 Lokich JJ *et al.* (1986) Doxorubicin/vinblastine and doxorubicin/cyclophosphamide combination chemotherapy by continuous infusion. *Cancer* **58**, 1020–3.

35 Vogelsang NJ *et al.* (1985) Phase I trial of an implanted, battery-powered, programmable drug delivery system for continuous doxorubicin administration. *J. Clin. Oncol.* **3**, 407–14.

36 Garnick MB *et al.* (1983) Clinical evaluation of long term continuous infusion of doxorubicin. *Cancer Treat. Rep.* **67**, 133–42.

37 Bowen J *et al.* (1981) Phase I study of adriamycin by 5-day continuous intravenous infusion. *Proc. Am. Assoc. Cancer Res.* **22**, 354 (C-84).

38 Lokich JJ *et al.* (1983) Constant infusion schedule for adriamycin: A phase I–II clinical trial of a 30-day schedule by ambulatory pump delivery system. *J. Clin. Oncol.* **1**, 24–8.

39 Vogelsang J *et al.* (1984) Continuous doxorubicin infusion using an implanted lithium battery-powered drug administration device system (DADS, Medtronic, Inc.). *Proc. Am. Soc. Clin. Oncol.* **3**, 263 (C-1030).

40 Legha SS *et al.* (1987) Anthracyclines. In: (Lokich JJ ed.), *Cancer Chemotherapy by Infusion*. MTP Press Ltd, Lancaster.

Prepared by Jayne Wood

EPIRUBICIN

1 General details

Approved name: Epirubicin.

Proprietary name: Pharmorubicin rapid dissolution, Pharmorubicin solution for injection.

Manufacturer or supplier: Pharmacia and Upjohn Ltd.

Presentation and formulation details:

▼ pharmorubicin rapid dissolution: sterile, pyrogen-free, red, freeze-dried powder in vials containing 10 mg, 20 mg and 50 mg of epirubicin hydrochloride with lactose and hydroxybenzoate. The inclusion of hydroxybenzoate 0.04% (which is a sub-preservative concentration) is to prevent gel formation which used to occur occasionally on reconstitution of pharmorubicin. Pharmorubicin has been replaced by pharmorubicin rapid dissolution.[1]

▼ pharmorubicin solution for injection: sterile, red, mobile solution in vials containing 10 mg, 20 mg and 50 mg of epirubicin hydrochloride as a 2 mg/ml solution in 0.9% sodium chloride.[2]

Storage and shelf-life of unopened container:

▼ pharmorubicin rapid dissolution: three years when protected from sunlight at room temperature.[3]

▼ pharmorubicin solution for injection: stored between 2 and 8°C the shelf-life is two years. Once removed from the refrigerator, the shelf-life is 48 hours. Use within 24 hours of first penetration of the rubber stopper.[3]

2 Chemistry

Type: A cytotoxic antibiotic consisting of an amino sugar, acosamine, linked through a glycosidic bond to the C7 of a tetracyclic aglycone, doxorubicinone.

Molecular structure: (8S,10S)-10-(3-amino-2,3,6-trtideoxy-α-L-arabino-hexo-pyranosyloxy)-8-glycoloyl-7,8,9,10-tetrahydro-6,8,11-trihydroxy-1-methoxynaphthacene-5,12-dione hydrochloride.

Molecular weight: 580.0.

Formula: $C_{27}H_{29}NO_{11}HCl$.

Solubility: Epirubicin is soluble in water for injections, 5% glucose and 0.9% sodium chloride.[4]

3 Stability profile

3.1 *Physical and chemical stability*

The manufacturer states that reconstituted solutions of epirubicin rapid dissolution are chemically stable for up to 48 hours at 2–8°C, or 24 hours at room temperature.[1] Epirubicin solution for injection is stable for 18 months at 2–8°C and for 48 hours at room temperature.[3] The literature indicates that epirubicin may be chemically stable for longer periods, although few data have been published.[5,6]

The stability of epirubicin depends on a number of factors. Degradation in aqueous solution is pH dependent. Epirubicin is also light-sensitive and adsorbs on to glass and certain plastics.

Effect of pH: Acid hydrolysis of epirubicin (pH below 4) which is shown in Figure 1, yields a red-coloured, water-insoluble aglycone, doxorubicinone, and a water-soluble amino sugar, acosamine.

At pH values above 4, the degradation pathway of epirubicin has not been elucidated. However, on addition to strongly alkaline solution a colour change from red to deep blue-purple is observed and rapid degradation occurs. Data on the degradation of epirubicin in alkaline solution have recently been published indicating that at pH 8.0 the main degradation product is 7,8,-dehydro-9,10-desacetyldaunorubicinone.[7] The structure of this compound is shown in Figure 2.

In alkaline solution, the rate of degradation of the anthracyclines is affected by structural differences in the aglycone portion of the molecule and is unaffected by structural differences in the amino sugar moiety. As epirubicin and doxorubicin possess the same aglycone their rates of degradation in alkaline solution are similar.[7]

Effect of light: Data on the kinetics of degradation of doxorubicin in fluorescent light have been published[8] but until recently there were no available data for epirubicin. Results from a study in which the rates of photodegradation of doxorubicin, daunorubicin and epirubicin were compared indicated that the rate of photodegradation of epirubicin was similar to doxorubicin. This suggests that photodegradation of epirubicin may be significant at concentrations below 100 µg/ml if solutions are exposed to light for sufficient time.[9] However, at higher concentrations, such as those used for cancer chemotherapy (at least 500 µg/ml), no special precautions are necessary to protect freshly prepared solutions of epirubicin from light.[9]

Effect of temperature: In a well-controlled study Beijnen *et al.*[7] reported that epirubicin was stable, in polypropylene tubes, in 5% glucose (pH 4.7) and 3.3% glucose with 0.3% sodium chloride (pH 4.4) for 28 days at 25°C, when stored in the dark. However, in 0.9% sodium chloride (pH 7.0) significant degradation occurred after eight days at the same temperature.[7]

Wood *et al.*[10] reported that epirubicin was stable for at least 43 days in PVC minibags in 5% glucose (pH 4.36) and 0.9% sodium chloride (pH 5.20) at 25 and 4°C. When dissolved in 0.9% sodium chloride (pH 6.47) epirubicin was stable for 24 days at 25°C and at least 43 days at 4°C. In the same study epirubicin was reported to be stable for at least 43 days, when reconstituted with water for injections and stored in polypropylene syringes at 4°C.

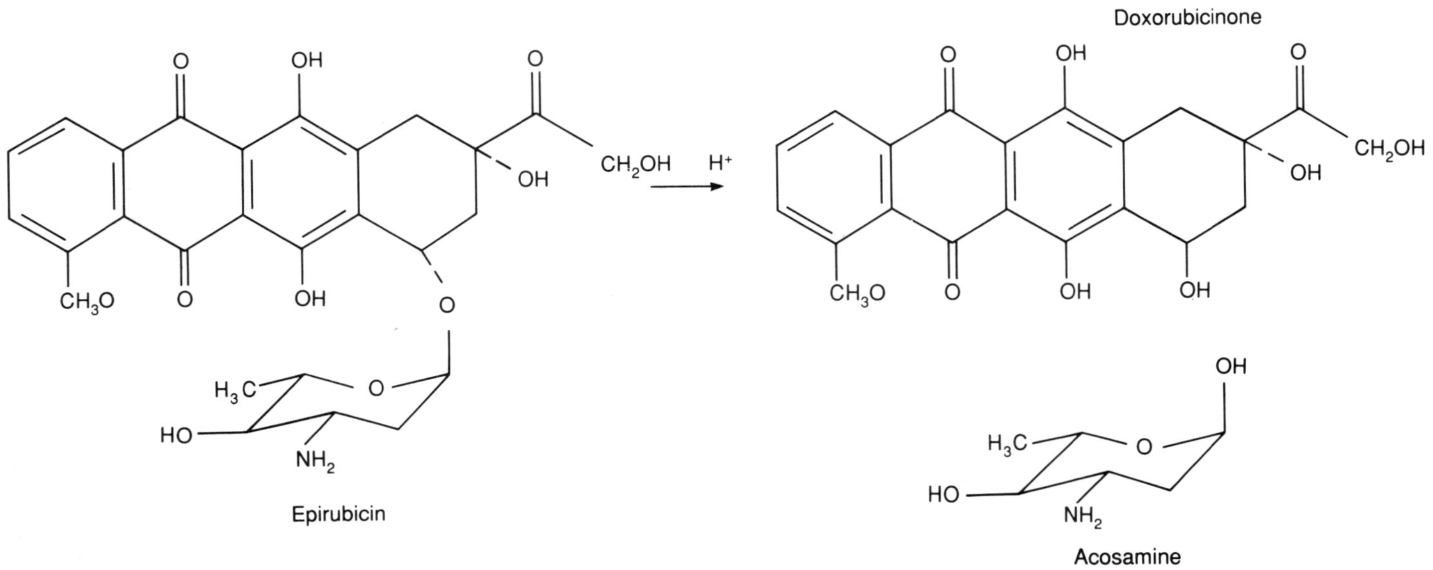

Figure 1: *Degradation pathway of epirubicin in acidic solution*

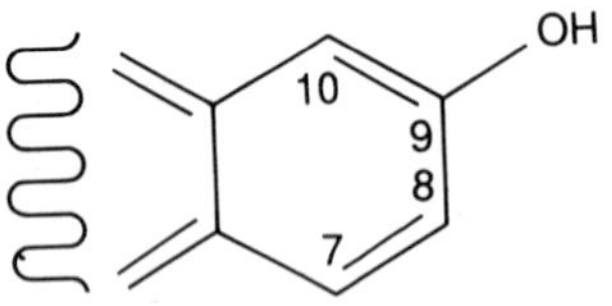

Figure 2: *Structure of 7,8--dehydro-9,10-desacetyldaunorubicinone[7]*

Adams *et al.*[11] reported that epirubicin (0.5 mg/ml and 1 mg/ml in 0.9% sodium chloride) was stable in plastic syringes (Braun Omnifix) for 28 days at 4 and 20°C. Dine *et al.*[12] reported that epirubicin (20 µg/ml in 5% glucose and 0.9% sodium chloride) was stable in PVC infusion bags (Macopharma Laboratories) for seven days at 4°C when protected from light.

De Vroe *et al.*[13] investigated the stability of epirubicin during storage and simulated continuous infusion. Adsorption to administration sets was also studied. Results showed that epirubicin (50 µg/ml) was stable in PVC, glass and high density polyethylene (HDPE) in 0.9% sodium chloride (pH 5.5) and 5% glucose (pH 4.26) for periods of 24 and 25 days respectively at 4°C. No adsorption on to infusion containers or administration sets was observed during simulated infusion. Infusion through an end-line filter (Pall ELD-96 LL) resulted in negligible loss of potency.

Two studies have investigated the effects of freezing epirubicin. In the first, epirubicin was reported to be stable for four weeks when frozen at –20°C in PVC minibags containing 0.9% sodium chloride.[6] In the second, epirubicin was observed to be stable for at least 43 days in PVC minibags in 5% glucose (pH 4.36) and 0.9% sodium chloride (pH 5.20 and 6.47) at –20°C.[10] Repeated freezing and re-thawing of these minibags at ambient temperature did not cause degradation.

Container compatibility: Epirubicin is compatible with polypropylene, PVC and glass.[10,13,14] Epirubicin adsorbs on to glass and polyethylene but not to siliconized glass or polypropylene.[10,14] However, in clinical practice, when epirubicin is used at concentrations of at least 500 µg/ml, adsorptive losses during storage and delivery are negligible.[10,13,14]

Compatibility with other drugs: Prolonged contact with any solution of alkaline pH should be avoided. Epirubicin should not be mixed with heparin as a precipitate may form.[1,2] The manufacturers recommend that epirubicin is not mixed with any other drugs.

3.2 Stability in clinical practice

Epirubicin is compatible with polypropylene, PVC and glass.[10,13,14] Epirubicin appears to be chemically stable in PVC minibags (100 µg/ml) for at least 28 days in 5% glucose and 0.9% sodium chloride at 4 and –20°C, and in polypropylene syringes (2 mg/ml) for at least 28 days at 4°C.[10] After reconstitution, vials of epirubicin (2 mg/ml) are stable for at least 14 days at 4°C.[14]

3.3 Stability in specialized delivery systems

Epirubicin (200 µg/ml to 1 mg/ml) is stable in 0.9% sodium chloride for at least 15 days in the Baxter Infusor at 4°C.[15]

4 Clinical use

Main indications: Epirubicin as a single agent has produced regression in a wide range of neoplastic conditions including breast, ovarian, gastric and colorectal carcinomas, lymphomas, leukaemias and multiple myeloma. Intravesical epirubicin has been found to be beneficial in the treatment of papillary transitional cell carcinoma of the bladder and in the prophylaxis of recurrences after transurethral resection. Epirubicin may be used in combination with other cytotoxic agents.[1,2]

Dosage and administration: Dosage is usually calculated on the basis of body surface area. For single agent intravenous therapy, the dose range most commonly used is 60–90 mg/m² every three weeks. The total dose for the cycle may be divided over two successive days. When epirubicin is used in combination therapy with other cytotoxics the dosage should be reduced. Dosage should also be reduced in hepatic impairment.[1] In moderate hepatic impairment (bilirubin 1.4 to 3 mg/100 ml) dosage should be reduced by 50%, and in severe impairment (bilirubin above 3 mg/100 ml) dosage should be reduced by 75%.

High doses: As a single agent in previously untreated small cell lung cancer at high doses 120 mg/m² on day one, every three weeks. For previously untreated non-small cell lung cancer (squamous, large cell and adenocarcinoma) 135 mg/m² on day one, or 45 mg/m² on days one, two and three, every three weeks.

Epirubicin can be administered intravenously on a weekly regimen, particularly for the palliative treatment of poor-risk patients for whom the toxicity of a conventional three-weekly regimen would be unacceptable. For these patients, the most commonly used dose is 20 mg per week.[1]

Epirubicin can be used intravesically to treat papillary transitional cell carcinoma of the bladder and carcinoma-in-situ. However, it should not be used to treat invasive bladder tumours which have penetrated the bladder wall, where systemic therapy or surgery is more appropriate. Epirubicin has also been used successfully intravesically as a prophylactic agent after transurethral resection of superficial tumours in order to prevent recurrences.

For therapy of papillary transitional cell carcinoma of the bladder weekly instillations of 50 mg in 50 ml of normal saline or water for injections are given for eight weeks. If local toxicity occurs (chemical cystitis) a dose reduction to 30 mg in 50 ml is advised. For carcinoma-in-situ the dose may be increased to 80 mg in 50 ml (depending on patient tolerance). For prophylaxis, weekly administration of 50 mg in 50 ml for four weeks is followed by monthly instillations for 11 months at the same dosage.

The solution should be retained intravesically for one hour. During the instillation, the patient should be rotated occasionally and should be instructed to void at the end of the instillation time.[1]

A cumulative dose of 900–1000 mg/m² should only be exceeded with extreme caution, as above this level the risk of irreversible congestive cardiac failure increases greatly. A lower cumulative dose of epirubicin is recommended for patients with prior or concomitant mediastinal radiation, or therapy with related anthracycline compounds such as doxorubicin, daunorubicin or anthracene derivatives.[1,2]

5 Preparation of injection

Reconstitution: The contents of the 10 mg vial are reconstituted with 5 ml of water for injections or 0.9% sodium chloride, the 20 mg vial with 10 ml, and the 50 mg vial with 25 ml of either of the same solvents. After addition of the diluent and gentle shaking, the contents, without inversion of the vial, will dissolve to produce a solution of 2 mg/ml.[1]

Bolus administration: Injection is only by the intravenous route. Epirubicin should **not** be injected intramuscularly or intrathecally. The reconstituted solution is given, over three to five minutes, via the tubing of a freely-running intravenous infusion of 0.9% sodium chloride. This technique minimizes the risk of thrombosis or perivenous extravasation, which can lead to severe cellulitis or vesication.[1,2] Administration of epirubicin by intra-arterial, intrapleural and intraperitoneal routes has been investigated in clinical trials.[16–18]

Intravenous infusion: Continuous infusion schedules of epirubicin have been investigated. At New York University, epirubicin has been given as a six-hour infusion.[19] At the MD Anderson Center, a 48-hour infusion of doxorubicin (60 to 70 mg/m²) has been compared with a 48-hour infusion of epirubicin (90 to 105 mg/m²).[20]

Extravasation: Potent vesicant (*see* Chapter 6).

6 Destruction of drug or contaminated articles

Incineration: 700°C.[3]

Chemical: 10% sodium hypochlorite (1% available chlorine)/24 hours.[1,2]

Contact with skin: Wash well with water, soap and water, or sodium bicarbonate solution. If the eyes are contaminated, immediate irrigation with 0.9% sodium chloride solution should be carried out.[1,2]

References

1 *ABPI Data Sheet Compendium 1995–96* (1995) DataPharm Publications Ltd, London, pp. 1304–5.
2 *ABPI Data Sheet Compendium 1995–96* (1995) DataPharm Publications Ltd, London, pp. 1305–7.
3 Pharmacia Ltd. Personal communication.
4 Anon. (1989). *The Extra Pharmacopoeia.* 30th edn. (JEF Reynolds ed.), Pharmaceutical Press, London, pp. 477–8.
5 Beijnen JH *et al.* (1985) Stability of anthracycline antitumour agents in infusion fluids. *J. Parenter. Sci. Technol.* **39**, 220–2.
6 Keusters L *et al.* (1986) Stability of solutions of doxorubicin and epirubicin in plastic minibags for intravesical use after storage at –20°C and thawing by microwave radiation. *Pharm. Weekbl. (Sci. Edn.)* **8**, 194–7.
7 Beijnen JH *et al.* (1986) Aspects of the degradation kinetics of doxorubicin in aqueous solution. *Int. J. Pharm.* **32**, 123–31.
8 Tavoloni N *et al.* (1980) Photolytic degradation of adriamycin. *J. Pharm. Pharmacol.* **32**, 860–2.
9 Wood MJ *et al.* (1990) Photodegradation of doxorubicin, daunorubicin and epirubicin measured by high-performance liquid chromatography. *J. Clin. Pharm. Ther.* **15**, 291–300.
10 Wood MJ *et al.* (1990) Stability of doxorubicin, daunorubicin and epirubicin in plastic syringes and minibags. *J. Clin. Pharm. Ther.* **15**, 279–89.
11 Adams PS *et al.* (1987) Pharmaceutical aspects of home infusion therapy for cancer patients. *Pharm. J.* April 11th, 476–8.

12 Dine T *et al.* (1992) Stability and compatibility of four anthracyclines: doxorubicin, daunorubicin, epirubicin and pirarubicin with PVC infusion bags. *Pharm. Weekbl. (Sci. Edn)* **14**(6), 365–9.

13 De Vroe C *et al.* (1990) A study on the stability of three antineoplastic drugs and on their sorption by IV delivery systems and end-line filters. *Int. J. Pharm.* **65**, 49–56.

14 Wood MJ (1989) MPhil. thesis, University of Aston, Birmingham, UK.

15 Baxter Healthcare Ltd. Personal communication.

16 Ferrazzi E *et al.* (1982) Preliminary phase II experience with 4'epidoxorubicin. In: (FM Muggia, CW Young, SK Carter eds), *Anthracycline antibiotics in cancer therapy*, Martinus Nijhoff, The Hague, p. 562.

17 Strocchi E *et al.* (1983) 4'Epidoxorubicin in locoregional therapy: Pharmacokinetic study after intrahepatic arterial and intraperitoneal administration. *Proc. 4th NCI-EORTC Symposium,* Brussels, Abst. 108.

18 Friedman MA, Ignoffo RJ (1984) Intra-arterial use of adriamycin. In: (M Ogawa, FM Muggia, M Rozencweig eds), *Adriamycin: Its expanding role in cancer treatment*, Excerpta Medica, Tokyo, p. 387.

19 Muggia FM, Green MD (1984) Special modes of administration: In: (Bonnadonna G. ed.), *Advances in anthracycline chemotherapy: Epirubicin.* Masson, Milano, pp. 149–52.

20 Bodey GP *et al.* (1983) Clinical trials with 4'epidoxorubicin. *Proc. 13th International Congress of Chemotherapy, Vienna,* part 215/23, Masson, Canada.

Prepared by Jayne Wood

ETOPOSIDE

1 General details

Approved name: Etoposide.

Proprietary name: Vepesid.

Manufacturer or supplier: Bristol-Myers Pharmaceuticals Ltd.

Presentation and formulation details: Glass vials containing 100 mg etoposide in 5 ml solution, 20 mg/ml. Each vial also contains: polyethylene glycol 300, ethyl alcohol, polysorbate 80, benzyl alcohol and citric acid.

Storage and shelf-life of unopened container: Five years from the date of manufacture when stored at room temperature and protected from light.

2 Chemistry

Type: Semi-synthetic podophyllotoxin derivative.

Molecular structure: 4-*o*-demethyl-1-1 *o*-(4,6-*o*-ethylidene-β-D-glucopyranosyl)-epi-podophyllotoxin.

Molecular weight: 588.6.

Solubility: Highly insoluble in water, soluble in organic solvents.[1] In dilutions with 0.9% sodium chloride, the concentration of etoposide should not exceed 0.25 mg/ml.[2] In other reports, however, it is suggested that concentrations up to 0.4 mg/ml are acceptable in clinical practice.[3,4] Occasional precipitation of drug has been reported in infusions where etoposide concentration exceeded 0.4 mg/ml.[4] Etoposide precipitation is unpredictable and depends not only on drug concentration but also on other physical factors.[5]

3 Stability profile

3.1 *Physical and chemical stability*

Etoposide degrades by hydrolytic cleavage of the glucopyranosyl moiety, or by epimerization to the *cis*-lactone.

Effect of pH: Maximum stability is found at 5.0.[6] The aglycone may hydrolyse in acid, while based-catalysed epimerization occurs in alkali.[6]

Effect of light: Etoposide should be protected from light during storage[2] and from strong daylight during administration.

Container compatibility: According to the manufacturers,[2] glass or PVC containers are suitable for etoposide infusion. However, a recent study[7] demonstrated significant leaching of DEHP plasticizer from a PVC medication reservoir into an infusion containing etoposide (0.4 mg/ml). DEHP concentrations in the 100 ml volume infusion after 24 hours at 37 and 8°C exceeded 100 µg/ml and 20 µg/ml respectively.[7] On this basis, EVA or glass containers may be preferable for etoposide administration.

Dilute infusions of etoposide are compatible with polypropylene syringes[8] but undiluted Vepesid injection has been implicated in the formation of hairline cracks in infusion devices constructed of plastics produced from the monomers acrylonitride, butadiene and styrene.[9] The effect on these plastics (known collectively as ABS plastic) has been attributed to the action of polyethylene glycol (PEG) 300, a solubilizing agent in the formulation. Caution should be exercised in the use of any plastic infusion device with undiluted etoposide injection.

Etoposide injection is incompatible with cellulose acetate membrane filters but is compatible with nylon or fluripore-type membranes.[10] Etoposide infusion is also compatible with the Pall ELD 96 pyrogen retentive 'set-saver' filter.[11]

Compatibility with other drugs: The manufacturer does not recommend mixing etoposide with any other drug.[2]

3.2 *Stability in clinical practice*

Etoposide infusions (0.4 mg/ml) in 5% glucose and in 0.9% sodium chloride are chemically stable for at least four days at room temperature.[5,12] As with an earlier report,[3] the stability of etoposide was not influenced by the type of container material (glass or PVC) or by normal room fluorescent lighting. One report however, has suggested that etoposide may be daylight-sensitive and is unstable beyond six hours in unprotected solutions.[4]

Polypropylene syringes containing etoposide infusion (1 mg/ml in water for injections) prepared for continuous infusion were chemically stable at 4 and 20°C for 28 days.[8] However, etoposide precipitated during administration and clinical use of concentrated infusions cannot be recommended.

Etoposide injection diluted with water to 10 mg/ml for oral use and filled into 5 ml plastic *oral* syringes (Burron Medical, model 0–5C) was stable for 22 days at ambient temperature (22°C) irrespective of lighting conditions employed.[13]

3.3 *Stability in specialized delivery systems*

With the exception of DEHP leaching, infusions of etoposide (0.4 mg/ml in 0.9% sodium chloride) stored in Graseby 9000 Series PVC Medication Cassettes were physically and chemically stable for 14 days at 8°C and seven days at 37°C.[7] These data suggest that by using medication reservoirs made of a plasticizer-free material, it would be possible to supply complete courses of etoposide infusion for ambulatory use.

4 Clinical use

Type of cytoxic agent: Mitotic inhibitor that arrests the cell cycle in the G_2 phase.

Main indications: Small cell carcinoma of the lung. Resistant non-seminomatous testicular carcinoma.

Dosage by injection: 60–120 mg/m² by intravenous infusion daily, for five consecutive days repeated every three to four weeks. Alternatively, 100 mg/m²/day on days one, two, three and five, every three to four weeks.

Oral: Twice the intravenous dose should be given on five consecutive days, every three to four weeks, myelosuppression permitting.

5 Preparation of the injection

Dilution: The injection should be diluted in 0.9% sodium chloride solution to give a maximum concentration of 0.25 mg/ml etoposide in the infusion.

Bolus administration: Not recommended.

Intravenous infusion: The dose should be given by infusion over not less than 30 minutes.

Extravasation: Irritant (*see* Chapter 6).

6 Destruction of drug or contaminated articles

Incineration: 1000°C.

Chemical: 10% sodium hypochlorite solution (1% available chlorine)/24 hours.

Contact with skin: Accidental exposure to etoposide may cause skin reactions. A soap and water wash should be employed.

References

1 Anon. (1982) *The Extra Pharmacopoeia*, 29th edn. (JEF Reynolds ed.), Pharmaceutical Press, London, pp. 208–9.
2 *ABPI Data Sheet Compendium 1995–96* (1995) DataPharm Publications Ltd, London, pp. 319–21.
3 Phillips NC, Lauper RD (1983) Review of etoposide. *Clin. Pharm.* **2**, 112–19.
4 Arnold AM (1979) Podophyllotoxin derivative VP16-213. *Cancer Chemother. Pharmacol.* **3**, 71–80.
5 Beijnen JH *et al.* (1991) Chemical and physical stability of etoposide and teniposide in commonly used infusion fluids. *J. Parenter. Sci. Technol.* **45**, 108–12.
6 Lidenberg WJM *et al.* (1985) Analysis and degradation kinetics of etoposide (VP16-213) in aqueous solution. *Pharm. Weekbl. Sci. Ed.* **1**, 291.
7 Sewell GJ, Priston MJ (1995) Stability and compatibility studies on a range of drug infusions in a new, multipurpose ambulatory pump. Presentation at National Quality Control Symposium (Aseptic Preparation Services) Coventry, UK, Sept. 27–28.

8 Adams PS *et al* (1987) Pharmaceutical aspects of home infusion therapy for cancer patients. *Pharm. J.* **238**, 476–8.

9 Schwinghammer TL, Reilly M (1988) Cracking of ABS plastic devices used to infuse undiluted etoposide injection (letter). *Am. J. Hosp. Pharm.* **45**, 1277.

10 Forrest SC (1984) Vepesid injection (letter). *Pharm. J.* **232**, 88.

11 Pall Biomedical, Portsmouth, UK (1995) Personal communication.

12 Trissel LA (1992) *Handbook on Injectable Drugs*, 8th edn. American Society of Hospital Pharmacists, Bethesda, Maryland, USA.

13 McLeod HL, Relling MV (1992) Stability of etoposide solution for oral use. *Am. J. Hosp. Pharm.* **49**, 2784–5.

Prepared by Graham Sewell

FLUDARABINE

1 General details

Approved names: Fludarabine, fludarabine phosphate, 2-fluoro-adrenine arabinoside-5-phosphate, 2-fluoro-ARA-AMP.

Proprietary name: Fludara.

Manufacturer or supplier: Schering Health Care Ltd.

Presentation and formulation details: 5 ml vials, each containing fludarabine phosphate 50 mg (equivalent to fludarabine 39.05 mg) as a sterile lyophilized cake. Vials also contain mannitol and sodium hydroxide to adjust pH.[1,2]

Storage and shelf-life of unopened container: When stored at room temperature below 30°C the vials have a shelf-life of 24 months.

2 Chemistry

Type: Antimetabolite.

Molecular structure: 9H-purine-6-amine, 2-fluoro-9-(5-*o*-phosphono-β-D-arabino-furanoeyl).

Molecular weight: 401.2.

Solubility: 9 mg/ml in water.

3 Stability profile

3.1 Physical and chemical stability

Fludarabine phosphate is chemically stable in solution, showing less than 2% decomposition in 16 days at room temperature in artificial light.[1,3]

Effect of pH: Chemically stable in solution between pH 4.5 and 8, with optimum pH of 7.6.[1]

Effect of temperature: At a concentration of 25 mg/ml in distilled water stored at room temperature (22–25°C) in normal laboratory light, fludarabine phosphate exhibited less than 2% decomposition in 16 days.[3]

Diluted to a concentration of 1 mg/ml in 5% glucose or in 0.9% sodium chloride, less than 3% decomposition occurred in 16 days at room temperature (22–25°C) under normal laboratory light.[3]

3.2 Stability in clinical practice

Although the manufacturer recommends that the contents of the vial should be used within eight hours of being reconstituted,[2] solutions of fludarabine phosphate 0.04 mg/ml in 5% glucose or 0.9% sodium chloride exhibited no losses over 48 hours, in glass or PVC, at room temperature or in the fridge.[1,3] At 1 mg/ml in these fluids, less than 3% decomposition was seen in 16 days at room temperature in artificial light.[1,3] For a review of the compatibility of fludarabine and a range of other drugs *see* Trissel[1] and Williams and Lokich.[4]

3.3 Stability in specialized delivery systems

No data available.

4 Clinical use

Type of cytotoxic: Antimetabolite.

Main indications: As a single agent treatment for B-cell chronic lymphocytic leukaemia unresponsive to, or relapsed after previous treatment with an alkylating agent.

Dosage: 25 mg/m² daily for five consecutive days in every 28 days. The cycle may be repeated up to six times.

5 Preparation of injection

Reconstitution: Add 2 ml water for injection to the contents of a vial and mix gently for 10–15 seconds.

Bolus administration: Dilute further to 10 ml with 0.9% sodium chloride.

Intravenous infusion: As an alternative to bolus administration the dose may be diluted in up to 100 ml 0.9% sodium chloride for infusion over 30 minutes.

Extravasation: Non-vesicant.

References

1 Trissel LA (1994) *Handbook on Injectable Drugs*, 8th edn. American Society of Hospital Pharmacists, Bethesda, Maryland, USA.
2 *ABPI Data Sheet Compendium 1995–96* (1995) DataPharm Publications Ltd, London, pp. 1609–10.
3 NCI Investigational Drugs, Pharmaceutical Data, National Cancer Institute, Bethesda, Maryland, USA.
4 Williams DA, Lokich J (1992) A review of the stability and compatibility of antineoplastic drugs for multiple drug infusion. *Cancer Chemother. Pharmacol.* **31**, 171–81.

Prepared by Tim Root

FLUOROURACIL

1 General details

Approved names: Fluorouracil, 5-fluorouracil.

Proprietary names: Fluoro-uracil.

Manufacturer or supplier: Faulding DBL Ltd.

Presentation and formulation details: Colourless to slightly yellow solution in rubber-capped clear glass vials (Onco-tain™) containing 25 mg/ml fluorouracil (10, 20 and 100 ml); solution in water for injections with sodium hydroxide for pH adjustment.

Storage and shelf-life of unopened container: The shelf-life is two years when stored at room temperature and protected from light.

2 Chemistry

Type: Fluorinated pyrimidine.

Molecular structure: 5-fluoro-2,4(1H,3H)pyrimidine-dione.

Molecular weight: 130.1

Solubility: 12.5 mg/ml in water; 6 mg/ml in ethanol.

3 Stability profile

3.1 Physical and chemical stability

Fluorouracil breakdown occurs by two routes: thermal and photochemical decomposition cause the opening of the pyrimidine ring between N3 and C4 and N1 and C5 to produce urea. Alkaline hydrolysis leads to the production of barbituric acid and uracil which further degrades to urea. The rate of alkaline hydrolysis increases rapidly above pH 9.0 so the injection is formulated within the pH range of 8.6–9.0. Although the drug is stable at acid pH, solubility is reduced.

The injection should be protected from strong daylight and temperatures above 25°C.

Container compatibility: Many studies have been made of container compatibility at various concentrations. At concentrations of 5–10 mg/ml, the drug has been shown to be stable for 16 weeks at 5°C in PVC containers. Similar and more concentrated solutions have been shown to be stable for up to 42 days at room temperature.[1,2,3] A small increase in concentration resulted from the loss of moisture. Likewise, solutions of 10 and 50 mg/ml have been shown to be stable in EVA containers for 28 days over a wide temperature range.[4]

Undiluted injection has been stored in a plastic syringe or glass vial without loss of potency.[5] Studies for the Exeter continuous chemotherapy infusion programme showed the undiluted injection to be stable for 28 days at 5 and 25°C in plastic syringes.[6]

Compatibility with other drugs: Fluorouracil has been shown to be compatible with bleomycin,[7] cyclophosphamide and methotrexate,[8] etoposide,[9] floxuridine,[10] ifosfamide,[9] heparin,[11] and metoclopramide.[12] Studies had indicated that fluorouracil could be mixed with calcium folinate.[13,14] However, recent work has indicated that a crystalline deposit forms in stored mixtures in less than four days[15,16] and, as a consequence, the manufacturers of calcium folinate are now stating that the two drugs should not be mixed.

Compatibility studies of mixing with other drugs briefly in a syringe, or in a simulated 'Y' site injection, have indicated compatibility with a number of drugs.[17-24] Compatibility with ondansetron appears to be concentration dependent.[25,26] Incompatibility is likely to be seen with acidic drugs, or drugs that are unstable in an alkaline environment, and has been demonstrated with carboplatin,[9] cisplatin,[27] cytarabine,[28] diazepam,[29] doxorubicin,[29] droperidol,[17] epirubicin,[30] filgrastim,[31] gallium nitrate,[32] and vinorelbine.[33]

3.2 Stability in clinical practice

Fluorouracil has been shown to be quite stable at alkaline pH values below 9.0 and when protected from strong daylight and high temperatures. In syringes, PVC and EVA containers, undiluted, or diluted in 0.9% sodium chloride, fluorouracil has been shown to be stable for at least 28 days. In glucose 5%, several studies have indicated prolonged stability, although one study found a loss of 10% in 43 hours,[34] and, although this may have been an adsorption effect, care should be taken in assigning an extended expiry for fluorouracil in glucose 5%.

The extended stability data that have been reported for mixtures with calcium folinate should be treated with caution since the recent discovery of crystalline deposits in such mixtures after short periods of storage. Mixtures for immediate intravenous infusion may be compatible, but are not recommended by the calcium folinate manufacturers.

3.3 Stability in specialized delivery systems

Stability of fluorouracil has been extensively studied in ambulatory pump reservoirs. Fluorouracil (DBL) 25 mg/ml is stable for at least 14 days at 4 and 37°C in the Parker Micropump.[35] Fluorouracil 50 mg/ml is stable for at least seven days during slow continuous administration at 25 and 37°C in the Deltec CADD-1 (Pharmacia), Cormed 11, Infumed 200 (Medfusion) and the Provider I.V., Model 2000 (Pancretic) devices.[35] Solutions of fluorouracil ranging from 5–42 mg/ml in 0.9% sodium chloride have been shown to be stable for at least 15 days in the Baxter Infusor when stored at 4°C.[35] Fluorouracil is also stable after refrigerated storage for 15 days, during administration through a seven day infusor or large volume intermate reservoir (Baxter).[35] Solutions of fluorouracil 12 mg/ml diluted in 5% glucose and stored in the infusor at 5°C have been shown less than 10% loss after storage for 16 weeks. Storage at 25°C, however, led to significant increases in drug concentration, indicating water evaporation.[1] Fluorouracil (DBL) 25 mg/ml has recently been reported to be stable for at least six months during storage in Medex reservoirs (65 and 150 ml capacity) at 5 or 25°C.[36]

4 Clinical use

Type of cytotoxic: Antimetabolite.

Main indications: Palliative treatment of a variety of carcinomas, both alone and in combination.

Dosage: Up to 15 mg/kg intravenously once weekly, maximum daily dose usually 1 g. Fluorouracil may be used as an induction once daily for five to seven days or in a three to four week cycle as part of combination therapy. It is also commonly used in conjunction with calcium folinate for colorectal cancer. 5–7.5 mg/kg by continuous intra-arterial infusion over 24 hours has also been used.

5 Preparation of injection

Dilution: May be administered undiluted or diluted as an infusion.

Bolus administration: Administer injection slowly (not less than 3–5 minutes) directly into the vein or via a fast-running drip.

Intravenous infusion: Dilute in 300–500 ml 5% glucose or 0.9% sodium chloride and administer over either 30–60 minutes, or over 4–24 hours if convenient.

Extravasation: Non-irritant.

6 Destruction of drug or contaminated articles

Incineration: 700°C.

Chemical: 10% sodium hypochlorite/24 hours.

Contact with skin: Wash thoroughly with soap and water.

References

1 Quebbeman EJ *et al.* (1984) Stability of fluorouracil in plastic containers used for continuous infusion at home. *Am. J. Hosp. Pharm.* **41**, 1153–6.
2 Vincke AE *et al.* (1989) Extended stability of 5-fluorouracil and methotrexate solutions in PVC containers. *Int. J. Pharm.* **54**, 181–9.
3 Allen VJ *et al.* (1988) Stability study of fluorouracil administered using a constant infusion pump. American Society of Hospital Pharmacists Meeting, **23**, 387.
4 Rochard EB *et al.* (1992) Stability of fluorouracil, cytarabine, or doxorubicin hydrochloride in ethylene vinylacetate portable infusion-pump reservoirs. *Am. J. Hosp. Pharm.* **49**, 619–23.
5 Sesin GP *et al.* (1982) Stability study of 5-fluorouracil following repackaging in plastic disposable syringes and multidose vials. *Am. J. Intraven. Ther. Clin. Nutr.* **9**, 23–5, 29–30.
6 Sewell GJ (1988) Cancer chemotherapy by infusion: drug stability and compatibility considerations. *Proc. Int. Symposium on Oncological Pharmacy Practice*, Rotorua, New Zealand, 253–78.
7 Dorr RT *et al.* (1982) Bleomycin compatibility with selected intravenous medications. *J. Med.* **13**, 121–30.
8 Lokich J *et al.* (1989) Cyclophosphamide, methotrexate and 5-fluorouracil in a three-drug admixture. *Cancer* **63**, 822–4.
9 Williams DA, Lokich J (1992) A review of the stability and compatibility of antineoplastic drugs for multiple-drug infusions. *Cancer Chemother. Pharmacol.* **31**, 171–81.

10 Anderson N *et al.* (1989) Combined 5-fluorouracil and floxuridine administered as a 14-day infusion. *Cancer* **63**, 825–7.

11 Barberi-Heyob M *et al.* (1995) Addition of heparin in 5-fluorouracil solution for portal vein infusion has no influence on its stability under clinically relevant conditions. *Anti-Cancer Drugs* **6**, 163–4.

12 Wang DP *et al.* (1995) Stability of fluorouracil-metoclopramide hydrochloride mixture. *Am. J. Health-Syst. Pharm.* **52**, 98–9.

13 Anderson N *et al.* (1989) A Phase 1 clinical trial of combined fluoropyrimidines with leucovorin in a 14-day infusion. *Cancer* **63**, 233–7.

14 Milano G *et al.* (1993) Long-term stability of 5-fluorouracil and folinic acid admixtures. *Eur. J. Cancer* **29A**, 129–32.

15 Adralan B, Flores MR (1993) A new complication of permanent indwelling central venous catheters using high dose fluorouracil and leucovorin. *J. Clin. Oncol.* **11**, 384.

16 Trissel LA *et al.* (1995) Incompatibility of fluorouracil with leucovorin calcium or levoleucovorin calcium. *Am. J. Health-Syst. Pharm.* **52**, 710–15.

17 Cohen MH *et al.* (1985) Drug precipitation within IV tubing: a potential hazard of chemotherapy administration. *Cancer Treat. Rep.* **69**, 1325–6.

18 Trissel LA, Martinez JF (1994) Physical compatibility of allopurinol sodium with selected drugs during simulated Y-site administration. *Am. J. Hosp. Pharm.* **51**, 1792–9.

19 Trissel LA *et al.* (1991) Visual compatibility of fludarabine phosphate with antineoplastic drugs, anti-infectives, and other selected drugs during simulated Y-site injection. *Am. J. Hosp. Pharm.* **48**, 2186–9.

20 Allen LV, Stiles ML (1981) Compatibility of various admixtures with secondary additives at Y-injection sites of intravenous administration sets. Part 2. *Am. J. Hosp. Pharm.* **38**, 380–1.

21 Woloschuck DMM *et al.* (1991) Stability and compatibility of fluorouracil and mannitol during simulated Y-site administration. *Am. J. Hosp. Pharm.* **48**, 2158–60.

22 Trissel LA, Martinez JF (1993) Melphalan physical compatibility with selected drugs during simulated Y-site administration. *Am. J. Hosp. Pharm.* **50**, 2359–63.

23 Trissel LA, Bready BB (1992) Turbidimetric assessment of the compatibility of taxol with selected other drugs during simulated Y-site injection. *Am. J. Hosp. Pharm.* **49**, 1716–19.

24 Trissel LA, Martinez JF (1994) Physical compatibility of piperacillin sodium plus tazobactam sodium with selected drugs during simulated Y-site administration. *Am. J. Hosp. Pharm.* **51**, 672–8.

25 Trissel LA *et al.* (1991) Visual compatibility of ondansetron hydrochloride with other selected drugs during simulated Y-site injection. *Am. J. Hosp. Pharm.* **48**, 988–92.

26 Leak RF, Woodford JD (1989) Pharmaceutical development of ondansetron injection. *Eur. J. Cancer Clin. Oncol.* **25** (Suppl. 1), S76–S69.

27 Stewart CF, Fleming RA (1990) Compatibility of cisplatin and fluorouracil in 0.9% sodium chloride injection. *Am. J. Hosp. Pharm.* **47**, 1373–7.

28 McRae MP, King JC (1976) Compatibility of antineoplastic, antibiotic and corticosteroid drugs in intravenous admixtures. *Am. J. Hosp. Pharm.* **33**, 1010–13.

29 Dorr RT (1979) Incompatibilities with parenteral and anticancer drugs. *Am. J. Intraven. Ther. Clin. Nutr.* **6**, 42, 45, 46, 52.

30 Adams PS *et al.* (1987). Pharmaceutical aspects of home infusion therapy for cancer patients. *Pharm. J.* **238**, 476–8.

31 Trissel LA, Martinez JF (1994) Physical compatibility of filgrastim with selected drugs during simulated Y-site administration. *Am. J. Hosp. Pharm.* **51**, 1907–13.

32 Lober CA, Dollard PA (1993) Visual compatibility of gallium nitrate with selected drugs during simulated Y-site injection. *Am. J. Hosp. Pharm.* **50**, 1208–10.

33 Trissel LA, Martinez JF (1994) Visual, turbidimetric, and particle-content assessment of compatibility of vinorelbine tartrate with selected drugs during simulated Y-site injection. *Am. J. Hosp. Pharm.* **51**, 495–9.

34 Benvenuto JA *et al.* (1981) Stability and compatibility of antitumor agents in glass and plastic containers. *Am. J. Hosp. Pharm.* **38**, 1914–18.

35 Baxter Healthcare (1992) Personal communication.

36 Faulding DBL Ltd (1995) Personal communication.

Prepared by Richard Needle

GEMCITABINE

1 General details

Approved name: Gemcitabine hydrochloride.

Proprietary name: Gemzar.

Manufacturer or supplier: Eli Lilly Ltd.

Presentation and formulation details: White to off-white lyophilized powder in glass vials containing gemcitabine hydrochloride equivalent to 200 mg or 1000 mg of gemcitabine. The vials also contain mannitol and sodium acetate.[1]

Storage and shelf-life of unopened containers: The shelf-life is two years when stored at room temperature (15–25°C) and protected from light.[2]

2 Chemistry

Type: Pyrimidine analogue.

Molecular structure: 2'-deoxy-2', 2'-difluorocytidine monohydrochloride.

Formula: $C_9H_{11}O_4N_3F_2$.

Molecular weight: 299.7.

Characteristics and solubility: A powder reconstitution produces a clear colourless to straw-coloured solution. Because of drug solubility limitations doses of $2500 \, mg/m^2$ and greater must be diluted in at least 1000 ml of 0.9% sodium chloride.

3 Stability profile

3.1 Physical and chemical stability

The lyophilized product is stable for 24 months when stored at room temperature (15–25°C).[2]

Compatibility with other drugs: There is no further information available.

3.2 Stability in clinical practice

The stability of solutions of gemcitabine has been investigated up to 48 hours when reconstituted with 0.9% sodium chloride. There was no significant decomposition of gemcitabine.[2] Solutions should not be refrigerated as crystallization will occur.[2]

3.3 Stability in specialized delivery systems

No information is available.

4 Clinical use

Type of cytotoxic: Pyrimidine antimetabolite which inhibits DNA replication and repair. Gemcitabine appears to be cell cycle specific for S phase, causing cells to accumulate at the G_1 S phase boundary.

Main indications: Palliative treatment of adult patients with locally advanced or metastatic non-small cell lung cancer.

Dosage: The recommended dose is 1000 mg/m² given by 30 minute intravenous infusion. This dose should be repeated once weekly for three weeks followed by a one week rest period. The four-week cycle is then repeated.

5 Preparation of injection

Reconstitution: Add at least 5 ml of 0.9% sodium chloride to the 200 mg vial or at least 25 ml to the 1 g vial. Shake to dissolve. The appropriate amount of drug may be administered as prepared or further diluted with 0.9% sodium chloride. Due to solubility considerations, the maximum concentration on reconstitution is 40 mg/ml. Solutions of reconstituted gemcitabine may be kept at room temperature (15–25°C).[2] Reconstituted solutions should be used as soon as possible and no later than six hours after reconstitution. Solutions should not be refrigerated as crystallization may occur.

Extravasation: No information available.

6 Destruction of drug or contaminated articles

Incineration: 700°C.

Chemical: 0.5 M sulphuric acid and 0.1 M potassium permanganate solution/two hours.

Contact with skin: Wash thoroughly with soap and copious amounts of water.

References

1 *Gemzar Data Sheet (Sept. 1995)* Eli Lilly and Co., Basingstoke, UK.
2 Eli Lilly and Co. (1995) Personal communication.

Prepared by Jeff Koundakjian

IDARUBICIN

1 General details

Approved name: Idarubicin.

Proprietary name: Zavedos.

Manufacturer or supplier: Pharmacia Ltd.

Presentation and formulation details: Sterile pyrogen-free, orange-red, freeze-dried powder in vials containing 5 mg and 10 mg idarubicin hydrochloride, with 50 mg and 100 mg lactose respectively.[1] Capsules (5 mg and 10 mg) are available for the treatment of patients in whom intravenous therapy cannot be employed.[2]

Storage and shelf-life of unopened container: Three years at room temperature protected from sunlight.[3]

2 Chemistry

Type: A cytotoxic antibiotic consisting of an amino sugar daunosamine, linked through a glycosidic bond to the C7 of a tetracyclic aglycone, 4-demethoxydaunorubicinone.

Molecular structure: (1S,3S)-3-acetyl-1,2,3,4,6,11-hexahydro-3,5,12-trihydroxy-6, 11-dioxo-1-naphthacenyl-3-amino-2,3,6-trideoxy-α-L-lyso-hexopyranoside.

Molecular weight: 533.97.

Formula: $C_{26}H_{27}NO_9HCl$.

Solubility: Idarubicin is sparingly soluble in water for injections, 5% glucose and 0.9% sodium chloride.[4]

3 Stability profile

3.1 Physical and chemical stability

The manufacturer states that the reconstituted solution is chemically stable for at least 48 hours at 2–8°C and 24 hours at room temperature.[1] Very few data on the long-term stability of idarubicin are available.

The stability of the anthracyclines is dependent on a number of factors, including the pH of the medium. They are also light-sensitive and adsorb on to glass and certain plastics.

Effect of pH: Acidic hydrolysis of idarubicin, which is shown in Figure 1, is expected to yield a red-coloured, water-insoluble aglycone, 4-demethoxydaunorubicinone, and a water-soluble amino sugar, daunosamine. The rate of cleavage of the glycosidic bond in acidic media is stongly dependent on structural modifications in the amino sugar moiety.[5] As daunorubicin and idarubicin both possess daunosamine as the sugar moiety, the rate of degradation of these analogues in acidic solution is expected to be similar. There are no published data to confirm this hypothesis.

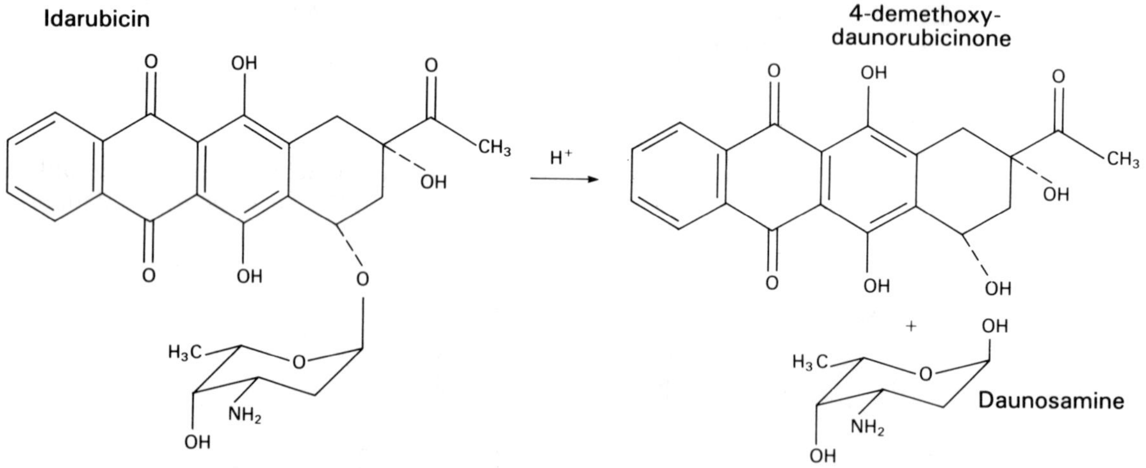

Figure 1: *Proposed degradation pathway for idarubicin in acidic solution*

In alkaline solution, the rate of degradation of the anthracyclines is affected by structural modifications in the aglycone portion of the molecule.[5] As idarubicin possesses a unique aglycone, 4-demethoxydaunorubicinone, its stability in alkaline media cannot be predicted from existing data for the other anthracyclines. The manufacturers recommend that prolonged contact of idarubicin with any solution of alkaline pH should be avoided as it will result in degradation.[1]

Effect of light: Data on the photodegradation of doxorubicin, daunorubicin and epirubicin have been published.[6,7] The rates of photodegradation of these three analogues have been reported to be similar and may be substantial at concentrations below 100 µg/ml if solutions are exposed to light for sufficient time.[7] Similarly, dilute solutions of idarubicin (10 µg/ml) are light-sensitive, undergoing some degradation when exposed to light for periods greater than six hours.[8] At higher concentrations, such as those used for cancer chemotherapy (at least 500 µg/ml), no special precautions are necessary to protect freshly prepared solutions of doxorubicin, daunorubicin and epirubicin from light.[6] The manufacturers suggest that idarubicin is treated in a similar fashion to these other anthracyclines and that no precautions are necessary to protect freshly prepared solutions of idarubicin from light.[3]

Effect of temperature: A review of the literature reveals one well controlled study, in which Beijnen et al.[9] reported that idarubicin was stable in polypropylene tubes, in 5% glucose (pH 4.7), 3.3% glucose with 0.3% sodium chloride (pH 4.4), lactated Ringer's (pH 6.8) and 0.9% sodium chloride (pH 7.0) for 28 days when stored in the dark at 25°C.

Haze formation: Idarubicin solutions in 0.9% sodium chloride exhibit a low level haze that is visible under high intensity light and measurable with a turbidimeter. Dilution of the drug from concentrations of 500 µg/ml to 1 mg/ml increases this haze until a maximum is reached at about 50 µg/ml. This haze appears to be normal for idarubicin in solution and is not an incompatibility.[10]

Container compatibility: Idarubicin is compatible with polypropylene, PVC and glass.[3] Doxorubicin, daunorubicin and epirubicin adsorb on to glass but not on to siliconized glass or polypropylene.[11,12] Therefore, idarubicin may behave in a similar manner. In clinical practice, when idarubicin is used at concentrations of at least 500 µg/ml, adsorptive losses during storage and delivery are expected to be negligible.

Compatibility with other drugs: Prolonged contact with any solution of alkaline pH should be avoided as it will result in degradation.[1] Idarubicin has been observed to be physically incompatible with acyclovir, ceftazidime, clindamycin, dexamethasone, etoposide, frusemide, gentamicin, hydrocortisone, imipenem/cilastin, lorazepam, methotrexate, mezlocillin, sodium bicarbonate, vancomycin and vincristine.[13] Idarubicin should not be mixed with heparin as a precipitate may form.[1] The manufacturer recommends that no other drugs are mixed with idarubicin.[1]

3.2 Stability in clinical practice

Idarubicin (100 µg/ml) appears to be chemically stable for at least 28 days in 5% glucose, glucose/saline admixtures and 0.9% sodium chloride at 25°C.[9] After reconstitution, vials of idarubicin should be refrigerated.[3]

3.3 Stability in specialized delivery systems

No data available.

4 Clinical use

Main indications: Remission induction in untreated adults with acute non-lymphocytic leukaemia (ANLL) or for remission induction in relapsed or refractory patients. Idarubicin is also indicated in acute lymphocytic leukaemia as second line treatment in adults and children. It may be used in combination regimens with other cytotoxic agents.[1]

Dosage: Dosage is usually calculated on the basis of body surface area. The manufacturer gives the following recommendations for the intravenous preparation:

▼ acute non-lymphocytic leukaemia: in adults, the dose schedule suggested is 12 mg/m² intravenously daily, for three days in combination with cytarabine. Another dosage schedule in which idarubicin has been used as a single agent and in combination is 8 mg/m² intravenously daily, for five days.

▼ acute lymphocytic leukaemia: as a single agent the suggested dose is 12 mg/m² intravenously daily, for three days in adults, and 10 mg/m² intravenously daily, for three days in children.

On the basis of the recommended intravenous dosage schedules, the total cumulative dose administered over two courses can be expected to reach 60–80 mg/m². Although a cumulative dosage limit cannot yet be defined, a specific cardiologic evaluation in cancer patients showed no significant modifications of cardiac function in patients treated with intravenous idarubicin at a mean cumulative dosage of 93 mg/m².[1]

▼ oral idarubicin: in ANLL patients in whom oral idarubicin is used the dose is 30 mg/m² daily, for three days as a single agent or between 15 and 30 mg/m² orally daily, for three days in combination with other antileukaemic agents. In advanced breast cancer the recommended dosage schedule as a single agent is 45 mg/m² orally, given either on a single day or divided over three consecutive days, to be repeated every three or four weeks based on haematological recovery. A maximum cumulative dose of 400 mg/m² for oral idarubicin is recommended.[2]

All of the above dosage schedules should, however, take into account the haematological status of the patient and the dosages of other cytotoxic drugs when used in combination. Idarubicin therapy should not be started in patients with severe renal and liver impairment or patients with uncontrolled infections. In a number of phase III trials, treatment was not given if bilirubin levels exceeded 2 mg/100 ml. With other anthracyclines, a 50% dosage reduction is generally employed if bilirubin levels are in the range of 1.2–2.0 mg/100 ml.[1]

5 Preparation of injection

Reconstitution: The contents of the 5 mg vial should be dissolved in 5 ml of water for injections and the 10 mg vial in 10 ml of the same solvent. After addition of the diluent and gentle shaking, the contents of the vial will dissolve to produce a solution of 1 mg/ml.[1]

Bolus administration: Administration is by the intravenous route only. The reconstituted solution should be given, over five to ten minutes, into the side arm of a freely-running intravenous infusion of 0.9% sodium chloride. This technique minimizes the risk of thrombosis or perivenous extravasation which can lead to severe cellulitis or necrosis.[1]

Intravenous infusion: The doses and duration of infusions of idarubicin that have been used in clinical trials range from 8 mg/m² to 16 mg/m² over four hours, 24 hours or 72 hours.[3,14–16]

Extravasation: Potent vesicant (*see* Chapter 6).

6 Destruction of drug or contaminated articles

Incineration: 700°C.[3]

Chemical: 10% sodium hypochlorite (1% available chlorine) solution/24 hours.[1]

Contact with skin: Wash well with water, or soap and water. If the eyes are contaminated, immediate irrigation with 0.9% sodium chloride should be carried out.[1]

References

1 *ABPI Data Sheet Compendium 1995–96* (1995) DataPharm Publications Ltd, London, pp. 1328–30.
2 *ABPI Data Sheet Compendium 1995–96* (1995) DataPharm Publications Ltd, London, pp. 1330–1.

3 Pharmacia Ltd. (1992) Personal communication.

4 *Idarubicin: Summary of preclinical studies up to March 1980* (1992) (MG Cagnasso ed.), Farmitalia Carlo-Erba Ltd.

5 Beijnen JH *et al.* (1986) Aspects of the degradation kinetics of doxorubicin in aqueous solution. *Int. J. Pharm.* **32**, 123–31.

6 Tavoloni N *et al.* (1980) Photolytic degradation of adriamycin. *J. Pharm. Pharmacol.* **32**, 860–2.

7 Wood MJ *et al.* (1990) Photodegradation of doxorubicin, daunorubicin and epirubicin measured by high-performance liquid chromatography. *J. Clin. Pharm. Ther.* **15**, 291–300.

8 Trissel LA (1994) *Handbook of Injectable Drugs*, 8th edn. American Society of Hospital Pharmacists, Bethesda, USA.

9 Beijnen JH *et al.* (1985) Stability of anthracycline antitumour agents in infusion fluids. *J. Parenter. Sci. Technol.* **39**, 220–2.

10 Trissel LA (1993) Idarubicin hydrochloride turbidity versus incompatibility. *Am. J. Hosp. Pharm.* **50**, 1134, 1137.

11 Bosanquet AG (1986) Stability of solutions of antineoplastic agents during preparation and storage for *in vitro* assays: II. Assay methods, adriamycin and the other antitumour antibiotics. *Cancer Chemother. Pharmacol.* **17**, 1–10.

12 Wood MJ (1989) MPhil. Thesis, University of Aston, Birmingham, UK.

13 Turowski RC, Durthaler JM (1991) Visual compatibility of idarubicin hydrochloride with selected drugs during simulated Y-site injection. *Am. J. Hosp. Pharm.* **48**, 2181–4.

14 Speth PAJ *et al.* (1986) Plasma and human leukaemic cell pharmacokinetics of oral and intravenous 4-demethoxydaunomycin. *Clin. Pharmacol. Ther.* **40**, 643–9.

15 Speth PAJ *et al.* (1989) Idarubicin *vs* daunorubicin: Pre-clinical and clinical pharmacokinetic studies. *Semin. Oncol.* **16** (Suppl.2), 2–9.

16 Vogler WR *et al.* (1988) A phase III trial comparing daunorubicin or idarubicin combined with cytosine arabinoside in acute myelogenous leukaemia (AML). Abstract of two symposia, *XXII Congress of the International Society of Haematology*, Milan, Italy.

Prepared by Jayne Wood

IFOSFAMIDE

1 General details

Approved names: Ifosfamide, iphosphamide, isophosphamide.

Proprietary name: Mitoxana.

Manufacturer or supplier: ASTA Medica Ltd.

Presentation and formulation details: White freeze-dried powder in glass vials containing 1 g or 2 g ifosfamide. Contains no excipients.

Storage and shelf-life of unopened container: Vials should be stored below 25°C, protected from light.[1] The intact vials are stable for at least five years at 22–25°C.[2]

2 Chemistry

Type: Nitrogen mustard.

Molecular structure: N,3-(2-chloroethyl)tetrahydro-2H-1,2,3 oxaphosphorin-2-amine.

Molecular weight: 261.1.

Solubility: In water: 1 in 10; in methylene chloride up to 1 g/ml and in carbon disulphide 15 mg/ml. Readily soluble in ethanol.

3 Stability profile

3.1 Physical and chemical stability

Ifosfamide is relatively stable after reconstitution.

Effect of pH: No information available.

Effect of light: Infusions should be protected from light during storage. Light protection during administration is not necessary.

Container compatibility: Compatible with glass, PVC and polypropylene containers.[3]

Compatibility with other drugs: Compatible with mesna (*see* mesna monograph page 368 for details). No further information is available.

Reconstitution of ifosfamide with water for injections containing benzyl alcohol (0.9%) results in the formation of two separate liquid phases.[4] Ifosfamide should, therefore, be reconstituted with unpreserved water for injections.

3.2 Stability in clinical practice

Reconstituted solutions are chemically stable for seven days at room temperature and for six weeks under refrigeration.[2,3] Ifosfamide infusion 50 mg/ml in 10 ml polypropylene syringes showed no drug loss over seven days at 4 and 20°C.[5] Combinations of ifosfamide (50 mg/ml) and mesna (40 mg/ml) in 10 ml syringes were stable for 28 days at 4 and 20°C.[5] Ifosfamide (50 mg/ml) and combinations of ifosfamide with mesna (each 50 mg/ml) showed no drug loss at 37°C over 24 hours.[6] In a further study,[7] ifosfamide in aqueous solution (either alone or mixed with mesna) was found to be stable for nine days when stored in a dark environment at 27°C.

Dilution of the reconstituted solution to ifosfamide concentrations of 16 and 0.6 mg/ml in the following intravenous infusion solutions resulted in 1–5% decomposition over seven days at room temperature and no decomposition over six weeks under refrigeration:[2]

5% glucose in Ringer's injection, lactated
5% glucose in 0.9% sodium chloride
glucose in water
Ringer's injection, lactated
0.45% sodium chloride
0.9% sodium chloride
1/6 M sodium lactate.

3.3 Stability in specialized delivery systems

Ifosfamide, 20, 40 or 80 mg/ml in 0.9% sodium chloride, or 80 mg/ml in water for injections, was reported to be stable for eight days at 35°C stored in 100 ml PVC medication cassettes (Pharmacia device).[8] Ifosfamide in combination with mesna (each 50 mg/ml) was stable for 24 hours at 37°C in Graseby 9000 Medication Cassettes.[6]

4 Clinical use

Type of cytotoxic agent: Alkylating agent of the nitrogen-mustard type, activated by hepatic microsomal enzymes to produce anti-tumour metabolites.

Main indications: Tumours of the lung, ovary, cervix, breast and testis and soft-tissue sarcoma. Ifosfamide also produces response in osteosarcoma, malignant lymphoma, carcinoma of the pancreas, head and neck tumours and acute leukaemias (except AML).

Dosage: Ifosfamide should not be used without the concurrent administration of mesna (*see* mesna monograph page 368).

The usual dose for each course is $8–10 \text{ g/m}^2$, equally fractionated as single daily doses over five days or alternatively, $5–6 \text{ g/m}^2$ (maximum of 10 g) administered as a 24 hour infusion. Courses are normally repeated at intervals of two to four weeks for intermittent therapy, or three to four weeks for 24 hour infusions. The white cell count should not be less than $4 \times 10^3/\text{mm}^3$ and the platelet count not less than $100 \times 10^3/\text{mm}^3$ before starting each course. Usually, four courses are given, but up to seven (six by 24 hour infusion) have been administered.

5 Preparation of injection

Reconstitution: The injection should be reconstituted to give a solution of approximately 8% (80 mg/ml) using:

▼ 12.5 ml water for injections with 1 g ifosfamide
▼ 25 ml water for injections with 2 g ifosfamide.

Bolus administration: Dilute to less than 4% and inject into the vein with the patient supine, or inject directly into a fast-running infusion.

Intravenous infusion: Infuse in 5% glucose, glucose-saline or 0.9% sodium chloride infusion over 30–120 minutes, or infuse over 24 hours in 3 × 1 l glucose-saline or 0.9% sodium chloride. Increased doses of mesna are recommended in children and in patients with urothelial damage from previous therapies (*see* mesna monograph page 368).

Extravasation: Non-irritant.

6 Destruction of drug or contaminated waste

Incineration: 1000°C.

Chemical: 2 N sodium hydroxide in dimethyl formamide/24 hours.

Contact with skin: Wash with water.

References

1 *ABPI Data Sheet Compendium 1995–96* (1995) DataPharm Publications Ltd, London, pp. 104–5.
2 Trissel LA *et al.* (1979) Investigational drug information: ifosfamide and semustine. *Drug Intell. Clin. Pharm.* **13**, 340–3.
3 Trissel LA *et al.* (1985) *Investigational drugs pharmaceutical data*. NCI, Bethesda, Maryland, USA.
4 Behme RJ *et al.* (1988) Incompatibility of ifosfamide with benzyl-alcohol-preserved bacteriostatic water for injections. *Am. J. Hosp. Pharm.* **45**, 627–8.
5 Adams PS *et al.* (1987) Pharmaceutical aspects of home infusion therapy for cancer patients. *Pharm. J.* **238**, 476–8.
6 Sewell GJ, Priston MJ, Allsopp M *et al.* (1994) Stability of drug infusions in ambulatory infusion devices. *Aust. J. Hosp. Pharm.* **24**, 102.
7 Radford JA *et al.* (1990) The stability of ifosfamide in aqueous solution and its suitability for continuous 7-day infusion by ambulatory pump. *Cancer Chemother. Pharmacol.* **26**, 144–6.
8 Munoz M *et al.* (1992) Stability of ifosfamide in 0.9% sodium chloride solution in water for injection in a portable IV pump cassette. *Am. J. Hosp. Pharm.* **49**, 1137–9.

Prepared by Graham Sewell

MELPHALAN

1 General details

Approved names: Melphalan, phenylalanine mustard, L-sarcolysine.

Proprietary name: Alkeran.

Manufacturer or supplier: Wellcome Medical Division.

Presentation and formulation details: 50 mg sterile anhydrous melphan BP (as the hydrochloride) in 20 ml vial; includes 20 mg povidone K12.[1] A 10 ml buffer solution with 60% v/v propylene glycol, sodium citrate and ethanol.[1]

Storage and shelf-life of unopened container: The shelf-life is three years when stored below 30°C and protected from light.

2 Chemistry

Type: Alkylating agent related to nitrogen mustard.

Molecular structure: 4-[bis(2-chloroethyl)amino]-L-phenylalanine.

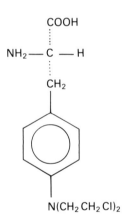

Molecular weight: 305.2 (base); 345.9 (hydrochloride).

Solubility: Practically insoluble in water, soluble in ethanol.

3 Stability profile

3.1 Physical and chemical stability

The reconstituted drug is relatively unstable. The rate of degradation is influenced by temperature, aqueous vehicle and pH.[2] The degradation products are also less water-soluble than melphalan and a precipitate may form on standing, especially in the reconstituted vial.[3] The reconstituted injection retains 90% of its initial potency for approximately 19 hours.

Effect of pH: The drug is most stable at pH 3.0, stability is slightly reduced at pH 5–7 but substantially reduced at pH 9.0. Data from Tabibi and Cradock[3] have quantified this effect as shown on the following page.

pH (buffer)	$t_{1/2}$
3.0	5.3 h
5.0	4.9 h
7.0	4.8 h
9.0	3.9 h

The addition of reconstituted injection to infusions will tend to acidify such solutions. The pH of infusions after adding melphalan injection (final concentration 40 µg/ml) are as follows:[2]

infusion fluid	pH
5% glucose	4.1
0.9% sodium chloride	4.2
Ringer's lactate	5.9

Effect of chloride ions: Studies have shown that chloride reduces the rate of hydrolysis of melphalan.[2,4-6] For example, $t_{90\%}$ of melphalan in 5% glucose is 1.5 hours and in 0.9% sodium chloride is 4.5 hours at 20°C. Hydrophobic interaction of melphalan with propylene glycol also contributes to greater stability.[6]

Studies[2] provide some evidence of the significance of storage temperature on rates of degradation. Increasing the temperature from 15 to 20°C raised the degradation rate by approximately 25% in various infusion fluids. Unfortunately no studies were conducted under refrigerated storage, but the manufacturer suggests the drug may precipitate on refrigeration.

Effect of light: No information available.

Degradation pathways: Melphalan is degraded to mono-hydroxy-melphalan (II), and then to di-hydroxy-melphalan (III).[3] The kinetics can be described as pseudo-first order (*see* Figure 1).[2,5]

Degradation products are said to be much less cytotoxic.[7]

Container compatibility: Melphalan is compatible with plastic containers, administration sets and plastic syringes.[7]

Compatibility with other drugs: Physical compatibility of melphalan, 0.1 mg/ml, was investigated with a wide range of drugs during simulated Y-site administration. Results indicate that malphalan, 0.1 mg/ml, is compatible with most drugs.[8]

3.2 Stability in clinical practice

Reconstituted vials must be used or further diluted within 30 minutes.[1] They can be further diluted in 0.9% sodium chloride and infused over two hours. The diluted drug should not be stored for longer than two hours at ambient temperature (refrigeration may cause precipitation). Melphalan is not absorbed by in-line filters.[9] It is also suggested that solutions of melphalan can be stored frozen in 0.9% sodium chloride for six months without undergoing significant degradation.[10] Melphalan, 0.2 mg/ml, in 0.9% sodium chloride infusion in PVC bags was stable (not more than 10% degradation) for up to 72 hours at –20°C, six hours at 4°C and three hours at room temperature (not greater than 26°C).[10] No precipitation was observed during storage at 4°C.[10] It was also reported that stability was greater in 3% sodium chloride, extending to 48 hours at 4°C and six hours at room temperature.[10] Solutions containing 2 mg/ml melphalan showed similar stability.[10]

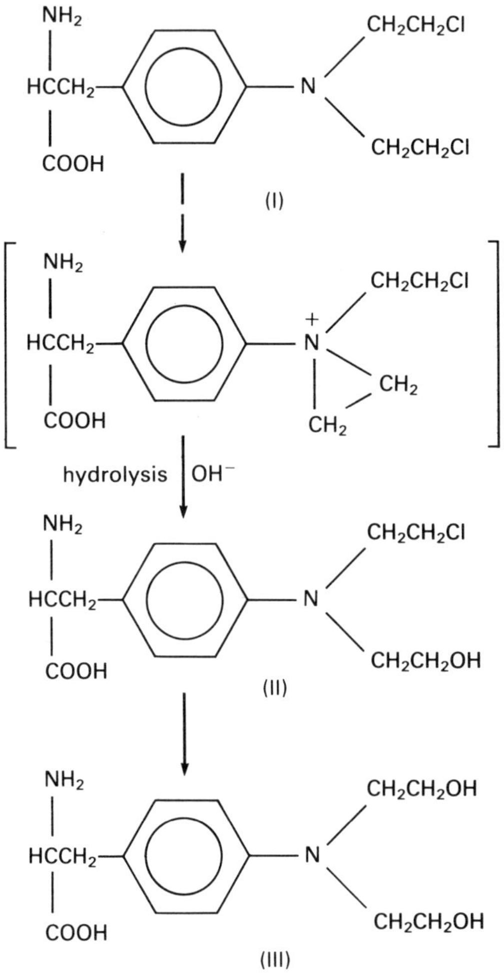

Figure 1: *Degradation of melphalan; first-step hydrolysis*

No special precautions are required to protect the injection from normal lighting conditions; however, exposure to strong daylight should be avoided.

3.3 Stability in specialized delivery systems

No data available.

4 Clinical use

Type of cytotoxic: Alkylating agent.

Main indications: Localized malignant melanomas; localized soft-tissue sarcoma of the extremities.

Dosage: Between 8 and 30 mg/m², administered intravenously every two to six weeks, or by regional perfusion of between 0.6 and 1.5 mg/kg (depending on the site) through the part of the body affected by the tumour.

5 Preparation of injection

Reconstitution: Add the contents of the diluent vial to the freeze-dried powder and immediately shake vigorously until solution is complete. The resulting solution contains 5 mg/ml anhydrous melphalan. Refrigeration of the solution should be avoided.[1]

Bolus administration: Inject within 30 minutes of preparation into the tubing of a fast-running infusion.

Intravenous infusion: Dilute only in 0.9% sodium chloride and infuse slowly over two hours.[9] Consult relevant literature for details and alternative methods of tissue perfusion.

Extravasation: Not very irritant (*see* Chapter 6).

6 Destruction of drug or contaminated articles

Incineration: 500°C.

Chemical: 5% sodium thiosulphate in sodium hydroxide solution/24 hours.

Contact with skin: Wash with water.

References

1 *ABPI Data Sheet Compendium 1995–96* (1995) DataPharm Publications Ltd, London, pp. 1913–16.
2 Flora KP *et al.* (1979) Application of a simple HPLC method for the determination of melphalan in the presence of its hydrolysis products. *J. Chromatogr.* **177**, 91–7.
3 Tabibi SE, Cradock JC (1984) Stability of melphalan in infusion fluids. *Am. J. Hosp. Pharm.* **41**, 1380–2.
4 Trissel LA (1992) *Handbook on Injectable Drugs*, 8th edn. American Society of Hospital Pharmacists, Bethesda, Maryland, USA.
5 Chang SY *et al.* (1978) Hydrolysis and protein binding of melphalan. *J. Pharm. Sci.* **67**, 682–4.
6 Chang SY *et al.* (1979) The stability of melphalan in the presence of chloride ions. *J. Pharm. Pharmacol.* **31**, 853–4.
7 Calmic Medical Division. Unpublished data.
8 Tissel LA, Martinez JF (1993) Physical compatibility of melphalan with selected drugs during simulated Y-site administration. *Am. J. Hosp. Phar.* **50**, 2359–63.
9 Bosanquet AG (1985) Stability of solutions of melphalan during preparation and storage for *in vitro* chemosensitivity assays. *J. Pharm. Sci.* **74**, 348–51.
10 Pinguet F *et al.* (1994) Effect of sodium chloride concentration and temperature on melphalan stability during storage and use. *Am. J. Hosp. Pharm.* **51**, 2701–4.

Prepared by Michael Allwood

METHOTREXATE

1 General details

Approved name: Methotrexate.

Proprietary name: Methotrexate injection.

Manufacturer or supplier: Lederle Laboratories Ltd, David Bull Laboratories Ltd (DBL).

Presentation and formulation details:

Methotrexate injection (Lederle): A clear, yellow, aqueous, isotonic solution containing methotrexate sodium equivalent to 50 mg/2 ml, 200 mg/8 ml, 500 mg/20 ml, 1 g/40 ml, 5 g/200 ml of methotrexate per vial, together with sodium chloride and sodium hydroxide or hydrochloric acid to adjust the pH to approximately 8.5. All formulations are preservative-free.

Methotrexate injection (DBL): A clear, yellowish solution of methotrexate in water for injections with sodium hydroxide to adjust pH to between 8 and 9. The lower strengths are made isotonic with sodium chloride. The 1 g in 10 ml and 5 g in 50 ml presentations do not contain sodium chloride and are slightly hypertonic. It is available in the following strengths and packs: 5 mg/2 ml, 50 mg/2 ml, 500 mg/20 ml, 1 g/10 ml, 5 g/50 ml. All solutions are preservative-free.

Storage and shelf-life of unopened containers: Methotrexate preparations (Lederle) should be stored at controlled room temperature (15–30°C) and protected from direct sunlight. All preparations have a shelf-life of two years from the date of manufacture.

Methotrexate injection (DBL) should be stored below 25°C. It should be protected from light and freezing. All preparations have a shelf-life of two years from the date of manufacture.

2 Chemistry

Type: 4-amino-N-methyl analogue of folic acid.

Molecular structure:

Molecular weight: 454.44.

Solubility: Practically insoluble in water. Dissolves in solutions of mineral acids and in dilute solutions of alkali hydroxides and carbonates.[1]

3 Stability profile

3.1 Physical and chemical stability

Methotrexate is relatively stable in aqueous solution provided the recommended storage conditions are observed. The compound is susceptible both to hydrolytic and photolytic degradation. The rate of hydrolytic degradation increases with increase in pH, with minimum degradation occurring between pH 6.6–8.2[2]

Degradation pathways: The major hydrolytic degradation compound is N-methyl-pteroylglutamic acid (methopterin). The major photolytic degradation compounds are *p*-aminobenzoylglutamic acid and 2-amino-4-hydroxypteridine-6-carboxylic acid.[3]

Effect of light: The drug is light-sensitive and forms a yellow precipitate on prolonged exposure to direct sunlight. Polypropylene and styrene acrylonitrile syringes provide better light protection than glass ampoules when the drug is stored under controlled light conditions at 25°C.[4] In all cases, no precipitate was observed over a seven day storage period. Samples stored in the dark showed no evidence of precipitation.[4]

McElnay *et al.*[5] studied the photodegradation of methotrexate 0.1% w/v in 0.9% w/v sodium chloride in three burette administration systems (a standard set, a 'light-protective' Amberset and a 'low adsorption' Sureset (Avon Medical)). Storage under normal lighting conditions (diffuse daylight/fluorescent tube room lighting) led to little change in drug concentration over the first 24 hours of storage although a decrease in concentration (maximum 12%) was noted in both the standard sets and Suresets by 48 hours. A much more rapid decrease in methotrexate concentration was demonstrated when the drug solution was exposed to sunlight. An 11% decline in methotrexate concentration occurred in the standard sets in seven hours (Suresets not investigated). The use of Ambersets, or wrapping the standard sets in tinfoil prevented photodegradation over this period. Storage in the administration tubing of all three sets under normal lighting conditions resulted in greater than 10% degradation within 12 hours in the standard sets and Suresets and within 48 hours in the light-protected Suresets and Ambersets. All these results were obtained for a static system and it is difficult to extrapolate them to the dynamic situation of an intravenous administration.

Effect of pH: Methotrexate is a bicarboxylic acid with a pK_a in the range 4.8–5.5.[6] Hence, it is essentially ionized at physiological pH. At pH values between 2.6 and 6.6, the drug is converted to the bicarboxylic acid which is relatively insoluble in aqueous solution and will precipitate. Commercially available injection is stabilized to approximately pH 8.4, however, dilution in acidic solutions may result in precipitation of the drug. For this reason, dilutions in 5% glucose should be checked carefully for evidence of precipitation.

Container compatibility: At a pH value of 8.4, methotrexate injection is largely ionized and, therefore, is unlikely to exhibit sorption phenomena.

McElnay *et al.*[5] found the sorption of methotrexate, 0.1% w/v in 0.9% w/v sodium chloride, stored in 'low sorption' Suresets and standard or Ambersets (Avon Medical) to be negligible, but were unable to explain the greater than 10% loss of drug when methotrexate was stored in light-protected polybutadiene and PVC tubing for 48 hours at room temperature. No other studies have shown significant sorption to PVC containers. The sorption of methotrexate in 5% glucose to the latex reservoir of Baxter infusors was also found to be negligible.[7]

Methotrexate 50 mg in 100 ml, 0.9% w/v sodium chloride was not absorbed by a 0.2 μm endotoxin-retentive and end-line filter (Pall Intravenous Set Saver, Pall Biomedical Ltd) when infused at a rate of 80 ml/hr.[8]

Although extraction into solution is possible, especially with plastic syringes, the extent and rate of leaching are likely to be low at room temperature.[9,10] It should be noted, however, that 2-mercaptobenzothiazole (a mercaptan present in the rubber plunger) is soluble in alkali and alkali carbonate solutions[11] and may leach into the alkaline methotrexate injection on prolonged storage in plastic syringes. Mercaptans may cause problems as analytical or toxicological contaminants.

Compatibility with other drugs: D'Arcy[12] found methotrexate to be chemically and physically incompatible with cytarabine, fluorouracil and prednisolone sodium phosphate. However, two other studies have shown the drug to be compatible and stable with cytarabine and fluorouracil under defined storage conditions. In the first study[13] the stability of cytarabine, methotrexate sodium and hydrocortisone sodium succinate admixtures was investigated. Two admixtures: (cytarabine 50 mg, methotrexate 12 mg (as the sodium salt) and hydrocortisone 25 mg (as the sodium succinate salt); and cytarabine 30 mg, methotrexate 12 mg (as the sodium salt) and hydrocortisone 15 mg (as the sodium succinate salt)) were prepared in one of four diluents (Elliott's B solution, 0.9% sodium chloride, 5% glucose and lactated Ringer's). The drugs were reconstituted according to manufacturers' instructions with the infusion fluid under test. After reconstitution, the drug solutions were mixed in the desired proportions and diluted to 12 ml with the respective infusion fluid. Each admixture was filtered through a 0.45 μm membrane filter and placed in a 12 ml disposable syringe (type of plastic not identified) and kept at $25 \pm 0.1°C$ in a water bath. Cytarabine and methotrexate were stable in the fluids studied for 24 hours at 25°C. Alteration in stability related to vehicles or drug concentration combinations was not evident and the stability of each of the drugs did not appear to be affected by the presence of the other two drugs. Hydrocortisone sodium succinate was found to be less stable in Elliott's B solution, with only 94.1% of the drug remaining in the first admixture, and 86% remaining in the second after 24 hours. Alkaline catalysis may explain the increased degradation of the drug in Elliott's B solution, which has a higher pH than the other vehicles. No precipitation was observed in either group of admixtures during eight hours at 25°C, although storage for several days resulted in some precipitation. The nature of the precipitate was not identified.

At the concentrations studied, cytarabine, methotrexate and hydrocortisone sodium succinate may be mixed in 0.9% sodium chloride, 5% glucose or lactated Ringer's and stored in plastic disposable syringes for up to 24 hours at 25°C. Admixtures in Elliott's B solution should be used within ten hours.

The second study[14] investigated the compatibility and stability of cyclophosphamide, methotrexate and 5-fluorouracil in a three-drug admixture. Cyclophosphamide (100 mg), methotrexate (1.5 mg), and 5-fluorouracil (500 mg) were reconstituted in a total volume of 60 ml of 0.9% sodium chloride. The solution was maintained at room temperature in PVC plastic reservoir bags (Lifecare 1500 System, Abbott). No significant loss of 5-fluorouracil or methotrexate was observed up to 14 days after reconstitution of the three-drug admixture. However, a 9.3% loss of cyclophosphamide was observed, accompanied by the appearance of a degradation product in the HPLC chromatogram after seven days. Control admixtures indicated that the cyclophosphamide and methotrexate were chemically incompatible and that there was a pH change in this admixture from 6.6 to 4.57. At this pH methotrexate stability is compromised.

Based on this information, it may be possible to administer cyclophosphamide, methotrexate and 5-fluorouracil as a three-drug admixture in an infusion pump, in the proportions reported, for up to seven days. However, solutions should be checked carefully for precipitation and such admixtures should not be used in implantable infusion pumps.

In addition, Trissel[15] lists a wide range of compatibility information. Although useful for reference purposes, much of the data relate to short-term physical compatibility of admixtures in the laboratory setting and are not applicable clinically.

3.2 Stability in clinical practice

Although the manufacturers do not recommend re-use of the methotrexate injection after opening, its relative stability in aqueous solution would suggest that, provided the injection is manipulated under aseptic conditions and is stored in the original container at 4–8°C in the absence of light once opened, chemical and physical stability will be preserved. In general, a shelf-life of one month at 4°C after opening would seem to be satisfactory.

Infusions: Information on the stability of the drug, when diluted in the recommended solutions for infusion, is variable. The manufacturers are limited by the terms of their product licences to recommend a maximum shelf-life of 24 hours at 25°C. However, a number of reports suggest that methotrexate is stable over a wide range of concentrations when stored in Viaflex (Baxter) containers for longer than 24 hours.[16–20] In particular, work carried out by Baxter Laboratories[17] indicated that, at a concentration of 1–10 mg/ml in 5% glucose and 1.25–12.5 mg/ml in 0.9% sodium chloride infusions, methotrexate is stable (<10% degradation) for up to one month at 4°C, and five days at 25°C when stored in both Baxter infusors and Viaflex minibags. More recent data[18] indicate that solutions of methotrexate ranging from 1.25–12.5 mg/ml reconstituted with 0.9% sodium chloride are chemically stable for at least 15 days in the Baxter infusor when stored at 4°C. However, due to lack of stability data at 33°C, the company advise that methotrexate is delivered using the half-day infusor only.

Further studies[19] on the stability of methotrexate 1.25–12.5 mg/ml in 0.9% sodium chloride, stored in both glass and PVC containers (Viaflex, Baxter), have shown that the drug is physically and chemically stable for up to 15 weeks at 4°C followed by one week's storage at room temperature.

Although there is some evidence that methotrexate infusion solutions prepared in Viaflex (Baxter) minibags can be frozen to –20°C and stored for at least three months without significant reduction in methotrexate concentration or change in pH,[20] the use of microwave ovens to thaw solutions prior to use should not be undertaken without careful validation of the thawing process.

Syringe storage: Methotrexate injection, at a concentration of 50 mg/ml or less, stored in sealed Monoject (Sherwood Medical) or Plastipak (Becton-Dickinson) plastic disposable syringes in the absence of light at a temperature not exceeding 25°C, is stable (<10% degradation) for a period of up to eight months.[4] Storage in Sabre (Gillette) and Steriseal (NI Ltd) syringes should not exceed 70 days.[4]

3.3 Stability in specialized delivery systems

Methotrexate, over the concentration range 0.33–10.0 mg/ml in 0.9% w/v sodium chloride stored in an implantable infusion pump (Model 400, Shiley Infusaid Inc.)

at 37°C, was found to be stable for up to 12 days.[21] The solutions were filtered through a 5 μm filter prior to addition to the pump.

Methotrexate (Lederle) at a concentration of 25 mg/ml in 0.9% sodium chloride stored in a Medication Cassette reservoir (Pharmacia Deltec) exhibited no evidence of degradation over seven days storage at 25°C and 14 days storage at 5°C.[22]

4 Clinical use

Type of cytotoxic: Antimetabolite.

Main indications: Meningeal leukaemia, choriocarcinoma, non-Hodgkin's lymphomas, solid tumours, severe psoriasis, rheumatoid arthritis unresponsive to conventional therapy.

Dosage and administration: Methotrexate injection may be given by the intramuscular, intravenous (bolus injection or infusion), intrathecal, intra-arterial or intraventricular routes. Subcutaneous administration of methotrexate has been evaluated.[23] Methotrexate administered by this route is well tolerated and well absorbed. Intra-tumour administration using implantable catheters and subcutaneous refillable pumps has also been investigated.[21]

Dosages vary considerably depending on the condition being treated and are based on the patient's body weight or surface area,[24,25] except in the case of intrathecal or intraventricular administration, when a maximum dose of 15 mg is recommended.

It must be noted that all preparations of methotrexate (Lederle) are suitable for intrathecal use, although it is recommended that only the low volume preparations are used to avoid possible confusion. Methotrexate injection (DBL), 500 mg/20 ml, 1 g/10 ml and 5 g/50 ml, are not suitable for intrathecal use. The 1 g/10 ml and 5 g/50 ml solutions are hypertonic.

High doses may cause the precipitation of methotrexate and its metabolites in the renal tubules. A high fluid throughput and alkalinization of the urine to pH 6.5–7.0 by the oral or intravenous administration of sodium bicarbonate (e.g. 5×625 mg tablets every three hours) or acetazolamide (500 mg orally four times a day) is recommended as a preventive measure.[24,25]

Doses greater than 100 mg should be given by intravenous infusion over a period not exceeding 24 hours. Lower doses may be given by rapid intravenous bolus injection over two to three minutes, or by infusion. The concentration of the final injection is not critical.

5 Preparation of injection

Dilution: The drug may be diluted in 0.9% sodium chloride, 5% glucose, glucose-saline, compound sodium chloride, compound sodium lactate infusions or Elliott's B solution.

Extravasation: Irritant, but does not cause tissue damage (*see* Chapter 6).

6 Destruction of drug or contaminated articles

Incineration: 1000°C.[26]

Chemical: None recommended.

Contact with skin: Wash with water and soothe any transient stinging with a bland cream. Irrigate eyes with copious amounts of water or saline. If significant quantities are inhaled or injected, calcium folinate cover should be considered.

References

1 Anon. (1993) *The Extra Pharmacopoeia*, 30th edn. (JEF Reynolds ed.), The Pharmaceutical Press, London.

2 Hansen J et al. (1983) Kinetics of degradation of methotrexate in aqueous solution. *Int. J. Pharm.* **16**, 141–52.

3 Chatterji DC, Gallelli JF (1978) Thermal and photolytic decomposition of methotrexate in aqueous solution. *J. Pharm. Sci.* **67**, 526–31.

4 Wright MP, Newton JM (1988) Stability of methotrexate injection in prefilled plastic disposable syringes. *Int. J. Pharm.* **45**, 237–44.

5 McElnay JC et al. (1988) Stability of methotrexate and vinblastine in burette administration sets. *Int. J. Pharm.* **47**, 239–47.

6 Bleyer WA (1978) The clinical pharmacology of methotrexate. New applications of an old drug. *Cancer* **41**, 36–50.

7 Bertocchio F et al. (1986) Study of the viability of an infusion system. *J. Pharm. Clin.* **5**, 331–9.

8 Stevens RF, Wilkins KM (1989) Use of cytotoxic drugs with an end-line filter: A study of four drugs commonly administered to paediatric patients. *J. Clin. Pharm. Ther.* **14**, 475–9.

9 Sherwood Medical Industries Ltd (1984) Personal communication.

10 Gillette UK Ltd (1984) Personal communication.

11 *The Merck Index*, 10th edn (1983) Merck and Co. Inc., Rathway, New Jersey, USA.

12 D'Arcy PF (1983) Reactions and interactions in handling anticancer drugs. *Drug Intell. Clin. Pharm.* **17**, 532–8.

13 Cheung Y et al. (1984) Stability of cytarabine, methotrexate sodium and hydrocortisone sodium succinate admixtures. *Am. J. Hosp. Pharm.* **41**, 1802–6.

14 Lokich J et al. (1989) Cyclophosphamide, methotrexate, and 5-fluorouracil in a three-drug admixture. Phase I trial of 14-day continuous ambulatory infusion. *Cancer* **63**, 822–4.

15 Trissel LA (1994) *Handbook on Injectable Drugs*, 8th edn. American Society of Hospital Pharmacists, Bethesda, Maryland, USA.

16 Roach M (1979) Methotrexate infusions. *Pharm. J.* **223**, 557.

17 Baxter Healthcare Ltd (1985) Information chart.

18 Baxter Healthcare Ltd (1992) Personal communication.

19 Vincke BJ et al. (1989) Extended stability of 5-fluorouracil and methotrexate solutions in PVC containers. *Int. J. Pharm.* **54**, 181–9.

20 Dyvik O et al. (1986) Methotrexate in infusion solutions: A stability test for the hospital pharmacy. *J. Clin. Hosp. Pharm.* **11**, 343–8.

21 Nierenberg D et al. (1991) Continuous intratumoral infusion of methotrexate for recurrent glioblastoma: A pilot study. *Neurosurgery* **28**, 752–61.

22 Landersjo L, Nyhammar E (1989) Stability and compatibility of methotrexate in medication cassettes. A study by Apoteksbolaget AB, Stockholm, Sweden.

23 Balis FM et al. (1988) Pharmacokinetics of subcutaneous methotrexate. *J. Clin. Oncol.* **6**, 1882–6.

24 *ABPI Data Sheet Compendium 1995–96* (1995) DataPharm Publications Ltd, London, pp. 797–800.

25 Methotrexate (DBL) Data Sheet, October 1993. Amended 18 January 1995.

26 Bristol Myers Pharmaceuticals Ltd (1985) Personal communication.

Prepared by Patricia Wright

MITOMYCIN

1 General details

Approved names: Mitomycin C, mitomycin X.

Proprietary name: Mitomycin C Kyowa.

Manufacturer or supplier: Kyowa Hakko UK Ltd.

Presentation and formulation details: Purple powder in vials containing 2 mg, 10 mg or 20 mg mitomycin C. Vials contain 24 mg sodium chloride/1 mg mitomycin.

Storage and shelf-life of unopened container: Four years at ambient temperature and protected from light.

2 Chemistry

Molecular structure: 1 S-(1,8,8a,8b)-6-amino-8-(aminocarbonyl)oxy methyl-1,1,2,-8,8a,8b-hexahydro-methoxy-5-methyl-azirino 2',3',4,7, pyrrolo 1,2-indole-4,7-dione.

Molecular weight: 349.

Solubility: Sparingly soluble in water.

3 Stability profile

3.1 Physical and chemical stability

Mitomycin C is relatively unstable in aqueous solution, showing losses of approximately 10% in seven days at 25°C.[1] In phosphate buffer, pH 7.4, losses of less than 5% in seven days were reported.[1] Stability is pH dependent and is greatest between pH 7 and 8.[2] Mitomycin is significantly less stable in acid conditions. A degradation rate constant of 5×10^{-6} s^{-1} at pH 4.9 and 20°C was reported.[2]

Degradation pathways: In alkali the 7 amino group is replaced by an hydroxyl group while the remainder of the mitosane skeleton remains intact.[2]

In acid the methoxy group is cleaved to form a 9-9a unsaturated bond.[2] Also the 1,2-fused aziridine ring is opened to give two isomeric compounds 1 and 2, with an hydroxyl group at position 1 and amino group at position 2.

1

2

Degradation rate is related to temperature after reconstitution. The reconstituted drug is significantly more stable at 2–6°C compared to ambient conditions. However, solubility is reduced substantially in the refrigerator and solutions containing 0.5 mg/ml in water for injections may precipitate at 2–6°C. The reconstituted drug should be protected from daylight, although light-induced degradation would not normally be a significant factor during bolus administration.

Container compatibility: There is no information to indicate that stability or compatibility are affected by storage in plastic syringes.

Infusion containers: Studies suggest that stability is not greatly influenced by the nature of the container in which the drug is diluted (glass bottles, PVC containers, Viaflex), when the dilution vehicle is 0.9% sodium chloride infusion.[3]

Administration sets: No information available. However, the studies would suggest that mitomycin does not adsorb significantly to standard administration sets.[3]

Compatibility with other drugs: Mitomycin 10–50 µg/ml in 0.9% sodium chloride may be mixed with bleomycin 20–30 IU, if used immediately, but compatibility depends on concentration.[4] Some degradation of bleomycin was reported, mitomycin stability was not assessed. Trissel reported studies suggesting that mitomycin may be physically compatible with a number of other drugs.[1]

3.2 Stability in clinical practice

Current guidelines from the UK supplier recommend that reconstituted vials are stable for 12 hours if stored at room temperature. Refrigeration may cause precipitation and is not, therefore, recommended. The drug may be further diluted, preferably in 0.9% sodium chloride. In 5% glucose, the diluted infusion should be used immediately, whilst it may be stored for not more than 12 hours in 0.9% sodium chloride. Few studies have been reported on stability after dilution in infusion fluids. One report[3] indicates that degradation is more rapid in 5% glucose than in 0.9% sodium chloride. The studies suggest an initial rapid fall (about 10–15%) in content after dilution. However, these studies have not been repeated and remain controversial.

The stability of mitomycin was also studied in 0.9% sodium chloride and 5% glucose, with or without buffering, stored in PVC containers.[5] The drug, at a concentration of 50 µg/ml, was unstable in both (unbuffered) vehicles. There was about 75% degradation in 5% glucose after 12 hours storage at room temperature. In contrast, if vehicles were phosphate-buffered to pH 7.8, mitomycin appeared to be stable for more than 120 days at 5°C. These results, however, have been questioned.[6] In a further study, unbuffered solutions in 0.9% sodium chloride were reported to be stable when stored at –30°C for at least 28 days.[7] Sorption to

PVC containers does not occur.[1,8] Mitomycin 0.5 mg/ml in water for injections, stored at 2–6°C, may precipitate.[1]

The most recent study indicates that solutions of mitomycin C dissolved in water for injections to give concentrations of 0.6 mg/ml stored in PVC (Urotainers™) bags protected from light were stable (less than 10% degradation) for four days at ambient temperature, or at least seven days at 4°C. Higher concentrations showed evidence of precipitation, especially at 4°C.[7] Solutions containing 0.6 mg/ml mitomycin C in 0.9% sodium chloride were stable for four days at 4°C.[7]

3.3 Stability in specialized delivery systems

No data available.

4 Clinical use

Type of cytotoxic: Anti-tumour antibiotic.

Main indications: Bladder, rectal and skin cancer.

Dosage: 4–10 mg (0.06–0.15 mg/kg) at one to six weekly intervals; up to 40–80 mg (2 mg/kg) cumulative doses have been given in some treatments.

5 Preparation of injection

Reconstitution: solutions are formed rapidly.
  2 mg vial + 5 ml water for injections or 20% glucose = 0.4 mg/ml
  10 mg vial + 10 ml water for injections or 20% glucose = 1 mg/ml
  20 mg vial + 20 ml water for injections or 20% glucose = 1 mg/ml
  May be stored for up to 12 hours at room temperature (do not refrigerate).[9]

Bolus administration: Inject slowly into a vein or slow-running drip at a rate of approximately 1 ml/min or more rapidly into a fast-running drip of 0.9% sodium chloride or 5% glucose. The stability of reconstituted drug in plastic syringes is not known.

Intravenous infusion: Dilute with 0.9% sodium chloride (use within 12 hours) or 5% glucose (use immediately) and infuse over one hour. Extended storage for four to seven days may be acceptable provided mitomycin C concentration does not exceed 0.6 mg/ml.[1]

Extravasation: Vesicant, very damaging (*see* Chapter 6).

6 Destruction of drug or contaminated articles

Incineration: 1000°C.

Chemical: 2–5% of hydrochloric acid or sodium hydroxide/12 hours.

Contact with skin: Very irritant, neutralize with several washes of sodium bicarbonate solution (8.4%) followed by soap and water; avoid hand creams.

References

1 Beijnen JH *et al.* (1990) Chemical stability of the anti-tumor drug mitomycin C in solutions for intravesical installation. *J. Parenter. Sci. Technol.* **44**, 332–5.

2 Beijner JH, Underberg WJM (1985) Degradation of mitomycin C in acidic conditions. *Int. J. Pharm.* **24**, 219–29.
3 Benuvento JA *et al.* (1981) Stability and compatibility of antitumour agents in glass and plastic containers. *Am. J. Hosp. Pharm.* **38**, 1914–18.
4 Dorr RT *et al.* (1982) Bleomycin compatibility with selected intravenous medications. *J. Med.* **13**, 121–30.
5 Quebberman EJ *et al.* (1985) Stability of mitomycin admixtures. *Am. J. Hosp. Pharm.* **42**, 1750–4.
6 Keller JH (1986) Stability of mitomycin admixtures. *Am. J. Hosp. Pharm.* **43**, 59–64.
7 Stole LML *et al.* (1986) Stability after freezing and thawing of solutions of Mitomycin C in plastic minibags for intravesical use. *Pharm. Weekbl. (Sci.)* **8**, 286–8.
8 Quebberman EJ, Hoffman NE (1986) Stability of mitomycin admixtures. *Am J. Hosp. Pharm.* **43**, 64.
9 *ABPI Data Sheet Compendium 1995–96* (1995) DataPharm Publications Ltd, London, pp. 760–1.

Prepared by Michael Allwood

MITOZANTRONE

1 General details

Approved name: Mitozantrone.

Proprietary name: Novantrone.

Manufacturer or supplier: Lederle Laboratories Ltd.

Presentation and formulation details: Vials containing mitozantrone dihydrochloride solution, equivalent to 2 mg/ml mitozantrone. Solutions of 20 mg in 10 ml, 25 mg in 12.5 ml and 30 mg in 15 ml are available. Each vial also contains: sodium chloride 0.8% w/v, sodium metabisulphate 0.01% w/v and sodium acetate/acetic acid buffer to approximately pH 3.[1]

Storage and shelf-life of unopened container: Store at controlled room temperature 15–25°C. Stable for two years from the date of manufacture.

2 Chemistry

Type: Anthracenedione.

Molecular structure: 1,4-dihydroxy-5,8-bis-2-(2-hydroxyethyl) amino ethylamine-9,10-anthraquinone dihydrochloride.

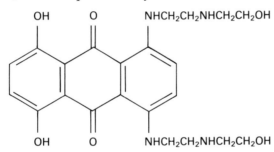

Molecular weight: 517.4.

Solubility: Water soluble.

3 Stability profile

3.1 Physical and chemical stability

Mitozantrone degrades by oxidation of the phenylenediamine moiety to the corresponding quinoneimine, which then hydrolyses to the quinone.[2]

Effect of pH: Stability is optimal in acidic conditions.

Effect of light: Vials of mitozantrone may precipitate under refrigerated storage. Exposure of vials to sunlight for one month has little effect on the potency or appearance of the product.

Container compatibility: Mitozantrone adsorbs on to glass but not on to polypropylene or PVC.[3,4]

Compatibility with other drugs: Unstable in alkaline infusions. The injection should not be mixed with infusions containing heparin as precipitation may occur.[1] Trissel[5] reported that hydrocortisone sodium phosphate or succinate may be compatible, but this may depend on the container.

3.2 Stability in clinical practice

Dilution to 5 mg/l in 0.9% sodium chloride or 5% glucose infusions produced solutions that were physically and chemically compatible, exhibiting no decomposition in 48 hours.[5] The Data Sheet[1] states that dilutions retain potency for 24 hours at room temperature. Polypropylene syringes containing mitozantrone diluted to 2 mg in 10 ml with water for injections (for use in continuous infusion schedules) were found to be stable for 14 days at 4 and 20°C[6] and for 24 hours at 37°C.[3] Studies on mitozantrone given as an intraperitoneal infusion demonstrated drug degradation in peritoneal fluid and concluded that the intraperitoneal route cannot be recommended for mitozantrone.[7]

3.3 Stability in specialized delivery systems

Mitozantrone infusions (0.2 mg/ml in water for injections) in PVC medication reservoirs (for use with an ambulatory infusion pump) were chemically and physically stable for 14 days at 4°C and under 'in-use' conditions at 37°C.[8] Mitozantrone infusions (0.1–0.5 mg/ml in 0.9% sodium chloride) in Single and Multiday Infusors (Baxter Healthcare) have been reported to be stable for two days at room temperature and for five days at 33°C.[9] Infusions containing 0.5 mg/ml mitozantrone in 0.9% sodium chloride have also been reported to be stable in the CADD Medication Cassette (Pharmacia Deltec) for ten days at 25°C or 14 days at 5°C.[10]

4 Clinical use

Type of cytotoxic: Antibiotic anti-tumour agent.

Indications: Advanced breast cancer, non-Hodgkin's lymphoma, adult acute non-lymphocytic leukaemia in relapse and paediatric leukaemia, hepatoma.

Dosage: As a single agent, 14 mg/m² (12 mg/m² in patients with low bone marrow reserves).

5 Preparation of injection

Dilute the required volume of mitozantrone solution to at least 50 ml in either 0.9% sodium chloride, 5% glucose or 0.18% sodium chloride and 4% glucose.

Bolus administration: Not recommended (mitozantrone must be diluted before administration).

Intravenous infusion: Mitozantrone infusion should be administered over not less than three minutes via the tubing of a freely-running intravenous infusion of the above fluids.

Extravasation: Mildly irritant (*see* Chapter 6).

6 Destruction of drug or contaminated articles

Incineration: 800°C.

Chemical: 40% sodium hypochlorite solution (4% available chlorine)/24 hours.

Contact with skin: Wash with water.

References

1 *ABPI Data Sheet Compendium 1995–1996* (1995) DataPharm Publications, London, pp. 808–10.

2 Reynolds DL *et al.* (1981) Clinical analysis for the antineoplastic agent 1,4-dihydroxy-5,8-bis-2(2-hydroxyethyl) aminoethyl-amino 9, 10-anthracenedione di-hydrochloride (NSC 301739) in plasma. *J. Chromatography* **222**, 225–40.

3 Sewell GJ *et al.* (1988) Pharmaceutical aspects of domiciliary continuous infusion chemotherapy. *Br. J. Cancer* **58**, 536.

4 Priston MJ, Sewell GJ (1994) Improved LC assay for the determination of mito-zantrone in plasma: analytical considerations. *J. Pharm. Biomed. Anal.* **12** (9), 1153–62.

5 Trissel LA *et al.* (1985) *Investigational Drugs, Pharmaceutical Data.* Pharmaceutical aspects of home infusion therapy for cancer patients. NCI, Bethesda, Maryland, USA.

6 Adams PS *et al.* (1987) Pharmaceutical aspects of home infusion therapy for cancer patients. *Pharm. J.* **328**, 476–8.

7 Sewell GJ, Priston MJ (1994) Pharmacokinetic and stability studies on mitozantrone injected into the peritoneal cavity. *Aust. J. Hosp. Pharm.* **24** (1), 99–100.

8 Northcott M *et al.* (1991) The stability of carboplatin, diamorphine, 5-fluorouracil and mitozantrone infusions in an ambulatory pump under storage and prolonged 'in-use' conditions. *J. Clin. Pharm. Ther.* **16**, 123–9.

9 Baxter Healthcare Ltd (1992) Personal communication.

10 Pharmacia Deltec (1991) Personal communication.

Prepared by Graham Sewell

MUSTINE

1 General details

Approved names: Chlormethine, mustine hydrochloride, mustagen, mechlorethamine hydrochloride, nitrogen mustard.

Proprietary name: Mustine hydrochloride for injection BP.

Manufacturer or supplier: Knoll Pharmaceuticals (Boots).

Presentation and formulation details: White lyophilized powder in 20 ml vial, containing 10 mg mustine hydrochloride with no excipients.

Storage and shelf-life of unopened container: Two years when stored at 2–15°C.

2 Chemistry

Molecular structure: 2-chloro-N-(2-chloroethyl)-N-methylethanamine hydrochloride.

$$H_3C - \overset{+}{\underset{H}{N}} \overset{CH_2-CH_2-Cl}{\underset{CH_2-CH_2-Cl}{<}}$$

Molecular weight: 192.5 (hydrochloride).

Solubility: Very soluble in water.

3 Stability profile

3.1 Physical and chemical stability

Degradation pathways: The degradation route of mustine hydrochloride (II) in dilute aqueous solution is shown below.

In aqueous solution mustine appears to lose alkylating activity relatively slowly. Alkylating activity arises from mustine together with compounds II and III in the degradation pathway. However, certain of these degradation products are either more carcinogenic than mustine, or may be more neurotoxic.[1,2] Kirk[1] has reviewed the conflicting reports in the literature concerning the rate of degradation of mustine in aqueous solution. It is pointed out that almost all studies were carried out using a test for alkylating activity which was not fully stability-indicating. Certain of the products of degradation have alkylating activity *in vitro*. However, an analysis of previous studies indicates that degradation is very pH-dependent,[3] the compound degrading rapidly in neutral or alkaline conditions. An unbuffered solution of mustine has a pH of 3–5 and will be more stable.

The study by Kirk[2] showed that solutions of mustine after reconstitution in 0.9% sodium chloride or water for injections (1 mg/ml) at room temperature, degrade by 8–10% in six hours, or by 3–6% at 4°C. Solutions diluted in 0.9% sodium chloride (18–36 µg/ml) exhibited 15% loss in six hours at room temperature, whilst in 5% glucose, about 11% loss was recorded.

Stability after reconstitution is decreased as the temperature is raised. Mustine is stable in the frozen state (–20°C) for four weeks, showing about 5% loss.[1,4]

Mustine does not appear to be unduly sensitive to light.

Container compatibility: Kirk[1] has shown that mustine does not appear to interact with styrene acrylonitrile syringes (Gillette) or PVC infusion containers.

Compatibility with other drugs: Incompatible with methohexital sodium.[5] No further information is available.

3.2 Stability in clinical practice

Reconstituted mustine injection (1 mg/ml) should be used within four hours at room temperature or six hours if stored in the refrigerator.[4] Mustine injection diluted in 500 ml of 0.9% sodium chloride should be administered within two hours, and dilutions in 500 ml of 5% glucose should be used within four hours.[1]

3.3 Stability in specialized delivery systems

No data available.

4 Clinical use

Type of cytotoxic: Alklyating agent.

Main indications: Hodgkin's disease (with other agents).

Dosage: Single dose of 0.4 mg/kg body weight or a course of four daily doses of 0.1 mg/kg body weight.

5 Preparation of injection

Reconstitution: To each vial add 10 ml water for injections or 0.9% sodium chloride. The resulting solution contains 1 mg/ml.

Bolus administration: Inject intravenously slowly (over two minutes) into the bolus site of a fast-running drip of 5% glucose or 0.9% sodium chloride (60 drops/minute).

Intravenous infusion: Add the required volume of reconstituted injection to 500 ml of 0.9% sodium chloride and infuse slowly over one to two hours.

Extravasation: Vesicant, very damaging (*see* Chapter 6).

6 Destruction of drug or contaminated articles

Incineration: 800°C.

Chemical:

Sodium hydroxide (SG1.5)	1 part	for
IMS	4 parts	48
Water	3 parts	hours.

(Prepare 24 hours before use.)

Contact with skin: Wash immediately with large amounts of water. Can be neutralized with sodium thiosulphate or sodium bicarbonate.

References

1 Kirk B (1986) Stability of reconstituted mustine injection BP during storage. *Br. J. Parenter. Ther.* **7**, 86–92.
2 Kirk B (1987) A study of the stability of aqueous solutions of mustine hydrochloride using colorimetric and HPLC assay techniques. *Proc. of Guild.* **23**, 47–52.
3 Friedman OM, Boger E (1961) Colorimetric estimation of nitrogen mustards in aqueous media. *Anal. Chem.* **33**, 907–10.
4 *ABPI Data Sheet Compendium 1995–96* (1995) DataPharm Publications Ltd, London, pp. 293–4.
5 Trissel LA (1994) *Handbook on Injectable Drugs,* 8th edn. American Society of Hospital Pharmacists, Bethesda, Maryland, USA.

Prepared by Michael Allwood

PACLITAXEL

1 General details

Approved name: Paclitaxel.

Proprietary name: Taxol.

Manufacturer or supplier: Bristol-Myers Squibb Pharmaceuticals Ltd.

Presentation and formulation details: A clear, pale straw-coloured, sterile solution, 6 mg/ml in a 5 ml vial. The vehicle is a 50 : 50 mixture of polyoxyethylated castor oil (Cremophor EL) and dehydrated alcohol USP and this solution *must* be diluted before administration.

Storage and shelf-life of unopened container: Unopened vials should be stored between 15–25°C and protected from light. Prepared solutions are stable for up to 27 hours.

2 Chemistry

Type: Paclitaxel is a taxane diterpenoid, or taxoid compound.

Molecular structure: 5β,20-Epoxy-1,2α,4,7β,10β,13α-hexahydroxytax-11-en-9-one 4,10-diacetane 2-benzoate 13-ester with (2R,3S)-N-benzoyl-3-phenylisoserine.

Molecular weight: 853.9.

Solubility: Insoluble in water; soluble in polyethoxylated castor oil and ethanol.

3 Stability profile

3.1 Physical and chemical stability

Paclitaxel is stable until expiry date if kept under the recommended storage conditions. It must be diluted prior to use. Solutions are stable for at least 27 hours at room temperature. The stability of paclitaxel has been determined in several studies.

The first stability study for paclitaxel concentrate diluted in infusion solutions indicated that no loss of potency occurred over a 24 hour period when a 0.03 mg/ml concentration was passed through a 0.22 µm filter and stored at room temperature.[1]

Waugh et al.[2] determined the stability of paclitaxel in various containers and infusion solutions. Paclitaxel was diluted in 0.9% sodium chloride and 5% glucose to clinically useful concentrations and stored in PVC infusion bags, polyolefin plastic containers and glass bottles. Solutions were kept at room temperature and filtered through a 0.2 µm membrane. The authors concluded that paclitaxel was visually and chemically stable for at least 24 hours under these conditions, a conclusion that has been confirmed by other studies.[3,4]

Chin et al.[5] have shown that paclitaxel solutions are stable for 48 hours at room temperature under normal fluorescent light. Xu et al.[6] have established that paclitaxel solutions remain stable for three days, at temperatures up to 32°C.

Paclitaxel has also been shown to maintain its potency for a period of three years when frozen at –15°C. Potency was confirmed following thawing every three months. Some turbidity was however observed in the formulation.[7]

Paclitaxel solutions may develop haziness upon standing. This has been attributed to the surfactant vehicle, as no paclitaxel precipitation or loss of potency has been observed.[2,8]

A similar haze develops if the solution is stored at –15°C, or refrigerated (2–8°C). This again redissolves on warming without loss of potency.[7]

3.2 Stability in clinical practice

If diluted in 5% glucose in a non-PVC infusion container (e.g. the glass bottle provided in the Support Pack or polyolefin bag), and stored at ambient temperature, a shelf-life of 48 hours may be assigned. The concentration after dilution in 5% glucose must not exceed 1.2 mg/ml paclitaxel.

Compatibility with containers: Paclitaxel solution is incompatible wth PVC bags and intravenous tubing. Because paclitaxel is not water soluble, it is formulated as a concentrated solution containing polyethoxylated castor oil and ethanol. The polyethoxylated castor oil can result in leaching of diethylphthalate (DEHP) plasticizers from PVC equipment, and therefore the preparation, storage and administration of diluted paclitaxel should be carried out using non-PVC equipment. Suitable containers for use with paclitaxel include glass bottles, semi-rigid polyolefin plastic bags and polypropylene containers.

Allwood[9] noted the use of PVC infusion containers and administration sets to administer paclitaxel infusion is discouraged because of the risk of DEHP extraction from PVC, and glass containers are recommended. However the author comments that PVC infusion containers have the advantage of ease and familiarity of handling and recently investigated likely exposure to DEHP by patients receiving paclitaxel. Total exposure levels were determined using tests simulating clinical practice based on Data Sheet recommendations. Paclitaxel vehicle was used which has been shown to behave identically to paclitaxel injections in terms of DEHP extraction. The vehicle was diluted in 500 ml glucose 5% in Viaflex at concentrations equivalent to 0.6 mg/ml and 1.2 mg/ml paclitaxel. Infusion commenced immediately after drug preparation. The total volume of infusion was collected and analysed for DEHP concentration using HPLC. The results indicated that, in these conditions, patients may receive from 10 mg to 30 mg DEHP from doses of 300 mg and 600 mg paclitaxel respectively.[10] These figures compared favourably with studies that have shown that the level of DEHP contained in stored blood may be as much as 50 mg/l and that patients may receive up to 128 mg DEHP per transfusion. The author noted that the likelihood of chronic exposure to DEHP is negligible in patients receiving paclitaxel on four to six occasions.[10]

3.3 Stability in specialized delivery systems

No information available.

4 Clinical use

Indications: Treatment of metastatic ovarian cancer where standard platinum therapy has failed, treatment of metastatic breast cancer where standard anthracycline-containing therapy has failed, or is inappropriate.

Dosage: All patients must be premedicated with corticosteroids, antihistamines and H_2 antagonists prior to paclitaxel administration. The recommended dose of paclitaxel is 175 mg/m² given as a three hour intravenous infusion, with a three week interval between courses. Subsequent doses should be reviewed according to patient tolerance.[11] Paclitaxel should not be readministered until the neutrophil count is at least $1.5 \times 10^9/l$ and the platelet count is at least $100 \times 10^9/l$. Patients who experience severe neutropenia (neutrophil count $<0.5 \times 10^9/l$ for seven days or more) or severe peripheral neuropathy should receive a dose reduction of 20% for subsequent courses.[11]

5 Preparation of injection

Preparation and administration: Paclitaxel must be diluted, using aseptic techniques, prior to infusion to reach a final concentration of 0.3–1.2 mg/ml.[11] Recommended diluents are 0.9% sodium chloride, 5% glucose, 0.9% sodium chloride and 5% glucose and 5% glucose in Ringer's injection. Paclitaxel should be administered using non-PVC containing equipment, through an in-line filter with a microporous membrane not greater than 0.22 μm. PVC containers must not be used. Paclitaxel should be administered under the supervision of a physician experienced in the administration of chemotherapeutic agents.

Extravasation: Irritant and potentially vesicant, in a similar manner to the vinca alkaloids (*see* Chapter 6).

6 Destruction of drug or contaminated articles

Disposal: Excess and waste materials should be placed in double sealed polythene bags and incinerated at a temperature above 1000°C. Liquid waste should be flushed with copious amounts of water.

Contact with skin or eyes: Wash immediately with copious amounts of water; seek medical attention as soon as possible.

References

1 Trissel LA *et al.* (1987) *NCI Investigational Drugs*, Taxol, Pharmaceutical data. National Cancer Institute, Bethesda, MD, USA.

2 Waugh WN *et al.* (1992) Stability, compatibility and plasticizer extraction of Taxol (NC-125973) injection diluted in infusion solutions and stored in various containers. *Am. J. Hosp. Pharm.* **48**, 1520–4.

3 *National Cancer Institute Clinical Brochure (revised)* (1991) Taxol NSC-125973. National Cancer Institute, Bethesda, MD, USA.

4 Data on file, Bristol Myers Squibb Ltd.

5 Chin A *et al.* (1994) Paclitaxel stability and compatibility in polyolefin containers. *A. Pharmacother.* **28**, 35–6.

6 Xu QA *et al.* (1994) *Stability of paclitaxel in 5% dextrose injection and 0.9% sodium chloride injection at various temperatures.* ASHP Annual meeting, Reno, Nevada, USA, Proceedings.

7 Bristol Myers Squibb Ltd (1996) Personal communication.

8 Pearson SD, Trissel LA (1993) Leaching of diethylphthalate from polyvinyl chloride containers by selected drugs and formulation components. *Am. J. Hosp. Pharm.* **50**, 1405–9.

9 Allwood MC (1994) Taxol and PVC. *Pharm. J.* **252**, 556.

10 Allwood MC, Martin H (1996) The extraction of diethylphthalate (DEHP) from polyvinyl chloride components of intravenous infusion containers and administration sets by paclitaxel injection. *Int. J. Pharmaceutics* **127**, 65–71.

11 *ABPI Data Sheet Compendium 1995–6* (1995) DataPharm Publications Ltd, London, pp. 324–6.

Prepared by Andrew Stanley

PENTOSTATIN

1 General details

Approved names: Co-vidarabine, deoxycoformycin, 2-deoxycoformycin, pentostatin.

Proprietary name: Nipent.

Manufacturer or supplier: Wyeth Lederle.

Presentation and formulation details: Vials containing a lyophilized, white powder, containing 10 mg pentostatin. Each vial also contains 50 mg mannitol and sodium hydroxide or hydrochloric acid to maintain pH at 7.0–8.2.[1]

Storage and shelf-life of unopened container: Store at 2–8°C. Unopened vials expire two years from the date of manufacture.[1]

2 Chemistry

Type: Antimetabolite, 2-deoxyadenosine derivative, inhibitor of adenosine deaminase.

Molecular structure:

Molecular weight: 268.3.

Solubility: Greater than 30 mg/ml in water.

3 Stability profile

3.1 Physical and chemical stability

Data on stability and compatibility of pentostatin with diluents and other drugs are limited. Hydrolytic degradation is important.

Effect of pH: Pentostatin is more stable under alkaline than acidic conditions. The pH range of maximum stability is about pH 6.5–11.5.[2] Solutions in water for injection have a pH of approximately 7–8.5.[2]

Effect of ionic strength: At pH 6–8, hydrolysis is independent of ionic strength of the solution.[3]

Container compatibility: It has been reported that pentostatin diluted in 5% glucose or 0.9% sodium chloride does not interact with PVC infusion containers or administration sets as evidenced by both visual and chemical analysis.[4]

Compatibility with other drugs: Pentostatin has been investigated for its compatibility under simulated Y-site injection conditions with a variety of other drugs: fludarabine phosphate (1 mg/ml),[5] ondansetron hydrochloride (1 mg/ml),[6] paclitaxel (1.2 mg/ml)[7] and sargramostim (10 µg/ml)[8] were all physically compatible with pentostatin (0.4 mg/ml) for four hours at 22°C under fluorescent light, and melphalan hydrochloride (0.1 mg/ml)[9] showed no sign of incompatibility, increased turbidity or particle content when mixed with pentostatin (0.4 mg/ml) for three hours at 22°C under fluorescent light.

3.2 Stability in clinical practice

Reconstituted 2 mg/ml pentostatin solutions in 0.9% sodium chloride[4,10] or water[10,11] are reported to be chemically and physically stable for at least 72 hours at room temperature (22–25°C), exhibiting 2–4% degradation.

It has been reported that when diluted further to a final concentration of 20 µg/ml, and stored at room temperature, pentostatin solutions in 0.9% sodium chloride[10,11] or lactated Ringer's solution[10] exhibit less than 5% degradation in the first 48 hours.

Solutions in glucose are less stable under the same conditions and show approximately 2% degradation at 24 hours, and as much as 8–10% loss over 48 hours.[10,11] Degradation in 5% glucose was even more marked (10% after 11 hours storage at 23°C) when a 2 µg/ml pentostatin solution was studied.[11] 20 µg/ml pentostatin solutions in 5% glucose, or 0.9% sodium chloride, have also been reported to exhibit no loss of potency when stored refrigerated for up to 96 hours.[10,11]

3.3 Stability in specialized delivery systems

No information available.

4 Clinical use

Type of cytotoxic agent: Antimetabolite, inhibitor of adenosine deaminase, an important enzyme in the recycling of purines which catalyses the irreversible deamination of adenosine and deoxyinosine. Cytotoxic action is probably linked to intracellular accumulation of deoxyadenosine triphosphate (dATP), with consequent inhibition of ribonucleotide reductase, depletion of other deoxynucleotides and inhibition of DNA synthesis.[12]

Main indications: Hairy cell leukaemia, including that resistant to α-interferon. Pentostatin has useful activity against a variety of other lymphoproliferative disorders including B cell chronic lymphocytic leukaemia, prolymphocytic leukaemia, adult T cell leukaemia/lymphoma and cutaneous T cell lymphomas refractory to conventional chemotheray.[12]

Dosage: In hairy cell leukaemia, 4 mg/m² every alternate week, continuing for at least two doses after remission has been achieved, or for a maximum of 12 months. A range of other dose schedules have been used in other conditions including doses of up to 30 mg/m² daily for 1–3 days in relapsed acute lymphoblastic leukaemia.[12]

5 Preparation of injection

Reconstitution: Each 10 mg vial of powder should be dissolved in 5 ml of water for injection. The appropriate quantity of reconstituted injection solution should be further diluted with 25–50 ml 5% glucose or 0.9% sodium chloride prior to infusion.

Bolus administration: Not recommended.

Intravenous infusion: The dose should be infused over 30–50 minutes.

Extravasation: Potentially irritant, though no extravasation injuries have been reported in clinical studies (*see* Chapter 6).

6 Destruction of drug or contaminated articles

Incineration: No recommendation is made regarding incineration temperature, though this is the preferred method of disposal.[1]

Chemical: Manufacturer recommends that 5% sodium hypochlorite solution is used to treat spills and wastes prior to disposal.[1]

Contact with skin or eyes: Contact with eyes would be expected to produce irritation, extent of percutaneous absorption is unknown. Contaminated skin or eyes should be washed with water immediately.[1]

References

1 Anon. (1994) *Lederle Laboratories guidelines on the handling and storage of Lederle pharmaceuticals. Nipent injection.* Lederle Laboratories, Gosport, UK.
2 Anon. (1995) *Stability/compatibilities of Lederle injectables. Nipent.* Lederle Laboratories, Gosport, UK.
3 Trissel LA (1994) *Handbook on Injectable Drugs*, 8th edn. American Society of Hospital Pharmacists, Bethesda, Maryland.
4 Anon. (1995) *American Hospital Formulary Service*, American Society of Hospital Pharmacists, Bethesda, Maryland.
5 Trissel LA *et al.* (1991) Visual compatibility of fludarabine phosphate with antineoplastic drugs, anti-infectives, and other selected drugs during simulated Y-site injection. *Am. J. Hosp. Pharm.* **48**, 2186–9.
6 Trissel LA *et al.* (1991) Visual compatibility of ondansetron hydrochloride with other selected drugs during simulated Y-site injection. *Am. J. Hosp. Pharm.* **48**, 988–92.
7 Trissel LA, Martinez JF (1993) Turbidimetric assessment of the compatibility of taxol with 42 drugs during simulated Y-site injection. *Am. J. Hosp. Pharm.* **50**, 200–304.
8 Trissel LA *et al.* (1992) The visual compatibility of sargramostim with selected chemotherapeutic drugs, anti-infectives, and other drugs during simulated Y-site injection. *Am. J. Hosp. Pharm.* **49**, 402–6.
9 Trissel LA, Martinez JF (1993) Melphalan physical compatibility with selected drugs during simulated Y-site injection. *Am. J. Hosp. Pharm.* **50**, 2359–63.
10 Anon. (1988, 1989, 1990) NCI investigational drug data. National Cancer Institute, Bethesda, Maryland.
11 Al-Razzak LA *et al.* (1990) Chemical stability of pentostatin (NSC-218321), a cytotoxic and immunosuppressive agent. *Pharm. Res.* **7**, 452–60.
12 Brogden RN, Sorkin EM (1993) Pentostatin. A review of its pharmacodynamic and pharmacokinetic properties, and therapeutic potential in lymphoproliferative disorders. *Drugs* **46**, 652–77.

Prepared by Tim Root

PLICAMYCIN

1 General details

Approved names: Plicamycin, mithramycin.

Proprietary name: Mithracin.

Manufacturer or supplier: Pfizer Ltd.

Presentation and formulation details: Yellow lyophilized powder in vial, containing 2.5 mg plicamycin. Contains 100 mg mannitol and disodium hydrogen phosphate to adjust pH to 7.0 after reconstitution.

Storage and shelf-life of unopened container: Shelf-life of two years when stored in a refrigerator at 2–8°C and protected from light; shelf-life of six months at room temperature.[1]

2 Chemistry

Type: Cytotoxic antibiotic.

Molecular structure:

Molecular weight: 1085.2.

Solubility: Soluble in water.

3 Stability profile

3.1 Physical and chemical stability

The dry powder is stable for six months at ambient temperature.[2] The drug in aqueous solution decomposes in acid or alkaline conditions. The pH of an aqueous solution (0.5 mg/ml) is 4.5–5.5, although the injection is buffered to pH 7. Losses of about 13% at pH 4–5 and ambient temperature after 24 hours have been reported.[3] Solutions at pH 5–7.5 are stable for at least two days at 2–6°C.[4]

Effect of light: The drug is described as relatively sensitive to light, and direct exposure to strong daylight should be avoided.

Degradation pathways: Acid hydrolysis (below pH 5.0) yields a number of degradation products, including chromomycinone D, mycarose, D olivose and D oliose.[3] The relative toxicity of these compounds is unknown.

Compatibility with containers: Compatible with PVC,[3] and with in-line filters (Ivex-2) during infusion.[5]

Compatibility with other drugs: Plicamycin will chelate metals, such as iron. No further information is available.

3.2 Stability in clinical practice

The drug is relatively stable after reconstitution with water for injections and may be stored for two days at 2–6°C. The drug may be further diluted in 5% glucose (other infusion fluids are not recommended), although some degradation may occur indicating storage is undesirable. Such dilutions are quite stable (less than 10% loss) for 24 hours at room temperature in either glass or PVC containers, or 48 hours at 2–6°C.[3] However, the presence of degradation products is undesirable, so it is recommended the diluted injection be used immediately. It is reported that plicamycin binds to cellulose acetate in-line filters, approximately 14% of the dose being removed during passage of a solution in 5% glucose through an in-line filter.[6]

3.3 Stability in specialized delivery systems

No data available.

4 Clinical use

Type of cytotoxic: Anti-tumour antibiotic.

Main indications: Refractory hypercalcaemia.

Dosage: 25 µg/kg/day for three to four day periods.

5 Preparation of injection

Dilution: Add 4.9 ml water for injections and shake to dissolve. The solution contains 500 µg/ml plicamycin. It may be stored for short periods at 2–6°C but this is not recommended by the manufacturer.

Bolus administration: Not recommended.

Intravenous infusion: The required volume of the reconstituted injection is added to 1 l of 5% glucose or 0.9% sodium chloride.[7] Inject slowly over four to six hours (200 ml/h). The infusion may be stored at 2–6°C for up to 24 hours.

Extravasation: Moderately damaging. There is no known antidote.

Application of moderate heat to the site of extravasation is recommended to disperse the drug and reduce discomfort (*see* Chapter 6).

6 Destruction of drug or contaminated articles

Incineration: 1000°C.

Chemical: 10% w/v trisodium phosphate (or 0.1 M sodium hydroxide).

Contact with skin: Wash affected area with copious amounts of water.

References

1 Longland PW, Rowbottom PC (1987) Stability at room temperature of medicines normally recommended for cold storage. *Pharm. J.* **238**, 147–51.

2 Wolfert RR, Cox RM (1975) Room temperature stability of drug products labelled for refrigeration storage. *Am. J. Hosp. Pharm.* **32**, 585–7.

3 Cheng CC, Kwang-Yeun Z (1972) Some antineoplastic antibiotics. *J. Pharm. Sci.* **61**, 4.

4 Bosanquet AG (1986) Stability of solutions of anti-neoplastic agents during preparation and storage for *in vitro* assays. II. Assay methods, Adriamycin and the other anti-tumour antibiotics. *Cancer Chemother. Pharmacol.* **17**, 1–10.

5 Karke M *et al.* (1983) Binding of selected drugs to a 'treated' in-line filter. *Am. J. Hosp. Pharm.* **40**, 1323–8.

6 Butler LD *et al.* (1980) Effect of in-line filtration on the potency of low-dose drugs. *Am. J. Hosp. Pharm.* **37**, 935–41.

7 *ABPI Data Sheet Compendium 1995–96* (1995) DataPharm Publications Ltd, London, pp. 1236–7.

Prepared by Michael Allwood

RALTITREXED

1 General details

Approved name: Raltitrexed.

Proprietary name: Tomudex.

Manufacturer or supplier: Zeneca Ltd.

Presentation and formulation details: Sterile lyophilized powder for intravenous injection containing 2 mg raltitrexed packed in 5 ml glass vials. Inactive ingredients are dibasic sodium phosphate heptahydrate, mannitol and sodium hydroxide.[1]

Storage and shelf-life of unopened container: The expiry time of raltitrexed is 18 months when stored at 2–8°C, protected from light.[1]

2 Chemistry

Type: A folate analogue belonging to a family of antimetabolites, with potent direct and specific inhibitory activity against the enzyme thymidylate synthase (TS).

Molecular structure: N-(5-[N-(3,4-dihydro-2-methyl-4-oxoquinazolin-6-ylmethyl)-N-methylamino]-2-thenoyl)-L-glutamic acid.

Molecular weight: 458.49.

Formula: $C_{21}H_{22}N_4O_6S$.

Solubility: Raltitrexed exhibits pH dependent solubility. At pH values greater than 5.5 the solubility of the compound increases rapidly to greater than 100 mg/ml in water.

3 Stability profile

3.1 Physical and chemical stability

Prior to reconstitution, raltitrexed is both chemically and physically stable when stored at 2–8°C, protected from light.[1] It is known that raltitrexed degrades by two mechanisms, hydrolysis and oxidation. Hence, the product is prepared as a freeze-dried powder in nitrogen-filled vials. Information on the kinetics of chemical stability of raltitrexed after reconstitution is not available.

Container compatibility: There is no evidence of sorption to PVC or polyethylene infusion containers during storage for 24 hours at 25°C.[2]

3.2 Stability in clinical practice

Raltitrexed injection may be reconstituted and diluted in 0.9% sodium chloride or 5% glucose. Solutions in the concentration range 0.2–20 mg/ml raltitrexed and stored at 25°C exposed to artificial light are stable for 24 hours.[1]

3.3 Stability in specialized delivery systems

No information available.

4 Clinical use

Main indications: Palliative treatment of advanced colorectal cancer.

Dosage and administration: The recommended adult dose is 3 mg/m² given as a single intravenous infusion. Dose escalation is not recommended since higher doses have been associated with an increased incidence of life-threatening toxicity.[1]

5 Preparation of injection

Reconstitution: The contents of the vial, containing 2 mg raltitrexed, should be reconstituted with 4 ml water for injections to produce a solution containing 0.5 mg/ml. Reconstituted solutions can be stored at 2–8°C for up to 24 hours.[1]

Bolus administration: Not recommended.

Intravenous infusion: The appropriate dose is diluted in 50–250 ml of either 0.9% sodium chloride or 5% glucose and administered by intravenous infusion over a period of 15 minutes.

Extravasation: There is clinical experience of extravasation, although perivascular tolerance studies in animals revealed no significant irritant reaction.[2]

6 Destruction of drug or contaminated articles

Incineration: 1000°C recommended.

Chemical: No information.

Contact with skin: Remove and destroy contaminated clothing. Wash skin immediately with water. If eyes are contaminated, irrigate with eyewash or clean water, holding eyelids apart, for at least ten minutes.[1]

References

1 *Tomudex Summary of Product Characteristics* (1995) Zeneca Pharma.
2 Zeneca Pharma data, on file.

Prepared by Andrew Stanley

THIOTEPA

1 General details

Approved names: Thiotepa, thiophosphoramide, TESPA, TSPA.

Proprietary name: Thiotepa.

Manufacturer or supplier: Lederle Laboratories Ltd.

Presentation and formulation details: Lyophilized powder, in vials containing thiotepa 15 mg.

Storage and shelf-life of unopened container: The injection has a shelf-life of 18 months when stored between 2 and 8°C.

2 Chemistry

Molecular structure: 1,1'1"-phosphinothioyldinetris-aziridine.

Molecular weight: 189.2.

Solubility: Soluble 1 in 8 in water; 1 in 2 in ethanol; 1 in 2 in chloroform; and 1 in 4 in ether.

3 Stability profile

3.1 Physical and chemical stability

The stability of thiotepa in aqueous solution is pH dependent; it is least stable in acid solutions. The acid-catalysed reaction of thiotepa in the presence of chloride ions yields a series of chloroethyl derivatives (I–III) according to the following scheme:[1]

In strong acid solutions and in aqueous solutions at elevated temperatures, thiotepa undergoes P-N cleavage and/or ring-opening to give the azaridinium ion (IV).[2] Thiotepa will also polymerize to form insoluble polymeric derivatives.

At 37°C in pH 4.2 buffer the rate constant for loss of thiotepa is 9.8×10^{-3}/minute giving a $t_{90\%}$ of ten minutes. At pH 7 degradation was much slower; no breakdown could be detected after two hours at 37°C but longer term data were not available.[3]

Any polymerization reaction is likely to be catalysed by light, reducing the stability of thiotepa.

Compatibility with other drugs: Thiotepa is incompatible in solutions with mitozantrone. When mitozantrone and thiotepa were mixed in 5% glucose in a 10 ml syringe and the solution stored at room temperature protected from light, 10% of the mitozantrone degraded within the first 24 hours and over 50% after seven days.[4]

3.2 Stability in clinical practice

The manufacturer indicates that the reconstituted solution has a shelf-life of one day when stored at 2–8°C.[5] If a precipitate forms, the reconstituted injection must be discarded. The reconstituted solution is in fact reported to be stable for 28 days at 2–8°C, or seven days at ambient temperature.[5] Solutions of thiotepa, 15 mg in 1.5 ml water for injections, are also reported to be stable when frozen for up to 28 days (temperature not specified).[5] (The previous formulation, containing sodium chloride and sodium bicarbonate, was stable for five days at 2–8°C.[6]) Thiotepa solutions reconstituted in water for injections and diluted into 0.9% sodium chloride or 5% glucose infusions to a final concentration of 0.5 mg/ml in PVC bags are stable for 14 days at 2–8°C, but losses are more than 10% in seven days at ambient temperature.[5]

When administered as a bladder irrigation it is recommended that up to 60 mg thiotepa in 60 ml sterile water is instilled and the solution retained in the bladder for up to two hours.[7] Thiotepa is, however, unstable in acidic urine at 37°C. At pH 5.5, $t_{90\%}$ is 70 minutes and, at pH 4.0, $t_{90\%}$ is 3.3 minutes, with only 2.1% of the initial dose of thiotepa remaining after two hours.[3]

3.3 Stability in specialized delivery systems

No data available.

4 Clinical use

Type of cytotoxic: Thiotepa is a polyfunctional alkylating agent. It releases ethylenimine radicals which disrupt the bonds of DNA.

Main indications: Adenocarcinoma of the breast and of the ovary; for controlling intracavity effusions secondary to diffuse or localized neoplastic disease of various serosal cavities; and for the treatment of superficial papillary carcinoma of the bladder.[5,6] Thiotepa has been effective against lymphosarcoma and Hodgkin's disease but is now largely superseded by other treatments. It has also been used also for the post-operative management of pterygium.[8,9]

Both thiotepa and its active metabolite, tepa, efficiently cross the blood–brain barrier. A phase II evaluation of thiotepa in paediatric CNS malignancies has been reported.[10]

Dosage: By rapid intravenous infusion, 0.3–0.4 mg/kg at one- to four-week intervals. By intracavity instillation, 10–65 mg in 20–60 ml sterile water. By intravesical administration, up to 60 mg in 30–60 ml sterile water.

5 Preparation of injection

Reconstitution: Reconstitution of the 15 mg vial with 1.5 ml water gives a 10 mg/ml solution. If the thiotepa has polymerized a precipitate will form on reconstitution. Precipitated solutions should be discarded. Large bore needles are recommended to minimize pressure and possible formation of aerosols.

Administration: Thiotepa may be given by intravenous, intra-arterial, intramuscular and intrathecal routes. For intracavity instillation first aspirate as much fluid as possible then instil the dose of thiotepa. The same tubing may be used for both aspiration and instillation.

For bladder instillation the patient is dehydrated for eight to 12 hours. The solution is instilled into the bladder and retained there for two hours.

Extravasation: Thiotepa is nonvesicant and non-irritant.

6 Destruction of drug or contaminated articles

Incineration: 800°C.

Chemical: Dilute in large quantities of boiling water.

Contact with skin: Wash off with water.

References

1 Maxwell J *et al.* (1974) Behaviour of an aziridine alkylating agent in acid solution. *Biochem. Pharmacol.* **23**, 168–70.

2 Zon G *et al.* (1976) Observations of 1,1′,1″ phosphinothioylidinetris-aziridine (thiotepa) in acidic and saline media. An ¹H-NMR study. *Biochem. Pharmacol.* **25**, 989–92.

3 Cohen GE *et al.* (1984) Effects of pH and temperature on the stability and decomposition of N,N′N″ triethylenethio-phosphoramide in urine and buffer. *Cancer Res.* **44**, 4312–16.

4 Cacek T, Weber R (1991) Visual and chemical stability of mitoxantrone mixed individually with vincristine, etoposide, thiotepa, metoclopramine and cytarabine in plastic syringes. *ASHP Midyear Clinical Meeting* **25**, 470E.

5 Lederle Laboratories. Personal communication.

6 Kirschembaum BE, Latiolais CJ (1976) Stability of injectable medications after reconstitution. *Am. J. Hosp. Pharm.* **33**, 767–91.

7 Uyas HM *et al.* (1987) Drug stability guidelines for a continuous infusion chemotherapy programme. *Hosp. Pharm.* **22**, 685–7.

8 Erlich D (1977) The management of pterygium. *Ophthal. Surg.* **8**, 23–30.

9 Olander K (1978) Management of pterygium: should thiotepa be used? *Ann. Ophthalmol.* **10**, 853–6.

10 Steinberg SM *et al.* (1993) A phase II evaluation of thiotepa in pediatric central nervous system malignancies. *Cancer* **72**, 271–5.

Prepared by Gerard Lee

TREOSULFAN

1 General details

Approved name: Treosulfan.

Proprietary names: Treosulfan injection.

Manufacturer or supplier: Medac Gesellschaft für Klinische Spezialpräparate mbH, Hamburg, Germany.

Presentation and formulation details: White crystalline powder in vials containing 1 g and 5 g treosulfan. No excipients are used in the formulation.

Storage and shelf-life of unopened container: Five years at room temperature.

2 Chemistry

Type: Bifunctional alkylating agent.

Molecular structure: (2S,3S)-threitol-1,4-bismethane sulphonate.

$$H_3C-SO_2-O-CH_2-\overset{\overset{\displaystyle OH}{|}}{\underset{\underset{\displaystyle H}{|}}{C}}-\overset{\overset{\displaystyle H}{|}}{\underset{\underset{\displaystyle OH}{|}}{C}}-CH_2-O-SO_2-CH_3$$

Formula: $C_6H_{14}O_8S_2$.

Molecular weight: 278.3.

Melting point: 101.5–105°C.

Solubility: 6% (water); 5.8% (0.9% sodium chloride); 5.5% (5% glucose); 2.5% (50% glucose).

3 Stability profile

3.1 Physical and chemical stability

Treosulfan is relatively stable after reconstitution and further dilution (0.9% sodium chloride or 5% glucose), the reconstituted drug is stable for five days at room temperature and ambient light.[1]

Degradation pathway: In alkaline media, treosulfan degrades to methanesulphonic acid and diepoxybutane. The transformation of treosulfan into epoxides is highly pH dependent. The transformation reaction to L-diepoxybutane via the corresponding monoepoxide has been demonstrated *in vitro*.[2] At pH values less than 6.0, practically no transformation of treosulfan occurs.

Effect of pH: Acidic media do not influence the stability of treosulfan. In alkaline media, treosulfan degrades to methanesulphonic acid and diepoxybutane.

Effect of light: Treosulfan is not light-sensitive.

Effect of temperature: Samples of treosulfan were stored in sealed ampoules in heating cabinets at 60°C. Deterioration of 1% was found after storage for three months.[3]

Container compatibility: Contact with intravenous infusion administration sets (Mc Gaw V 1428 Metriset, Transcodan administration set, Avon A 100 blood administration set) does not seem to affect a treosulfan solution. The content of treosulfan is unaltered after four hours. There is no rise in the content of acidic degradation products.[4] Contact with ethylvinylacetate infusion bags does not affect the reconstituted treosulfan solution after storage for five days under ambient light.[5]

Compatibility with other drugs: No information available.

3.2 Stability in clinical practice

After reconstitution with water for injections, the resulting 50 mg/ml solution is chemically stable in the vial and may be stored for five days at room temperature (ambient light). The solution can be further diluted in 5% glucose or 0.9% sodium chloride infusions and the resulting solution is stable for the same time.

3.3 Stability in specialized delivery systems

No information available.

4 Clinical use

Type of cytotoxic: Treosulfan is a bifunctional alkylating agent which has been shown to possess antineoplastic activity in the animal tumour screen and in clinical trials.

Mechanism of action: The activity of treosulfan is due to the formation of epoxide compounds *in vivo*.[6]

Main indications: For the treatment of all types of ovarian cancer, either supplementary to surgery or palliatively. Some uncontrolled studies have suggested activity in a wider range of neoplasms. Because of a lack of cross-resistance reported between treosulfan and other cytotoxic agents treosulfan may be useful in any neoplasm refractory to conventional therapy.

Dosage and administration: Injection 5–15 g intravenously every one to three weeks, depending on blood count and concurrent chemotherapy. Single injections of up to 15 g have been given with no serious adverse effects. Doses up to 3 g have been given intraperitoneally.

Treatment should not be given if the white blood cell count is less than 3000/µl, or the thrombocyte count less than 100 000/µl. A repeat blood count should be made after an interval of one week, when treatment may be restarted if haematological parameters are satisfactory. Lower doses of treosulfan should be used if other cytotoxic drugs or radiotherapy are being given currently. Treatment is initiated as soon as possible after diagnosis.

5 Preparation of injection

Reconstitution: The contents of each infusion bottle should be dissolved in 20 ml (1 g) or 100 ml (5 g) water for injection, respectively. A transfer needle may be used for this purpose.

To avoid solubility problems during the dissolution of treosulfan the following stages should be adopted:

▼ solvent, water for injection, is warmed to a maximum of 30°C
▼ treosulfan is removed carefully from the inner surface of the infusion bottle by shaking. This procedure is very important, because moistening of powder that sticks to the surface results in caking. In cases where caking does occur the bottle has to be shaken vigorously, until the cake is dissolved
▼ one side of either a double-sided cannula or an adapter is put into the rubber stopper of the water bottle or bag. The treosulfan bottle is then put on the other end of the cannula or the adapter with the bottom on top. The whole construction is turned around and the water let run into the lower bottle while the bottle is shaken gently.

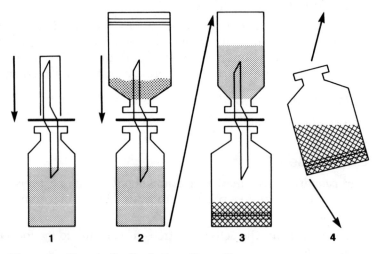

Figure 1: *Steps in the dissolution of treosulfan*

If the above procedures are followed, the whole dissolution procedure should take not longer than two minutes.

Bolus administration: Doses up to 5 g treosulfan may be given as a bolus injection. Larger doses should be administered as an intravenous infusion, at a rate of 5 g every 15–30 minutes.

Infusion: Solutions originally reconstituted with water for injections may be further diluted with either 5% glucose or 0.9% sodium chloride infusion.

Extravasation: Care should be taken in administration of the injection to avoid extravasation into tissues since this will cause local pain and tissue damage. If extravasion does occur, the injection should be discontinued immediately and any remaining portion of the dose should be introduced into another vein (*see* Chapter 6).

6 Destruction of drug or contaminated articles

Incineration: 1000°C.

Chemical: None reported.

Contact with skin: Wash with cold water.

Contact with eyes: If the eyes are contaminated irrigate immediately with 0.9% sodium chloride.

References

1 Medac GmbH Hamburg. Personal communication. Stability after reconstitution and storage in glass containers. Data on stability of treosulfan in various injection fluids. Unpublished information.
2 Feit PW, Rastrup-Andersen N (1970) Studies on epoxide formation from (2S,3S)-threitol 1,4-bismethanesulfonate. The preparation and biological activity of (2S,3S)-1,2-epoxy-3,4-butanediol 4-methanesulfonate. *J. Am. Chem.* **13**, 1173–5.
3 Medac GmbH Hamburg. Personal communication. Stability studies at higher temperatures. Unpublished information.
4 Medac GmbH Hamburg. Personal communication. Solubility and compatibility of treosulfan substance in various intravenous infusions. Compatibility of treosulfan substance with administration sets for intravenous infusions. Unpublished information.
5 Medac GmbH Hamburg. Personal communication. Stability after reconstitution and storage in ethylvinylacetate-infusion bags. Unpublished information.
6 *ABPI Data Sheet Compendium 1995–96* (1995) DataPharm Publications Ltd, London, pp. 964–5.

Prepared by Andrew Stanley

VINBLASTINE

1 General details

Approved names: Vinblastine, vincaleukoblastine.

Proprietary name: Velbe (Lilly).

Manufacturer or supplier: Eli Lilly & Co. Ltd, Lederle Laboratories Ltd, Faulding DBL Ltd.

Presentation and formulation details: Lyophilized powder containing 10 mg vinblastine sulphate. This is supplied with 10 ml aqueous diluent containing 90 mg sodium chloride and 0.2 ml benzyl alcohol (Lilly, Lederle, DBL), or as a solution of 10 mg/ml lyophilized powder (DBL).

Storage and shelf-life of unopened container: The injection has a shelf-life of three years when stored between 0 and 6°C. The solution shelf-life is 18 months.

2 Chemistry

Type: Vinca alkaloid.

Molecular structure: Vincaleukoblastine.

Molecular weight: 811.0 (vinblastine sulphate: 909.0).

Solubility: The base is insoluble in water; soluble in ethanol and chloroform. The sulphate salt is soluble 1 in 10 water; 1 in 1200 ethanol; 1 in 50 chloroform. pK_a: 5.4, 7.4.

3 Stability profile

3.1 Physical and chemical stability

Degradation pathways: Aqueous solutions of vinblastine are less stable at lower pH values, 4-desacetylvinblastine is the primary degradation product at pH 2.[1]

More recent studies indicate that the hydrolytic decomposition pathways for vinblastine are more complex. Below pH 1.5 and above pH 10.5, desacetylvinblastine has been confirmed as the major degradation product. However, between pH 2.5 and 7.0, the amount of desacetylvinblastine found was negligible and at least three other degradation products were detected.[2] Studies on 1 mg/ml solutions of vinblastine sulphate at pH 4.5–5.0 identified up to six breakdown products. The major degradents were tentatively identified as 19'-oxo-vinblastine and an isomer of vinblastine, but none of the decomposition products were positively categorized. From the data at 25, 37 and 55°C, $t_{90\%}$ values were estimated to be 16.6 days at 37°C, 150 days at 25°C and 10.7 years at 5°C.[3]

When exposed to direct incandescent light, decomposition is accelerated. At 25°C, the $t_{90\%}$ is approximately seven days and at 30°C, solutions of vinblastine sulphate had lost 10% of their potency after slightly more than one day.[4] The major degradation products were different from those identified in thermal degradation studies but the same pattern of products was identified in both cases.

Vinblastine base is practically insoluble in water and can precipitate from solutions of vinblastine sulphate above pH 6.

Container compatibility: No loss of potency was detected in solutions of vinblastine sulphate (10 mg/ml) stored for 30 days in polypropylene syringes at 4°C or room temperature.[5] There was no significant loss of potency when vinblastine sulphate solution (10 mg in 50 ml) in 5% glucose or 0.9% sodium chloride was filtered through a 0.22 µm cellulose ester membrane filter.[6]

No losses of vinblastine (2.5 mg/10 ml) could be detected to nylon, polysulphone or cellulose ester filters when using a syringe pump driver to deliver the drug. There was, however, significant adsorption to the Pall ELD96 activated nylon filter. A 30–40% loss of potency was detected during the first 30 minutes of infusion with the concentration only returning to its initial value after two to three hours.[7]

Losses of 24% occurred in 24 hours at 37°C from a 1 mg/ml solution of vinblastine sulphate in bacteriostatic 0.9% saline in an Infusaid implantable pump; in 12 days losses totalled 48%. Similar solutions in glass vials exhibited no losses after 24 hours and 20% loss after 12 days at 37°C.[8]

Vinblastine has been shown to be adsorbed on to PVC tubing and cellulose proprionate burette chambers. Up to 48% loss was found from a 3 µg/ml solution stored for 48 hours in PVC tubing and up to 20% loss of potency was found in similar solutions stored in cellulose proprionate burette chambers for 48 hours.[9] These results were obtained for a static system and it is difficult to extrapolate them to the dynamic situation of an intravenous administration. Significant losses are likely to occur, however, in PVC administration sets. The adsorption losses did not occur in polybutadiene tubing or methacrylate butadiene styrene burettes.[9]

Compatibility with other drugs: Trissel reports studies suggesting that vinblastine may be compatible with a number of drugs.[10]

3.2 Stability in clinical practice

The reconstituted injection is chemically stable for at least 28 days at 4°C and at 25°C,[3] provided it is protected from light. When stored at 37°C in the dark, the shelf-life of the reconstituted injection is 14 days. In direct incandescent light, the injection is chemically stable for seven days at room temperature.[4]

No degradation was detected in vinblastine solution 20 µg/ml in 0.9% sodium chloride, 5% glucose and in Ringer's lactate, stored in polypropylene tubes in the dark, after 21 days at 4°C. At 25°C there was a 2–3% degradation of vinblastine in the three infusion solutions after 21 days.[11]

3.3 Stability in specialized delivery systems

A 7% degradation has been observed in vinblastine solution ranging from 0.015–0.5 mg/ml in 0.9% sodium chloride after storage for 21 days at 4°C + five days at 33°C in a Baxter infusor. However, the study confirms that degradation is reduced to 5% after ten days of storage at 4°C, followed by five days at 33°C.[12] Vinblastine solution can therefore be stored for ten days at 4°C in Baxter infusor prior to being delivered through a one or five-day infusor.

4 Clinical use

Type of cytotoxic: Vinblastine arrests mitosis at the metaphase and inhibits RNA synthesis.

Main indications: Vinblastine is used in combination with other chemotherapeutic agents for treatment of metastatic testicular carcinoma, Hodgkin's and non-Hodgkin's lymphoma, neuroblastoma, histiocytosis X, mycosis fungoides, Kaposi's sarcoma, advanced breast carcinoma and choriocarcinoma.

Dosage: Usually 4–8 mg/m² weekly. Weekly injections starting at 3.7 mg/m² and rising by increments of 1.85 mg/m² up to a maximum of 18.5 mg/m², or until the white cell count has fallen to 3000/mm³.[13]

5 Preparation of injection

Reconstitution: Reconstitution of the 10 mg vial with 10 ml of sterile diluent gives a 1 mg/ml solution.

Bolus administration: Intravenously, directly into a vein or into the tubing of a running infusion, over a one-minute period.

Intravenous infusion: Vinblastine has been given as a continuous five-day infusion (1.4–2.0 mg/m²/day[14]). Infusions should be administered through a central line.

Since death has resulted from inadvertent intrathecal administration, it is recommended that syringes containing this product, should be labelled 'WARNING – VINBLASTINE FOR INTRAVENOUS USE ONLY'.[15]

Constant ambulatory intravenous infusion has been investigated using a tunnelled subclavian catheter and the Cor-med ML6 infusion pump[16] and the Travenol infusor system.[17] There are, however, insufficient data to draw reliable conclusions from this work.

Extravasation: Moderate to severe (*see* Chapter 6).

6 Destruction of drug or contaminated articles

Incineration: 1000°C.

Chemical: 10% sodium hypochlorite/24 hours.

Contact with skin: Wash with copious amounts of water.

References

1 Burns JH (1972) *Analytical Profiles of Drug Substance*, Vol. 1. Academic Press, Orlando, Florida, USA, 443pp.

2 Vendrig DEMM *et al.* (1988) Degradation kinetics of vinblastine sulphate in aqueous solutions. *Int. J. Pharm.* **43**, 131–8.

3 Black J *et al.* (1988) Studies on the stability of vinblastine sulphate in aqueous solution. *J. Pharm. Sci.* **77**, 630.

4 Black J *et al.* (1988) Stability of vinblastine sulphate when exposed to light. *Drug Intell. Clin. Pharm.* **22**, 634.

5 Ireland D *et al.* (1990) The chemical stability of cytarabine and vinblastine injections. *Br. J. Pharm. Pract.* **12**, 53–4.

6 Butler LD *et al.* (1980) Effect of in-line filtration on the potency of low-dose drugs. *Am. J. Hosp. Pharm.* **37**, 935.

7 Francomb MM *et al.* (1994) Adsorption of vincristine, vinblastine, doxorubicin and mitozantrone to in-line intravenous filters. *Int. J. Pharmaceutics* **103**, 87–92.

8 Keller JH, Ensminger WD (1982) Stability of cancer chemotherapeutic agents in totally implanted drug delivery systems. *Am. J. Hosp. Pharm.* **39**, 1321.

9 McElany JC *et al.* (1988) Stability of methotrexate and vinblastine in burette administration sets. *Int. J. Pharm.* **47**, 239–47.

10 Trissel LA (1994) *Handbook on Injectable Drugs*, 8th edn. American Society of Hospital Pharmacists, Bethesda, Maryland, USA.

11 Beijnen JH *et al.* (1989) Stability of vinca alkaloid anticancer drugs in three commonly used infusion fluids. *J. Parenter. Sci. Technol.* **43**, 84–7.

12 Baxter Healthcare Ltd. Personal communication.

13 Anon. (1986) *Physicians Desk Reference*, 40th edn. Medical Economics Company, Oradell, New Jersey, USA.

14 Yap HY *et al.* (1980) Vinblastine given as a continuous five-day infusion in the treatment of refractory advanced breast cancer. *Cancer Treat. Rep.* **64**, 279.

15 *ABPI Data Sheet Compendium 1995–96* (1995) DataPharm Publications Ltd, London, pp. 893–5.

16 Lokich J *et al.* (1982) The delivery of cancer chemotherapy by constant venous infusion. *Cancer* **50**, 2731.

17 Akokoshi MP *et al.* (1987) Safety and reliability of the Travenol Infusor. *J. Pharm. Technol.* (Mar/Apr), 65.

Prepared by Gerard Lee

VINCRISTINE

1 General details

Approved names: Vincristine, leurocristine.

Proprietary name: Oncovin (Lilly).

Manufacturer or supplier: Faulding DBL Ltd, Eli Lilly & Co. Ltd, Lederle Laboratories Ltd.

Presentation and formulation details: Lyophilized powder containing lactose in the following proportions of vincristine to lactose: 1–10 mg, 2–20 mg, 5–50 mg*. Supplied with 10 ml of diluent containing 90 mg sodium chloride and 0.2 ml benzyl alcohol (Lilly, Lederle*, DBL).

1 ml, 2 ml and 5 ml (DBL) vials containing vincristine sulphate 1 mg/ml in solution with mannitol 100 mg/ml, methylhydroxybenzoate 1.8 mg/ml and propylhydroxybenzoate 0.2 mg/ml (Lilly), or preservative-free (DBL); also available in prefilled syringes containing 1 mg in 1 ml, 2 mg in 2 ml (DBL).

Storage and shelf-life of unopened containers: When stored at 2–8°C, the lyophilized powder has a shelf-life of three years and the solution has a shelf-life of two years in vials or 18 months in syringes.

2 Chemistry

Type: Vinca alkaloid.

Molecular structure: 22-oxo-vincaleukoblastine (sulphate salt).

Molecular weight: 825.1 (vincristine sulphate: 923).

Solubility: Sulphate salt: 1 in 2 of water; 1 in 600 of ethanol; 1 in 30 of chloroform.
pK_a: 5.0, 7.4.

3 Stability profile

3.1 Physical and chemical stability

When vincristine sulphate was incubated at 37°C in 0.2 M glycine buffer containing 1% bovine serum albumin, five degradation products could be detected.[1] The major breakdown product was confirmed as 4-deacetyl vincristine. The remaining degradants were postulated to be an isomer of vincristine and of the 4-deacetyl derivative, 4-deacetyl-3-deoxy vincristine and N-formyl-leurosine. The degradation products were formed to the extent of 14%, 44% and 56% of the parent vincristine after incubating at 37°C for 72 hours at pH 4.0, 7.4, and 8.8 respectively.

Studies on the degradation kinetics of vincristine sulphate at 80°C, pH 2–11, indicate that vincristine is most stable at pH 4.8 and that its stability is comparable to that of vinblastine.[2] A half-life of 136 hours is given for vincristine in solutions at pH 4.8 and 80°C, with an activation energy of 70–80 kJ/mol, but the data are not easily extrapolated to temperatures of 25°C and below.

The reconstituted injection has a pH of 3.5–5.5. Precipitation can occur at alkaline pHs.

Container compatibility: No losses to plastic containers or syringes have been reported. After filtration through a 0.22 μm cellulose ester filter, 6.5% of a 1 mg/50 ml solution in 5% glucose and 12% of a 1 mg/50 ml solution in 0.9% sodium chloride was bound to the filter.[3] Vincristine sulphate, 1.5 mg in 3 ml, when injected as a bolus through a 0.22 μm nylon filter, and after flushing the filter with 10 ml normal saline, showed losses of 10% of the vincristine to the filter.[4]

No losses of vincristine (0.25 mg/10 ml) could be detected to nylon, polysulphone or cellulose ester filters when using a syringe pump driver to deliver the drug. Significant absorption was found however to the Pall ELD 96 filter. A 30–40% loss of potency could be seen in the first 30 minutes of the infusion, with the concentration only returning to its initial value after two to three hours.[5]

Compatibility with other drugs: Trissel reports studies suggesting that vincristine may be compatible with a number of drugs.[6]

3.2 Stability in clinical practice

The manufacturers recommend that the reconstituted injection be discarded after 14 days in the fridge.[7,8] The injection solution has a shelf-life of 18 months at 2–6°C[7,9] and so solutions with a pH of 3.5–5.5 would be expected to be equally stable. The reconstituted injection is chemically stable for 30 days when stored at 2–6°C.[9]

No degradation was detected in vincristine solution 20 μg/ml in 0.9% sodium chloride injection, 5% glucose injection and Ringer's lactate injection when stored at 4°C for 21 days in polypropylene tubes in the dark.[10] At 25°C there was a 5% loss of vincristine in 5% glucose injection after 21 days but losses in the other two infusion solutions were insignificant.

There was no evidence of physical or chemical incompatibility between vincristine and mitozantrone mixed together in 5% glucose solution contained in 10 ml plastic syringes and stored, protected from light, at room temperature for seven days.[10,11] Admixtures of doxorubicin and vincristine (1.88–2.37 mg/ml and 0.033–0.053 mg/ml respectively) are stable for at least seven days at 37°C in 0.9% sodium chloride injection, or 0.45% sodium chloride and 2.5% glucose injection.[12]

3.3 Stability in specialized delivery systems

Solutions of vincristine ranging from 0.04 to 0.2 mg/ml, reconstituted with 0.9% sodium chloride, have been shown to be chemically stable for ten days in a Baxter infusor when stored at room temperature.[13] However, due to the lack of stability data at 33°C, only half-day infusors should be used.[13] A mixture containing vincristine sulphate, 0.036 mg/ml and doxorubicin hydrochloride, 1.67 mg/ml, in 0.9% sodium chloride infusion, stored in either Deltec system (Pharmacia Upjohn Ltd) or Infusor (Baxter Healthcare Ltd) reservoirs has been shown to be stable for seven days at 4°C followed by four days at 35°C.[14]

4 Clinical use

Type of cytotoxic: Vincristine blocks mitosis with metaphase arrest by binding to tubulin and inhibiting the assembly of microtubules. It is M-phase specific.

Main indications: Vincristine is used, principally in combination chemotherapy regimens, against Hodgkin's and non-Hodgkin's lymphomas, acute lymphocytic leukaemia, lymphosarcoma, reticulum cell sarcoma, rhabdomyosarcoma, neuroblastoma, Wilms' tumour, advanced breast carcinoma and small-cell lung carcinoma. It has modest to moderate activity in many other malignancies.[15]

Dosage: 1.4 mg/m² weekly, up to a maximum of 2 mg. In children weighing less than 10 kg, 0.05 mg/kg weekly is used. Due to the narrow therapeutic range, the dose should be individually adjusted.

5 Preparation of injection

Reconstitution: Add 1 ml of diluent to a 1 mg vial, 2 ml to a 2 mg vial and 5 ml to a 5 mg vial to give a 1 mg/ml solution.

Bolus administration: By bolus injection or into the tubing of a running intravenous infusion. As it is vesicant, care must be taken to avoid extravasation during administration.

Intravenous infusion: Vincristine has been administered by continuous infusion[15,16] with reported higher blood concentrations and increased tumour response at a dose of 0.5 mg/m² daily for five days in three-week cycles.[16,17]

Since death has resulted from inadvertent intrathecal injection, it is recommended that syringes containing this product should be labelled 'WARNING – VINCRISTINE FOR INTRAVENOUS USE ONLY'.[7]

Extravasation: Moderate to severe (*see* Chapter 6).

6 Destruction of drugs or contaminated articles

Incineration: 1000°C.

Chemical: 5% sodium hypochlorite/24 hours.

Contact with skin: Wash with copious amounts of water.

References

1 Sethi VS, Thimmaiah KN (1985) Structural studies on the degradation products of vincristine dihydrogen sulphate. *Cancer Res.* **45**, 5386–9.

2 Vendrig DEMM *et al.* (1989) Degradation kinetics of vincristine sulphate and vindesine sulphate in aqueous solutions. *Int. J. Pharm.* **50**, 189–96.

3 Butler LD *et al.* (1980) Effect of in-line filtration on the potency of low-dose drugs. *Am. J. Hosp. Pharm.* **37**, 935–41.

4 Ennis CE *et al.* (1983) *In vitro* study of in-line filtration of medications commonly administered to paediatric cancer patients. *J. Parenter. Enter. Nutr.* **7**, 156–8.

5 Francomb MM *et al.* (1994) Adsorption of vincristine, vinblastine, doxorubicin and mitozantrone to in-line intravenous filters. *Int. J. Pharm.* **103**, 87–92.

6 Trissel LA (1994) *Handbook on Injectable Drugs*, 8th edn. American Society of Hospital Pharmacists, Bethesda, Maryland, USA.

7 *ABPI Data Sheet Compendium 1995–96* (1995) DataPharm Publications Ltd, London, pp. 882–4.

8 David Bull Laboratories. Data Sheet: *Vincristine sulphate.*

9 Vegenbery FR, Souney PF (1983) Stability guidelines for routinely refrigerated drug products. *Am. J. Hosp. Pharm.* **40**, 101–2.

10 Beijnen JH *et al.* (1989) Stability of vinca alkaloid anticancer drugs in three commonly used infusion fluids. *J. Parenter. Sci. Technol.* **43**, 84–7.

11 Cacek T, Weber R (1990) Visual and chemical stability of mitoxantrone mixed individually with vincristine, etoposide, thiotepa, metoclopramide and cytarabine in plastic syringes. *ASHP Midyear Clinical Meeting* **25**, P-47OE.

12 Beijnen JH *et al.* (1986) Stability of intravenous admixtures of doxorubicin and vincristine. *Am. J. Hosp. Pharm.* **43**, 3022–7.

13 Baxter Healthcare Ltd. Personal communication.

14 Nyhammar EJ *et al.* (1996) Stability of doxorubicin hydrochloride and vincristine sulfate in two portable infusion-pump reservoirs. *Am. J. Health-Syst. Pharm.* **53**, 1171–3.

15 Smith BD Antitumour update: Vinca alkaloids and epipodophyllotoxins. *Hosp. Formul.* **22**, 363–73.

16 Jackson DV *et al.* (1984) Intravenous vincristine infusion. *Cancer* **48**, 2559–664.

17 Jackson DV *et al.* (1981) Pharmacokinetics of vincristine infusion. *Cancer Treat. Rep.* **65**, 1043–8.

Prepared by Gerard Lee

VINDESINE

1 General details

Approved names: Vindesine, desacetyl vinblastine amide.

Proprietary name: Eldisine.

Manufacturer or supplier: Eli Lilly & Co. Ltd.

Presentation and formulation details: Lyophilized powder consisting of 5 mg vindesine sulphate with 25 mg mannitol. Supplied with 5 ml sterile diluent containing sodium chloride 9 mg/ml and 2% benzyl alcohol adjusted to pH 4.2–4.5 with hydrochloric acid or sodium hydroxide.[1]

Storage and shelf-life of unopened container: When stored between 2 and 6°C, the injection has a shelf-life of three years.

2 Chemistry

Type: Vinca alkaloid and synthetic derivative of vinblastine.

Molecular structure: 3-(aminocarbonyl)-O-deacetyl-3-de(methoxy-carbonyl)-vincaleukoblastine.

Molecular weight: 753.9 (vindesine sulphate: 852).

Solubility: The sulphate salt is freely soluble in water. pK_a: 5.4, 7.4.

3 Stability profile

3.1 Physical and chemical stability

In studies on the stability of vindesine in buffered serum albumin solution, Thimmaiah *et al.* have found that, when vindesine sulphate (500 mg in 10 ml) is incubated at 37°C in 0.2 M glycine buffer containing 1% bovine serum albumin, two degradation products can be detected.[2] These were tentatively identified as an eneamine/ether derivative of vindesine (I) and 3'4'-epoxyvindesine-N-oxide (II) (see Figure 1).

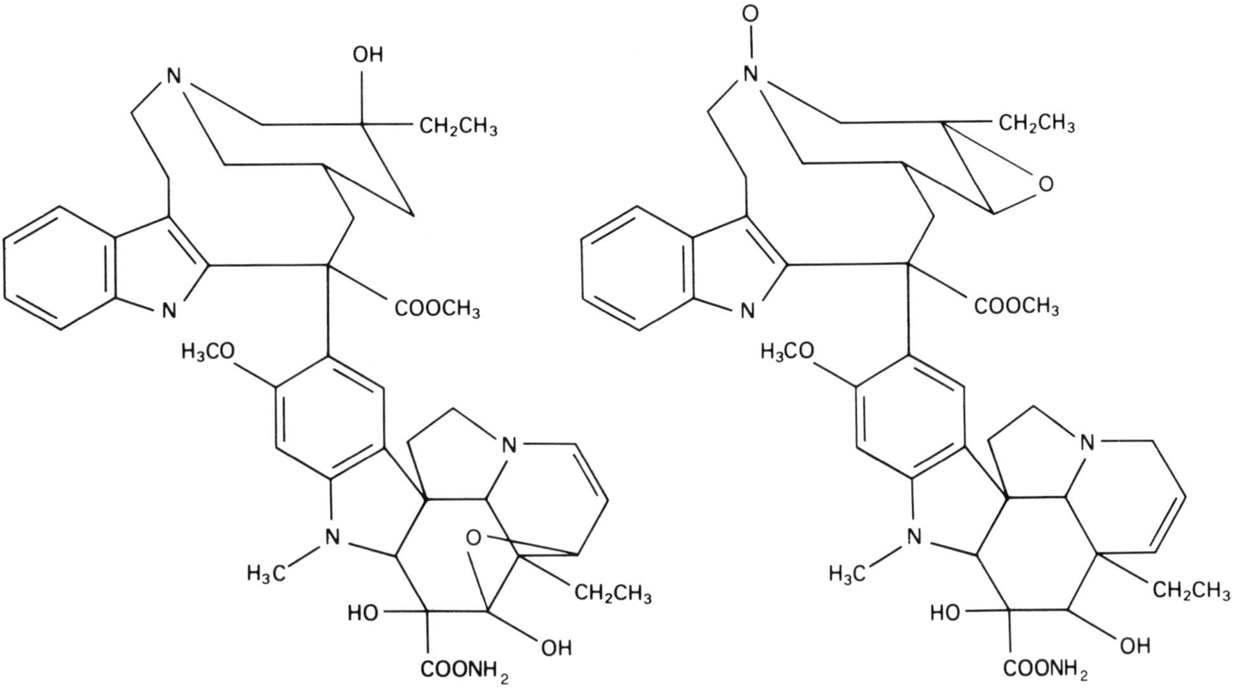

Figure 1: *Two major degradation products of vindesine incubated at 37°C in 0.2 M glycine buffer*

The degradation products were formed to an extent of about 11, 34 and 39% of the parent vindesine after 72 hours incubation at 37°C at pH 4.0, 7.4 and 8.8 respectively.

Investigations of the degradation kinetics of vindesine sulphate at 80°C in the pH range 2–11 indicate it is most stable at pH 1.9 and that it is more stable than vinblastine and vincristine in aqueous solution.[3] A half-life of 690 hours is quoted for vindesine at 80°C and pH 1.9 with an activation energy of 124 kJ/mol, but the data are not easily extrapolated to temperatures of 25°C and below.

Studies of the cell killing efficiency of vindesine solutions used in the human tumour clonogenic assay indicate a deterioration of cytotoxic activity for solutions stored in glass at low concentrations.[4] The lethal efficacy of 60 µg/ml solutions decreased to almost zero when tested after one, two and three weeks storage; a 225 µg/ml solution retained its lethal activity throughout the three-week period. The original reconstituted injection (1 mg/ml), stored in glass under the same conditions, retained its cytotoxic activity when diluted to the test concentrations. This would indicate that the loss of efficacy at low concentrations is not due to chemical inactivation but is more likely a result of sorptive losses to the glass vial.

The reconstituted injection has a pH of 4.2–4.5. Precipitation can occur at alkaline pHs.

Container compatibility: No incompatibilities have been reported with PVC containers and plastic syringes. There is evidence of sorptive losses of 60 µg/ml solutions in borosilicate glass vials.[4]

Compatibility with other drugs: No further information available.

3.2 Stability in clinical practice

The reconstituted injection is chemically stable for at least 30 days when stored at 4°C.[1] No degradation was detected in vindesine solution 20 µg/ml in 0.9% sodium chloride injection, 5% glucose injection or Ringer's lactate injection when stored for 21 days at both 4°C and 25°C in polypropylene tubes in the dark.[5]

3.3 Stability in specialized delivery systems

No data available.

4 Clinical use

Type of cytotoxic: Vindesine causes metaphase arrest by binding to tubulin, a substructure of the microtubular spindle apparatus. This leads to inhibition of tubulin polymerization which interrupts mitosis and leads to cell death.[6] For a complete review of the antineoplastic activity of vindesine *see* Cersosima *et al.*[6]

Main indications: Acute lymphoblastic leukaemia, chronic myelogenous leukaemia in blast crisis, malignant melanoma and advanced breast carcinoma.

Dosage: 3–4 mg/m^2 weekly as a bolus injection, or by four hour[7] or 48 hour infusion.[8] For fuller details of dosage regimens *see* Cersosima *et al.*[6]

5 Preparation of injection

Reconstitution: Reconstitute the 5 mg vial with 5 ml sterile diluent, to give a 1 mg/ml solution.

Bolus administration: Inject reconstituted preparation into the tubing of a fast running intravenous drip.

Intravenous infusion: Prepare in 5% glucose or 0.9% sodium chloride injections. Multielectrolyte infusion solutions, such as lactated Ringer's, are not recommended because of the possibility of precipitation, but this is not a problem for concentrations of less than 20 µg/ml.[5]

Since death has resulted from inadvertent intrathecal administration, it is recommended that syringes containing vindesine should be labelled 'WARNING – VINDESINE SULPHATE FOR INTRAVENOUS USE ONLY'.[4]

Extravasation: Moderate to severe. 1000 units of hyaluronidase in 20 ml saline may aid recovery (*see* Chapter 6).

6 Destruction of drug or contaminated articles

Incineration: 1000°C.

Chemical: 10% sodium hypochlorite/24 hours.

Contact with skin: Wash with copious amounts of water.

References

1 *ABPI Data Sheet Compendium 1995–96* (1995) DataPharm Publications Ltd, London, pp. 861–4.
2 Thimmaiah KN *et al.* (1990) Chemical characterisation of the *in vitro* degradation products of vindesine sulphate. *Microchem. J.* **42**, 115–20.
3 Vendrig DEMM *et al.* (1989) Degradation kinetics of vincristine sulphate and vindesine sulphate in aqueous solution. *Int. J. Pharm.* **50**, 189–96.
4 Yang L-Y, Drewinko B (1985) Cytotoxic efficacy of reconstituted and stored anti-tumour agents. *Cancer Res.* **45**, 1511–15.
5 Beijnen JH *et al.* (1988) Stability of vinca alkaloid anticancer drugs in three commonly used infusion fluids. *J. Parenter. Sci. Technol.* **43**, 84–7.
6 Cersosima RJ *et al.* (1983) Pharmacology, clinical efficacy and adverse effects of vindesine sulphate, a new vinca alkaloid. *Pharmacotherapy* **3**, 259–68.
7 Ettinger LJ *et al.* (1982) Vindesine – phase II study in childhood malignancies: A report for cancer and leukaemia group. *Med. Pediatr. Oncol.* **10**, 35–44.
8 Mathe G *et al.* (1981) Phase II clinical trials with hematogical malignancies. *Anticancer Res.* **1**, 1–10.

Prepared by Gerard Lee

The following monographs on cytokines represent those available on the UK market licensed for use in oncology. The list below contains other cytokines under investigation or awaiting licences in the UK. Many are already available in the US.

Chemical group	Approved name	Company or producer
Hu-r-GM-CSF	Sargramostim	Schering-Plough, Sandoz Immunex
Hu-r-M-CSF	–	Eurocetus, Biogen, Immunex, Bristol-Myers Squibb
Interleukin 3	–	Biogen, Eurocetus, Schering-Plough Immunex, Sandoz
Tumour necrosis factor	–	Knoll
Interferon α-2c	–	Boehringer Ingelheim
Interferon beta (natural source)	Ferono	Serono, Ferono, Bioferon
Interferon beta (recombinant source)	–	Bristol-Myers Squibb, Boehringer Ingelheim, Eurocetus, Interpharm, Roche, Schering-Plough, Wellcome
Interferon gamma (recombinant source)	–	Biogen
Interleukin 1*	–	Sandoz
Interleukin 6	–	Sandoz
Interleukin 11*	–	Sandoz
Stem cell factor*	–	Sandoz
PIXY 321 (a GM-CSF/IL 3 fusion protein)	–	Wyeth
Stem cell protector MIP 1α (BB 10,010)	–	British Biotechnology

* Reference has been made to these products by Vose and Armitage[1] as being close to clinical practice; however it has proved impossible to source the drugs.

The following table lists the drugs that are commercially available but not licensed for oncological use.

Chemical group	Approved name	Company or producer
Interferon β (powder for reconstitution 300 μg 96 million units per vial)	[Betaferon]	[Schering-Plough]
Interferon γ-1b (200 μg/ml 0.5 ml vials)	[Immukin]	[Boehringer Ingelheim]

Reference

1 Vose JM, Armitage JO (1995) Clinical applications of haematopoietic growth factors. *J. Clin. Oncol.* **13**, 1023–35.

BCG IMMUNOTHERAPEUTIC (MERIEUX UK LTD)

1 General details

Approved name: BCG immunotherapeutic.

Proprietary name: ImmuCyst.

Manufacturer or supplier: Merieux UK Ltd.

Presentation and formulation details: A white freeze-dried powder in glass vials containing 81 mg (dry weight) of Bacillus Calmette-Guérin (BCG) and 5% w/v monosodium glutamate. Vials of diluent contain, in 3 ml, approximately 0.85% w/v sodium chloride, 0.025% w/v Tween 80, 0.06% w/v sodium dihydrogen phosphate and 0.25% w/v disodium hydrogen phosphate. The product and diluent contain no preservative.

Storage and shelf-life of unopened container: The product and diluent should be stored at 2–8°C. At no time should the freeze-dried BCG immunotherapeutic be exposed to sunlight; direct or indirect. Exposure to artificial light should be kept to a minimum.

2 Chemistry

BCG immunotherapeutic is made from a culture of the Connaught strain of Bacillus Calmette-Guérin, which is an attenuated strain of living bovine tubercle bacillus, *Mycobacterium bovis*. The bacilli are lyophilized and are viable on reconstitution. When plated on culture media, the progenitor of each colony is termed a 'colony-forming unit' (CFU); each CFU is composed of at least one viable bacillus and may comprise of several bacilli, some of which may be viable and some non-viable. At the time of manufacture, the reconstituted product contains 6.6–19.2×10^8 CFU per dose and when used before the expiry date stated on the vial, the number of CFU per dose will be not less than 1.8×10^8.

3 Stability profile

3.1 Physical and chemical stability

No information available.

Effect of pH: No information available.

Effect of light: At no time should the product be exposed to sunlight; direct or indirect. Exposure to artificial light should be kept to a minimum.[1]

3.2 Stability in clinical practice

The product should be used immediately after reconstitution. An unavoidable delay between reconstitution and administration should not exceed two hours. Any reconstituted product that exhibits flocculation or clumping that cannot be dispersed with gentle shaking should not be used.[2]

4 Clinical use

Type of cytotoxic: BCG immunotherapeutic promotes a local acute inflammatory and sub-acute granulomatous reaction with histiocytic and leukocytic infiltration in the urothelium and lamina propria of the bladder. The local inflammatory effect is associated with an elimination or reduction of superficial cancerous lesions of the bladder. The exact mechanism by which this is accomplished is unknown, but the anti-tumour effect appears to be T-lymphocyte dependent.[3]

Indication: BCG immunotherapeutic is indicated for the treatment of superficial transitional cell carcinoma of the bladder.

Dosage: One dose consists of one vial of reconstituted material further diluted in sterile, preservative-free 0.9% sodium chloride. The treatment schedule consists of six weekly intravesical instillations. The exact number of instillations necessary to achieve an optimum response remains unknown. Most patients who respond will do so with six to 12 instillations.

5 Preparation of injection

Reconstitution: Preparation should take place in a biocontainment cabinet using full aseptic procedures. Handle as infectious material and do not remove the rubber stoppers from the vials. The contents of one vial should be reconstituted with one vial of diluent. The vial should only be shaken gently until a fine, even suspension is obtained. Once reconstituted, the content of the vial needs to be further diluted aseptically with 50 ml 0.9% sodium chloride before administration.

Administration: Intravesical instillation.

Warnings and precautions: The product contains viable attenuated mycobacteria so it must be handled as infectious material. In the event of BCG immunotherapeutic being accidentally injected, medical advice needs to be sought.

6 Destruction of drug or contaminated articles

Disposal: All equipment, contaminated packaging and cleaning materials should be disposed of by incineration, as with all other biohazardous waste.

Contact with skin: No information available.

References

1 *Product Data Sheet*, Connaught Laboratories Ltd.
2 Connaught Laboratories Ltd (1995) Personal communication.
3 Mikkelsen DJ, Ratliff TL (1989) Mechanisms of action of intravesical bacillus Calmette-Guérin for bladder cancer. *Urol. Oncol.* **3**, 195–211.

Prepared by Helen Streeter

BCG (EVANS MEDICAL LTD)

The author and editors note that BCG is also available in the UK from Evans Medical Ltd. It should be noted that this product is not licensed for the treatment of superficial bladder cancer, but does receive widespread usage in the UK.

1 General details

Approved name: Evans BCG.

Manufacturer or supplier: Evans Medical Ltd.

Presentation and formulation details: Two strengths of Evans BCG (intradermal and percutaneous) are produced for vaccination purposes against tuberculosis. **Only the high strength (percutaneous) version of Evans BCG is appropriate for intravesical administration when used in the treatment of superficial bladder cancers.** The intradermal strength is ten times less potent than the high strength (percutaneous) version of Evans BCG.

2 Chemistry

Evans BCG contains a live attenuated bovine strain of *Mycobacterium tuberculosis*, now known as the Evans strain (previously called 'Glaxo strain').

3 Stability profile

The manufacturer indicates that the product is stable for four hours after reconstitution.[1]

4 Clinical use

Dosage: The dose per instillation currently used is 1×10^9 to 5×10^9 colony-forming units (CFU).[1] The dose is referred to in CFU, as the clinical activity of BCG is a function of the CFU value. The dose should **not** be determined by 'mg wet weight', as this measurement depends on the manufacturer's technique of production and varies from one manufacturer to another.[2]

Each individual patient instillation dose is provided by either 20×1 ml vials of Evans percutaneous (high strength) BCG (containing 50 to 250×10^6 CFU per vial) or 1×25 ml vial of Evans percutaneous (high strength) BCG (containing 1 to 5×10^9 CFU per vial). $20 \times 50 = 1000$, $20 \times 250 = 5000$, therefore 20×1 ml vials contain the same total number of CFUs as 1×25 ml vial.

Evans percutaneous BCG for intravesical instillation is prepared according to the instructions given below. The instillation is freshly prepared in 50–100 ml of normal saline no more than four hours before use.[2,3]

▼ Between 50 and 100 ml of BCG suspension are instilled into the catheterized bladder and the catheter withdrawn. The patient retains the BCG suspension for one hour (and for up to a total of two hours if possible); in the first hour the patient is requested to lie for 15 minutes in each of the supine, right lateral, prone and left lateral positions to ensure that as much of the bladder epithelium as possible is exposed to the BCG suspension.

▼ The BCG suspension is then voided from the bladder. Care must be taken to destroy the voided live BCG organisms and to clean with antiseptic any parts of the patient's body splashed with the BCG suspension.

Every precaution should be taken in catheterization, and if trauma or bleeding per the urethra occurs, the urologist is strongly advised to postpone therapy for at least one week to avoid risk of systemic BCG infection.

5 Preparation of injection

Reconstitution: The freeze-dried powder is reconstituted with 0.9% sodium chloride. 1 ml is added to each of the 20, 1 ml vials. However, it is only necessary to add 18 ml to the 25 ml 'multidose vial'. Rotate/swirl the vials gently to suspend the powder. Do not shake.[2] Withdraw the reconstituted vaccine into the syringe and add to the sodium chloride bladder instillation.

6 Destruction of drug or contaminated articles

Destruction: Destroy any remaining (unused) BCG suspension by mixing with 200–2000 ppm free chlorine. For example, Milton diluted 1 in 10 = 2000 ppm. Allow to stand for 15 minutes. Flush into a drain with plenty of water.[2]

Some manufacturers have recommended that urine voided for six hours after instillation should be disinfected with an equal volume of 5% hypochlorite solution (e.g. undiluted household bleach) and allowed to stand for 15 minutes before flushing. Others recommend that for 24 hours after instillation, the toilet bowl should be washed out with bleach after each urination.[3]

Eyes: Irrigate with water for at least ten minutes. Obtain medical attention.

Skin: Wash thoroughly with soap and water. If the product has entered an open wound, or if accidental ingestion has occurred, obtain medical attention.

Ingestion/inhalation: Give water to drink. Allow to rest in fresh air. Obtain medical attention.

Spillage: Tackle spillages and/or breakages wearing protective equipment as described above. Absorb major spillages on to inert material (e.g. sand), then transfer into labelled, sealable containers suitable for holding broken glass. Dispose of in accordance with local and national regulations. Wash site of spillage with 1% hypochlorite solution (or free chlorine, minimum of 200 ppm) followed by detergent solution.

References

1 Anon. (1993) Evans BCG for superficial bladder cancer.
2 Evans Medical Ltd. Personal communication.
3 Brosman SA (1992) Bacillus Calmette-Guérin immunotherapy: techniques and results. *Urol. Clin. North Am.* **19** (3), 557–64.

Prepared by Helen Streeter and Andrew Stanley

INTERFERON α-2A

1 General details

Approved name: Interferon α-2a(rbe).

Proprietary name: Roferon-A, Roferon-A solution for injection.

Manufacturer or supplier: Roche Products Ltd.

Presentation and formulation details: Roferon-A vials: sterile powder for reconstitution in single dose vials, containing 19×10^6 IU of lyophilized interferon α-2a(rbe), 9 mg sodium chloride and 5 mg human serum albumin (European Pharmacopoeia) included as a stabilizer. The solution is reconstituted prior to use by addition of 1 ml of sterile water for injections BP, supplied as solvent.[1,2]

Roferon-A solution for injection: each vial contains 3, 4.5, 6, 9 or 18 million units of interferon α-2a(rbe) with ammonium acetate, sodium chloride, 1% benzyl alcohol (as preservative), polysorbate 80, acetic acid, sodium hydroxide and water for injection BP. The sodium content totals 0.123 mmol/l and the solutions are human serum albumin free.[2]

The 3, 4.5, 6 and 9 million unit vials contain a total volume of 1 ml, the 18 million unit vials have a volume of 3 ml, giving a strength of 6×10^6 IU/ml. (An 18 million unit in 1 ml vial is expected shortly.)[2]

Storage and shelf-life of unopened container: Unopened vials of lyophilized powder expire three years from the date of manufacture when stored between 2 and 8°C.[1] Unopened vials of interferon α-2a(rbe) solution have an expiry date two years after the date of manufacture, when stored between 2 and 8°C.

2 Chemistry

Interferon α-2a(rbe) is a recombinant interferon. It is a highly purified, sterile non-glycosylated protein containing 165 amino acids with two disulphide bridges between residues 1 and 98 and between 29 and 138.[3] It is produced by recombinant DNA technology using a genetically engineered *Escherichia coli* strain containing DNA that codes for the human protein. It differs from other recombinant interferons by the fact that amino acid 23 is a lysine group and amino acid 34 is a histidine group.

Interferon α-2a(rbe) has been shown to possess many of the activities of 'natural' human α-interferon. It has antiviral, antiproliferative and immunomodulatory actions.[4]

Molecular weight: Approximately 19 000.

Solubility: Interferon α-2a(rbe) is freely soluble in water.

Molecular structure: This is shown on the following page.

3 Stability profile

3.1 Physical and chemical stability

Reconstituted vials should not be used after more than 24 hours storage in a refrigerator (2–8°C) or two hours at room temperature. Reconstituted vials of 3×10^6 IU and 18×10^6 IU interferon α-2a(rbe) in 1 ml of water for injections, frozen immediately after reconstitution to –20°C have shown no physical degradation

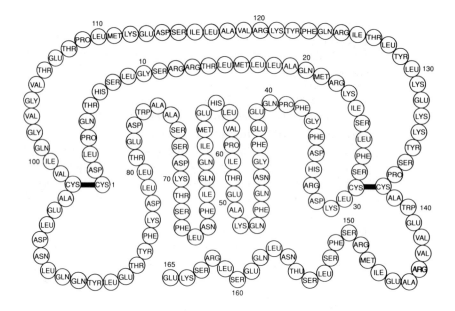

or loss of chemical activity on thawing at one month.[5] Interferon α-2a(rbe) is sensitive to heat, light and atmospheric oxygen.

Compatibility with other drugs: Data are not available concerning interferon α-2a(rbe) and other compounds, therefore the manufacturer recommends that it is not mixed with other drugs.

3.2 Stability in clinical practice

The recommended maximum storage temperature for interferon α-2a(rbe) vials is 25°C.[2] However, the vials appear stable for up to one month at –20°C when frozen immediately after reconstitution. Reconstituted vials should not be used after more than 24 hours storage in a refrigerator (2–8°C) or two hours at room temperature. The interferon α-2a(rbe) solution for injection is chemically and bacterially stable for 30 days from opening if stored between 2 and 8°C, protected from light.[1]

4 Clinical use

Type of cytotoxic agent: Activator of natural killer cells.

Main indications: Interferon α-2a is licensed for use as a single agent in the treatment of hairy-cell leukaemia, chronic phase Philadelphia chromosome positive chronic myelogenous leukaemia, cutaneous T-cell lymphoma. It is also indicated for recurrent or metastatic renal cell carcinoma and AIDS-related Kaposi's sarcoma in patients without history of opportunistic infection. Interferon α-2a is also licensed for the treatment of chronic active hepatitis B and chronic hepatitis C.[1]

Dosage: The following can be administered by subcutaneous or intramuscular injection:

▼ hairy-cell leukaemia: induction dose: 3 MIU daily for 16–24 weeks, followed by maintenance therapy of 3 MIU, three times per week

▼ chronic myelogenous leukaemia: induction dose: 3 MIU daily escalated to 9 MIU daily over 84 days. Maintenance therapy at 9 MIU daily (optimal) to 9 MIU three times weekly (minimum), for a maximum of 18 months, or until complete haematological response. In complete haematological responders continue therapy to achieve cytogenetic response

▼ cutaneous T-cell lymphoma: induction dose: 3 MIU daily escalated to 18 MIU daily over 84 days. Maintenance therapy at the maximum tolerable dose (maximum 18 MIU) three times weekly

▼ renal cell carcinoma: induction dose: 3 MIU daily escalated to 36 MIU daily over 84 days. Maintenance therapy at 18–36 MIU three times weekly (doses over 18 MIU to be given by intramuscular injection only)

▼ AIDS-related Kaposi's sarcoma: induction dose: 3 MIU daily escalated to 36 MIU daily over 84 days. Maintenance therapy at maximum tolerable dose (maximum 36 MIU) three times weekly.

▼ chronic hepatitis B: 2.5–5.0 MIU/m^2 three times weekly for 4–6 months, with dose escalation permissible if markers of viral replication do not decrease after one month of treatment.

▼ chronic hepatitis C: 6 MIU three times weekly for three months, followed by 3 MIU three times weekly for a further three months in responding patients (those showing normalization of ALT)

▼ follicular non-Hodgkin's lymphoma: interferon α-2a(rbe) should be administered concomitantly to a conventional chemotherapy regimen (such as the combination of cyclophosphamide, prednisone, vincristine and doxorubicin) according to a schedule such as 6 MIU/m^2 given subcutaneously or intramuscularly from day 22 to day 26 of each 28-day cycle.

5 Preparation of injection

Reconstitution: The content of roferon-A vials should be reconstituted with 1 ml of water for injections (supplied as the solvent) and swirled gently. Vigorous shaking should be avoided.

Bolus administration: $2–15 \times 10^6$ IU/m^2 by subcutaneous injection.

Intravenous infusion: Not recommended due to poor drug stability.

Extravasation: Not irritant; no recommendations available (*see* Chapter 6).

6 Destruction of drug or contaminated articles

Disposal: Excess interferon α-2a(rbe) solution may be disposed of into a drain with copious amounts of water. All other waste, including contaminated packaging or cleaning materials and used protective clothing must be placed with clinical waste for incineration.[6] When dealing with broken vials, disposable gloves, eye protection and a face mask should be worn.[6]

Contact with skin: Remove contaminated clothing and wash skin thoroughly with soap and water. If the eyes are contaminated, irrigate with water and obtain medical advice.[6]

References

1 American Product Information Sheet (1992) *Am. J. Hosp. Pharm.* **49**, 550–2.
2 *ABPI Data Sheet Compendium 1995–96* (1995) DataPharm Publications Ltd, London, pp. 1471–4.
3 Wetzel R (1981) Assignment of the disulphide bonds of leukocyte interferon. *Nature* **189**, 606–7.
4 Baron S *et al.* (1991) The interferons: Mechanisms of action and clinical applications. *JAMA* **266**, 1375–83.
5 Roche Products Ltd. Personal communication.
6 Interferon of alfa-2a(rbe) (1991) *COSHH Safety Data Sheet*, prepared by Roche Products Ltd.

Prepared by Andrew Stanley

INTERFERON α-2B

1 General details

Approved name: Interferon α-2b(rbe).

Proprietary name: Intron A.

Manufacturer or supplier: Schering-Plough Ltd.

Presentation and formulation details: Intron A is available as lyophilized powder for reconstitution or as a ready made solution. Vials of lyophilized powder are supplied containing 3, 5, and 10×10^6 IU of interferon α-2b(rbe) per vial. Reconstitution should occur just prior to administration by the addition of 1 ml sterile water for injection (supplied as diluent). Interferon α-2b(rbe) 3, 5 and 10×10^6 IU lyophilized powder also contains amino-acetic acid, mono and dibasic sodium phosphate and human albumin.

Vials of intron A solution are supplied containing 10 and 25×10^6 IU of interferon α-2b(rbe) per vial. These are multidose preparations and the solution contains 5×10^6 IU of interferon α-2b(rbe) per ml. Interferon α-2b(rbe) solution also contains methyl and propyl parabens, amino-acetic acid, mono and dibasic sodium phosphate and human albumin. 10×10^6 IU = 0.05 mg interferon α-2b(rbe) protein.[1]

Storage and shelf-life of unopened container: Store in the refrigerator. The shelf-life is three years from the date of manufacture.

2 Chemistry

Type: Interferon α-2b(rbe) is a recombinant interferon. It is a highly purified, sterile, non-glycosylated single chain protein containing 165 amino acids with two disulphide bridges between residues 1 and 98, and 29 and 138.[2] It is produced by recombinant DNA technology using a genetically engineered *Escherichia coli* strain containing DNA that codes for the human protein. It differs from other recombinant interferons by the fact that amino acid 23 is an arginine group and amino acid 34 is a histidine group.

Molecular structure:

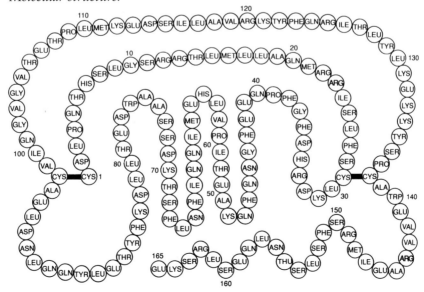

Molecular weight: Approximately 20 000.

Solubility: Interferon α-2b(rbe) is freely soluble, strengths up to 10×10^6 IU/ml are all isotonic when diluted with 1 ml of water for injections. Up to 60×10^6 IU will dissolve in 1 ml of water for injections.[2]

3 Stability profile

Interferon α-2b(rbe) degrades by cleavage of disulphide bridges. The liberated sulphydryl groups form oligomers (dimers and trimers) with other monomers. It is believed that only one disulphide bridge is required for biological activity.

3.1 Physical and chemical stability

Interferon α-2b(rbe) lyophilized powder is not photosensitive[2] and is generally unstable after reconstitution. Solutions of interferon α-2b(rbe) should be stored in the refrigerator at 2–8°C.

Effect of pH: Interferon α-2b(rbe) is most stable in the pH range 6.9–7.5.[2]

Container compatibility: No adsorption has been found to occur on to the surface of polypropylene syringes. At low concentrations of less than 0.1×10^6 IU/ml, interferon may bind to PVC, however this is believed to be a non-significant interaction.[2]

Compatibility with other drugs: Interferon α-2b(rbe) powder should only be reconstituted with water for injections, however, it is known to be compatible with 0.9% sodium chloride, Ringer's solution and lactated Ringer's (Hartmann's) solution; however, it is incompatible with glucose solutions.

3.2 Stability in clinical practice

When reconstituted with 1 ml water for injections per vial up to 10×10^6 IU an isotonic solution is produced which is stable for 24 hours at 2–8°C.[1]

Qualitative gradient-elution HPLC studies[3] on the degradation of aqueous solutions of interferon α-2b(rbe) lyophilized powder at a concentration of 430 000 IU/ml have shown significant degradation over five days storage at 4°C, with measurable degradation products appearing after 48 hours. At 37°C, degradation product peaks were observed after four hours.

However, interferon α-2b(rbe) has been shown to be stable for infusion over a 24-hour period[2] if the following criteria are strictly adhered to:

▼ temperature not greater than 25°C
▼ concentration of interferon α-2b greater than 1×10^6 IU/ml
▼ infusion container is glass or PVC (Viaflex).

The stability of interferon α-2b(rbe) can be summarized:[2–6]

Presentation	Temperature (°C)	Stability period
Lyophilized powder in vials	2–8	3 years
Lyophilized powder in vials	15–25	28 days
Reconstituted solutions in vial or syringe	2–8	28 days
Reconstituted solutions in vial	15–25	14 days
Reconstituted solutions in syringe	15–25	24 hours
Reconstituted solution frozen (including four freeze–thaw cycles)	–20	56 days
Reconstituted solution frozen	–80	1 year
Reconstituted solution 100 million units in 50 ml (2 million units/ml) in water for injections in a bladder Urotainer	4	21 days
Solution in vial	2–8	2 years
Solution in vial	15–25	4 weeks

4 Clinical use

Type of cytotoxic agent: Activator of natural killer cells.

Indications: Interferon α-2b(rbe) is licensed within the UK for use in the treatment of chronic myelogenous leukaemia, multiple myeloma (maintenance therapy), low grade non-Hodgkin's lymphoma (adjunctive with chemotherapy), hairy-cell leukaemia, AIDS-related Kaposi's sarcoma (in patients without history of opportunistic infection), genital warts (condylomata acuminata), chronic active hepatitis B and chronic hepatitis C.[1] Non-licensed indications (for which there are large research programmes) include malignant melanoma, renal cell carcinoma and superficial bladder cancer.

Dosage:

▼ chronic myelogenous leukaemia: the recommended daily dose is 4 to 5×10^6 IU, administered subcutaneously daily. When the white blood cell count is controlled, the dosage may be administered three times a week (on alternate days)

▼ multiple myeloma: maintenance therapy – in patients who are in plateau phase following induction chemotherapy. May be administered as monotherapy, subcutaneously, at a dose of 3×10^6 IU/m^2 three times a week (on alternate days)

▼ non-Hodgkin's lymphoma: adjunctive with chemotherapy. May be administered subcutaneously at a dose of 5×10^6 IU three times per week (on alternate days), for a duration of 18 months

▼ hairy-cell leukaemia: the recommended dose is 2×10^6 IU/m^2, administered three times a week (every other day). The normalization of one or more haematological variables begins with one month of therapy. Improvement in all three haematological variables (granulocyte count, platelet count and haemoglobin level) may require six months or more

▼ AIDS-related Kaposi's sarcoma: the optimal dosage is not yet known. Efficacy has been demonstrated at a dose of 30×10^6 IU/m^2 three to five times a week, subcutaneously or intramuscularly. Lower doses (i.e. 10 to 12×10^6 IU/m^2/day) also have been used without apparent loss of efficacy.

▼ condylomata acuminata: the lesion or lesions to be injected should be cleaned first with a sterile alcohol pad. The intralesional injection should be made at the base of the lesion using a fine needle (30 gauge). Inject 0.1 ml of reconstituted solution containing 1×10^6 IU into the lesion three times per week on alternate days, for three weeks. As many as five lesions can be treated at one time. The maximum total dose administered each week should not exceed 15×10^6 IU

▼ chronic active hepatitis B: the optimal schedule of treatment has not yet been established. The dosage is usually in the range of 2.5 to 5×10^6 IU/m^2 of body surface area administered subcutaneously three times a week for a period of four to six months

▼ chronic hepatitis C/non-A, non-B: the recommended dose is 3×10^6 IU administered subcutaneously three times a week, for up to 18 months.

5 Preparation of injection

Intron A lyophilized powder should be reconstituted with 1 ml water for injections (or for condylomata acuminata with sufficient to produce a concentration of 1×10^6 IU/0.1 ml). The vials should be swirled gently. Vigorous shaking should be avoided. Intron A ready-made solution is supplied at a concentration of 5×10^6 IU/ml in vials of 10×10^6 IU and 25×10^6 IU.

Bolus administration: 2–30×10^6 IU/m^2 injected subcutaneously.

Intravenous infusion: Not recommended due to poor drug stability, unless interferon α-2b(rbe) is being used as part of a high dose protocol, when adherence to the infusion stability criteria and conditions should be observed.

Extravasation: Non-irritant, no recommendations available.

6 Destruction of drug or contaminated articles

Disposal: Excess interferon α-2b(rbe) solution may be disposed of into a drain with copious amounts of water. All other waste, including contaminated packaging or cleaning materials and used protective clothing must be placed with clinical waste for incineration. When dealing with broken vials, disposable gloves, eye protection and a dusk mask should be worn.

Contact with skin: Remove contaminated clothing and wash skin thoroughly with soap and water. If the eyes are contaminated, irrigate with water and obtain medical advice.

References

1 *Data Sheet Compendium 1995–96* (1995) DataPharm Publications Ltd, London, pp. 1640–3.
2 Schering Corporation, USA. Personal communication.
3 Palmer AJ *et al.* (1988) Qualitative studies on interferon alfa-2b in prolonged continuous infusion regimes using gradient elution high performance liquid chromatography. *J. Clin. Pharm. Ther.* **13**, 225–31.

4 Merigan TC *et al.* (1978) Preliminary observations on the effect of human leukocyte interferon in non-Hodkin's lymphoma. *N. Engl. J. Med.* **199**, 1449–54.

5 Swada T *et al.* (1979) Preliminary report on the clinical use of human leukocyte interferon in neuroblastoma. *Cancer Treat. Rep.* **63**, 2111.

6 Schepart B *et al.* (1995) Long-term stability of Interferon alfa-2b diluted to 2 million units/ml. *Am. J. Health Syst. Pharm.* **52**, 2128–30.

Prepared by Andrew Stanley

INTERFERON α-N1

1 General details

Approved name: Interferon α-n1(Ins).

Proprietary name: Wellferon.

Manufacturer or supplier: Wellcome Medical Division, UK.

Presentation and formulation details: Wellferon is a clear colourless solution in single dose vials, containing 3×10^6, 5×10^6 or 10×10^6 IU of purified human lymphoblastoid interferon formulated in 1 ml Tris-glycine, buffered saline, with albumin solution (European Pharmacopoeia) at a concentration of 1.5 mg/ml as a stabilizer.

Storage and shelf-life of unopened container: Unopened vials expire three years from the date of manufacture when stored between 2–8°C.

2 Chemistry

Interferon α-n1(Ins) is a highly purified blend of natural human α-interferons, obtained from human lymphoblastoid cells following induction with Sendai virus. The final product has a purity of at least 95% and contains no detectable DNA (less than 10 pg of Namalwa cell DNA/ml).

Wellferon resembles human leukocyte interferon in that it is a mixture of natural α subtypes; at least 22 have been detected. It also differs from recombinant α-interferon preparations made from bacteria or other genetically engineered cells which contain only a single subtype.[1]

Molecular structure: Not available.

Molecular weight: Approximately 19 000.

Solubility: Interferon α-n1(Ins) is supplied as a solution.

3 Stability profile

3.1 Physical and chemical stability

No information is available.

Effect of pH: No information is available.

Effect of light: Interferon α-n1(Ins) is sensitive to photodegradation and should therefore be protected from light.[1]

3.2 Stability in clinical practice

Due to lack of information, it is only possible to recommend immediate use of interferon α-n1(Ins) after withdrawing the appropriate dose, followed by speedy disposal of any residue.

4 Clinical use

Main indications: Interferon α-n1(Ins) is licensed for use as a single agent in the treatment of hairy-cell leukaemia,[1] and for the treatment of adults with chronic active hepatitis B, who have markers for viral replication.

Dosage:

▼ hairy-cell leukaemia: for remission induction, the dose recommended is 3×10^6 IU given daily by intramuscular or subcutaneous injection; the latter being more convenient for patient self-administration. After initial improvement in peripheral haematological indices (commonly 12–16 weeks), the dose may be administered thrice weekly. Prolonged treatment for six months or more may be required to clear hairy cells from the bone marrow

▼ chronic active hepatitis B infection: a 12-week course of thrice-weekly intramuscular or subcutaneous injections of $10–15 \times 10^6$ IU (up to 7.5×10^6 IU/m² body surface area) is generally recommended. Longer periods of treatment for up to six months at lower doses ($5–10 \times 10^6$ IU thrice weekly, or up to 5×10^6 IU/m²) have been employed and may be preferred for patients who do not tolerate higher doses.[1]

Other uses (not currently licensed in the UK) are for chronic myeloid leukaemia[2] and chronic hepatitis C (non-A, non-B).

5 Preparation of injection

Reconstitution: Not applicable.

Bolus administration: $2–7.5 \times 10^6$ IU/m² injected subcutaneously, or by deep intramuscular injection.

Intravenous infusion: Not recommended.

Extravasation: Non-irritant; no recommendations available (*see* Chapter 6).

6 Destruction of drug or contaminated articles

Disposal: Excess interferon solution may be disposed of into a drain with copious amounts of water. All other waste, including contaminated packaging or cleaning materials and used protective clothing must be placed with clinical waste for incineration. When dealing with broken vials, disposable gloves, eye protection and a dust mask should be worn.

Contact with skin: Remove contaminated clothing and wash skin thoroughly with soap and water. If the eyes are contaminated, irrigate with water and obtain medical advice.

References

1 *ABPI Data Sheet Compendium 1995–96* (1995) DataPharm Publications Ltd, London, pp. 1971–3.
2 Allan NC *et al.* (1995) (on behalf of the UK MRC trials group) UK MRC randomised, multicentre trial of interferon alpha-n1 for CML: improved survival irrespective of cytogenetic response. *Lancet* **345**, 1392–7.

Prepared by Andrew Stanley

INTERLEUKIN 2

1 General details

Approved name: Aldesleukin (Proleukin)

Manufacturer or supplier: Eurocetus (UK) Ltd.

Presentation and formulation details: Aldesleukin is a sterile, white lyophilized powder for parenteral use containing 1.2 mg (18×10^6 IU/mg) aldesleukin, a recombinant human interleukin-2 (rIL-2), supplied in glass vials (5 ml).

When reconstituted with 1.2 ml water for injections BP, each vial delivers 1 ml solution containing 18×10^6 IU (1 mg) aldesleukin, 50 mg mannitol and 0.2 mg sodium dodecyl sulphate, buffered with sodium phosphates to a pH of 7.5 (range 7.2–7.8).

Storage and shelf-life of unopened container: Unopened vials expire two years from the date of manufacture when stored at 2–8°C.

2 Chemistry

Aldesleukin is produced by recombinant DNA technology using an *Escherichia coli* strain which contains a genetically engineered modification of the human IL-2 gene. This modified recombinant human IL-2 differs from native IL-2 in the following ways:

▼ the molecule is not glycosylated because it is derived from *Escherichia coli*
▼ the molecule has no N-terminal alanine
▼ the molecule has serine substituted for cysteine at amino acid position 125.

The two amino acid changes result in a more homogeneous IL-2 product. The biological activities of aldesleukin and native human IL-2, a naturally occurring lymphokine, are similar; both regulate the immune response. The administration of aldesleukin has been shown to reduce both tumour growth and spread. The exact mechanism by which aldesleukin-mediated immunostimulation leads to anti-tumour activity is not yet known.

Molecular structure:

Des-alanyl-1, serine-125 human interleukin-2; recombinant interleukin-2

```
                          10
Pro-Thr-Ser-Ser-Ser-Thr-Lys-Lys-Thr-Gln-Leu-Gln-Leu-Glu-His-Leu-
      20                                  30
Leu-Leu-Asp-Leu-Gln-Met-Ile-Leu-Asn-Gly-Ile-Asn-Asn-Tyr-Lys-Asn-
                    40
Pro-Lys-Leu-Thr-Arg-Met-Leu-Thr-Phe-Lys-Phe-Tyr-Met-Pro-Lys-Lys-
  50                          60
Ala-Thr-Glu-Leu-Lys-His-Leu-Gln-Cys-Leu-Glu-Glu-Glu-Leu-Lys-Pro-
                        70                            80
Leu-Glu-Glu-Val-Leu-Asn-Leu-Ala-Gln-Ser-Lys-Asn-Phe-His-Leu-Arg-
                              90
Pro-Arg-Asp-Leu-Ile-Ser-Asn-Ile-Asn-Val-Ile-Val-Leu-Glu-Leu-Lys-
    100                            110
Gly-Ser-Glu-Thr-Thr-Phe-Met-Cys-Glu-Tyr-Ala-Asp-Glu-Thr-Ala-Thr-
              120
Ile-Val-Glu-Phe-Leu-Asn-Arg-Trp-Ile-Thr-Phe-Ser-Gln-Ser-Ile-Ile-
Ser-Thr-Leu-Thr
```

Molecular weight: Approximately 15 600.

Solubility: Aldesleukin is freely soluble in water.

3 Stability profile

3.1 Physical and chemical stability

Store vials of lyophilized aldesleukin (rIL-2) in a refrigerator at 2–8°C. Reconstituted or diluted aldesleukin may be stored at refrigerated and at room temperature (2–30°C).

As rIL-2 is not glycosylated it is less water soluble (more lipophilic) when compared with endogenous IL-2. The more lipophilic properties of rIL-2 make it necessary to use sodium dodecyl sulphate (SDS) during the production and formulation of aldesleukin. SDS is a surface active compound which reversibly binds to rIL-2 and brings the lipophilic molecule into solution. In a solution of reconstituted IL-2, there is an equilibrium between rIL-2-bound SDS and free SDS. The capability for SDS to keep rIL-2 in solution is dependent on the concentrations of SDS and rIL-2. The addition of human serum albumin (HSA) is not needed when the reconstituted IL-2 is further diluted (with 5% glucose) to rIL-2 concentrations of between 100 and 1000 μg/ml, because the SDS concentration is high enough to keep the rIL-2 in solution within this concentration range.

It is also not advisable to use HSA, because its addition to rIL-2 at these high concentrations will result in the binding of HSA to SDS, which disturbs the sensitive equilibrium between the free SDS and the rIL-2-bound SDS. This can result in the precipitation of rIL-2.

However, when the solution is further diluted to concentrations below 100 μg/ml, the addition of HSA (0.1%) is necessary to prevent precipitation of rIL-2.

Human serum albumin should be added and mixed with 5% glucose injection prior to the addition of IL-2; it is added to protect against loss of bioactivity.

Container compatibility: IL-2 should be administered using infusion bags or syringes composed of one of the following materials: polypropylene syringes (e.g. Becton-Dickinson Plastipak or Sherwood Monoject), polyvinylchloride bags (e.g. Viaflex), polyolefine bags (e.g. PAB-Excel), or glass bottles.

Extension sets composed of polyethylene or standard administration sets can be used.

In-line filters should not be used when administering interleukin.

Effect of light: No information is available.

Effect of pH: Stable between pH 7.2–7.8. With time interleukin undergoes hydrolysis outside this range.

Compatibility with other drugs: Reconstitution and dilution procedures other than those recommended may result in incomplete delivery of bioactivity and/or formation of biologically inactive protein.

The use of bacteriostatic water for injections, or 0.9% sodium chloride should be avoided because of increased aggregation. Interleukin should not be mixed with other drugs.

3.2 Stability in clinical practice

Due to the unstable nature of IL-2, it must be used within 24 hours of preparation and stored refrigerated (2–8°C) until use.

4 Clinical use

Main indications: Used in the treatment of metastatic renal cell carcinoma, but excluding those patients in whom *all* the following three prognostic factors are present:

▼ a performance status of ECOG 1 or greater
▼ more than one organ with metastatic disease sites
▼ a period of less than 24 months between initial diagnosis of primary tumour and the date the patient is evaluated for IL-2 treatment.

Dosage: Full details of dosage recommendations for each of the licensed indications are provided in the manufacturer's data sheet.[1] Aldesleukin has also been extensively investigated in renal cell carcinoma, melanoma and colorectal tumours using subcutaneous administration schedules to try to minimize the side-effects of the rIL-2.[2]

5 Preparation of injection

Reconstitution: Each vial of IL-2 for injection should be reconstituted with 1.2 ml of water for injections. The diluent should be directed against the side of the vial to avoid excess foaming and the contents swirled gently until completely dissolved. Do not shake. The resulting solution should be a clear, colourless liquid. When reconstituted as directed, each ml contains 18×10^6 IU (1 mg) aldesleukin.

Extravasation: Non-irritant; however may cause local capillary leak syndrome and/or local tissue reaction (*see* Chapter 6).

6 Destruction of drug or contaminated articles

Disposal: Excess IL-2 solution may be disposed of into a drain with copious amounts of water. All other waste, including contaminated packaging or cleaning materials and used protective clothing must be placed with clinical waste for incineration. When dealing with broken vials, disposable gloves, eye protection and a dust mask should be worn.

Contact with skin: Remove contaminated clothing and wash skin thoroughly with soap and water. If the eyes are contaminated, irrigate with water and obtain medical advice.

References

1 *UK Data Sheet January 1992*. Eurocetus (UK) Ltd.
2 Eurocetus (UK) Ltd. Personal communication.

Prepared by Andrew Stanley

This section has been created to present in monograph form those therapeutic compounds that are licensed and have an impact on the practice of oncology pharmacy.

Whilst the editors acknowledge the existence of the following support therapies, it has not proved possible to construct meaningful monographs due to a lack of information.

Molgramostin rGM-CFS
Octreotide
Tropisetron

Other drugs being used in a support or adjuvant therapy context, but either not licensed for this specific use or under development are α and β epoetin for cytotoxic induced anaemia, and the L-isomer of folic acid.

AMIFOSTINE

1 General details

Approved name: Amifostine.

Proprietary names: Ethyol, WR2721, Gammaphos MCS 298962.

Manufacturer or supplier: The product licence is held by US Bio-sciences Inc. Amifostine is supplied by Schering-Plough Ltd.

Presentation and formulation details: Amifostine is supplied as a sterile lyophilized powder. Each vial contains 500 mg of amifostine anhydrous and 500 mg of mannitol.[1,2]

Storage and shelf-life of unopened container: Two years stored at 2–8°C.[1]

2 Chemistry

Type: Amifostine is a pro-drug that is non-reactive with electrophilic groups of chemotherapeutic agents.

Molecular structure: 5-2 (3 aminopropylamino) ethyl phosphoric acid.

$$NH_2-CH_2-CH_2-CH_2-NH(CH_2)_2 \; S-\overset{\displaystyle OH}{\underset{\displaystyle OH}{P}}=O$$

Molecular weight: 214.2.

Molecular formula: $C_5H_{15}N_2O_3PS$.

Solubility: Amifostine is soluble in water, 0.9% sodium chloride and phosphate buffer pH 7.0.[1]

3 Stability profile

3.1 Physical and chemical stability

Solutions containing amifostine 500 mg/10 ml 0.9% sodium chloride are stable for eight hours at room temperature (15–25°C), or 24 hours under refrigeration 2–8°C.[1,3]

Effect of pH: The pH of the reconstituted solution is in the range of 6–8.

Effect of light: No information available.

Container compatibility: Amifostine has been shown to be compatible with glass and PVC infusion containers.[1]

3.2 Stability in clinical practice

Amifostine 50 mg/ml is stable in 0.9% sodium chloride for eight hours at 15–25°C, and 24 hours at 2–8°C.[1,3]

4 Clinical use

Amifostine is dephosphorylated by the enzyme alkaline phosphatase to the active free thiol S[(aminopropyl) amino] ethanethiol.

Dephosphorylation occurs more rapidly in normal tissue than in bulky tumour masses because tumour masses are relatively hypovascular and the interstitial pH of tumours is relatively acidic and thereby kinetically unfavourable to the capillary-associated alkaline phosphatase. The dephosphorylated metabolite readily enters non-cancerous cells by facilitated diffusion, providing protection against oxygen-based radicals and electrophilic reactive drugs, such as alkylating agents and aquated organoplatinum anticancer drugs, by donating H^+ from its nucleophilic-free sulphydryl group, thus deactivating reactive cytotoxic agents.[4]

It is licensed at a dose of $910\,mg/m^2$ for the reduction of neutropenic-related risk of infection due to combined cyclophosphamide–cisplatinum therapy in patients with advanced fed. intern. gynea. onc. (FIGO) stage III or IV ovarian carcinoma.[2] It is administered once daily as a 15 minute intravenous infusion, starting 30 minutes prior to chemotherapy, with agents given by short infusions. Arterial blood pressure should be monitored carefully during amifostine administration.[2]

5 Preparation of injection

Preparation of injection: The contents of the 500 mg vial are dissolved by adding 9.5 ml 0.9% sodium chloride and gently shaking the contents of the vial to produce a solution containing 500 mg in 10 ml (50 mg/ml). To prepare the intravenous infusion the required volume of the reconstituted solution is added to 100–200 ml of 0.9% sodium chloride in a glass or PVC infusion container.[2]

References

1 Schering-Plough UK. Personal communications.
2 *Ethyol Data Sheet 1994*, Schering-Plough Ltd.
3 *Investigators' brochure – Ethyol* (1995) Schering-Plough Ltd.
4 *Ethyol (Amifostine) for the prevention of chemotherapy induced toxicity. Product Monograph* (1994) Schering-Plough Ltd.

Prepared by Andrew Stanley

CALCIUM FOLINATE

1 General details

Approved names: Calcium folinate, Leucovorin calcium.

Proprietary names: Lederfolin, Refolinon, Rescufolin, Wellcovorin.

Manufacturer or supplier: Cyanamid, Pharmacia, Nordic, Faulding/DBL, Wellcome USA.

Presentation and formulation details: Lyophilized powder for reconstitution in glass vials, or solution in water for injections in ampoules or vials. Solutions also contain sodium chloride, and pH is adjusted to somewhere between 6.5 and 8.5 (dependent on manufacturer), using sodium hydroxide or hydrochloric acid.

Storage and shelf-life of unopened container: Lyophilized powder for reconstitution has a shelf-life of three years when stored between 15–30°C. Solution has a shelf-life of 18 months or two years when stored between 2–8°C, and protected from light.

2 Chemistry

Molecular structure: Calcium N-[4-(2-amino-5-formyl-5,6,7,8-tetrahydro-4-hydroxy-pteridin-6-ylmethylamino)benzoyl]-L(+)glutamate.

Molecular weight: 511.5.

Solubility: Very soluble in water; practically insoluble in alcohol.

3 Stability profile

3.1 Physical and chemical stability

Calcium folinate degradation occurs by two routes: hydrolysis, or a conversion reaction. The main products of hydrolysis are 5-formyl tetrahydropteridin-6-carboxylic acid and N-(p-aminobenzoyl) glutamic acid, which undergoes further hydrolysis to p-aminobenzoic acid and glutamic acid. The conversion reaction involves the exchange of the formyl group from the N^5 nitrogen of the pteridinyl moiety, to the N^{10} nitrogen of the p-aminobenzoylglutamic acid group, to produce N^{10} formylfolic acid.[1] Hydrolysis occurs in acid pH, particularly at less than pH 5.

Compatibility with infusion fluids: Calcium folinate is compatible with sodium chloride, glucose, and compound sodium lactate infusion fluids and is stable in both glass and PVC containers.[1,2]

Compatibility with other drugs: Calcium folinate has been shown to be compatible with cisplatin, with or without floxuridine,[3] and with floxuridine alone.[4,5] Studies had indicated that calcium folinate could be mixed with fluorouracil.[5,6] However, recent work has indicated that a crystalline precipitate forms in stored mixtures in less than four days[7,8] and as a consequence, manufacturers now state that calcium folinate should not be mixed with fluorouracil.

Compatibility studies of mixing with other drugs briefly in a syringe, or in a simulated Y-site injection, have indicated compatibility with a number of drugs.[9–12] Incompatibility was seen with droperidol[9] and foscarnet.[13]

3.2 Stability in clinical practice

Stored at room temperature or refrigerated, and protected from light, calcium folinate has been shown to be stable for 96 hours at a concentration of 1.0–1.5 mg/ml in 0.9% sodium chloride or 5% glucose. Lower concentrations appear to be less stable, and are therefore not suitable for extended expiry.[1]

The extended stability data that have been reported for mixtures with fluoropyrimidines should be treated with caution since the recent discovery of crystalline deposits in mixtures with fluorouracil. Mixtures for immediate intravenous infusion may be compatible, but are not recommended by the manufacturers.

3.3 Stability in specialized delivery systems

No data available.

4 Clinical use

Type of pharmaceutical: An essential co-enzyme. It is the calcium salt of a formyl derivative of tetrahydrofolic acid, the metabolite and active form of folic acid.

Main indications:

▼ to diminish the toxicity and counteract the action of folate antagonists such as methotrexate in cytotoxic therapy (calcium folinate rescue)
▼ to enhance the effects of fluorouracil cytotoxic therapy.

Dosage:

▼ for calcium folinate rescue, normal dosage is for up to 150 mg to be given in divided doses over 24–28 hours, starting at 8–24 hours after the methotrexate dose
▼ for enhancing the effect of fluorouracil, doses of between 20 and 200 mg/m² are given prior to doses of fluorouracil.

5 Preparation of injection

Dilution: Should be reconstituted with water for injection.

Bolus administration: Doses of 15–30 mg may be administered as intravenous or intramuscular injections.

Intravenous infusion: May be diluted in sodium chloride, glucose, or compound sodium lactate infusions, and administered over not less than 3–5 minutes because of the calcium content.

6 Destruction of drug or contaminated articles

Calcium folinate is non-hazardous and can be handled and disposed of as a non-cytotoxic pharmaceutical.

References

1 Lecompte D *et al.* (1991) Stability study of reconstituted and diluted solutions of calcium folinate. *Pharm. Ind.* **1**, 90–4.

2 Benvenuto JA *et al.* (1981) Stability and compatibility of antitumour agents in glass and plastic containers. *Am. J. Hosp. Pharm.* **38**, 1914–18.

3 Williams DA, Lokich J (1992) A review of the stability and compatibility of anti-neoplastic drugs for multiple-drug infusions. *Cancer Chemother. Pharmacol.* **31**, 171–81.

4 Smith JA *et al.* (1989) Stability of floxuridine and leucovorin calcium admixtures for intraperitoneal administration. *Am. J. Hosp. Pharm.* **46**, 985–9.

5 Anderson N *et al.* (1989) A phase 1 clinical trial of combined fluoropyrimidines with leucovorin in a 14-day infusion. *Cancer* **63**, 233–7.

6 Milano G *et al.* (1993) Long-term stability of 5-fluorouracil and folinic acid admixtures. *Eur. J. Cancer.* **29A**, 129–32.

7 Adralan B, Flores MR (1993) A new complication of permanent indwelling central venous catheters using high dose fluorouracil and leucovorin. *J. Clin. Oncol.* **11**, 384.

8 Trissel LA *et al.* (1995) Incompatibility of fluorouracil with leucovorin calcium or levoleucovorin calcium. *Am. J. Health-Syst. Pharm.* **52**, 710–15.

9 Cohen MH *et al.* (1985) Drug precipitation within IV tubing: A potential hazard of chemotherapy administration. *Cancer Treat. Rep.* **69**, 1325–6.

10 Trissel LA, Martinez JF (1994) Physical compatibility of filgrastim with selected drugs during simulated Y-site administration. *Am. J. Hosp. Pharm.* **51**, 1907–13.

11 Trissel LA, Martinez JF (1994) Physical compatibility of piperacillin sodium plus tazobactam sodium with selected drugs during simulated Y-site administration. *Am. J. Hosp. Pharm.* **51**, 672–8.

12 Min DI *et al.* (1992) Visual compatibility of tacrolimus with commonly used drugs during simulated Y-site injection. *Am. J. Hosp. Pharm.* **49**, 2964–6.

13 Lor E, Takagi J (1990) Visible compatibility of foscarnet with other injectable drugs. *Am. J. Hosp. Pharm.* **47**, 157–9.

Prepared by Richard Needle

DEXRAZOXONE

1 General details

Approved name: Dexrazoxone.

Proprietary names: Zinecard, ADR-529, ICRF-187.

Manufacturer or supplier: Pharmacia, Upjohn.

Presentation and formulation details: Sterile white, to off-white, lyophilized powder in vials containing either 250 mg or 500 mg dexrazoxone; pH-adjusted with hydrochloric acid.

Each vial is supplied with a vial of diluent containing M/6 sodium lactate injection USP in vials of 25 ml (accompanying 250 mg vials) and 50 ml (accompanying 500 mg vials), where each ml of diluent contains 18.6 mg anhydrous sodium lactate in water for injection, pH being adjusted with sodium hydroxide, and/or hydrochloric acid.[1]

Storage and shelf-life of unopened container: Two years stored at 15–30°C.

2 Chemistry

Type: Dexrazoxone is a cyclic derivative of edetic acid (EDTA).[2]

Molecular structure: 4,4'-(1-methyl-1,2,-ethanediyl) bis [2,6-piperazinedione].

Molecular weight: 268.28.

Molecular formula: $C_{11}H_{16}N_4O_4$.

Solubility: Dexrazoxone is only sparingly soluble in water.

3 Stability profile

3.1 Physical and chemical stability

The reconstituted solution at a concentration of 10 mg/10 ml is reported to be stable for six hours when stored at 2–8°C.[3,4]

Effect of pH: No information is available. However, the molecule is likely to be sensitive to extremes of pH.

Effects of temperature: Dexrazoxone shows significant degradation at temperatures above 8°C, with a maximum stability of six hours at 15–30°C.[3]

3.2 Stability in clinical practice

The reconstituted solution may be diluted with either 0.9% sodium chloride or 5% glucose to a concentration of 1.4–5.0 mg/ml and should be refrigerated if not to be used immediately, with a practical life including refrigeration of six hours, at temperatures up to 30°C.

4 Clinical use

Dexrazoxone at a ratio of 10 : 1 (e.g. 500 mg/m² of dexrazoxone to 50 mg/m² of doxorubicin) is licensed for reducing the incidence and severity of cardio-myopathy associated with doxorubicin administration in women with metastatic breast cancer, who have received a cumulative dose of 300 mg/m² and who, in the opinion of their physician, would benefit from continuation of their doxorubicin therapy. It should be administered by slow intravenous bolus injection, or intravenous infusion after completing the infusion of dexrazoxone, and prior to a total elapsed time of 30 minutes after initiating doxorubicin therapy.[1-3]

5 Preparation of injection

Preparation of injection: Dexrazoxone must be reconstituted with the diluent supply (0.167 M sodium lactate injection) to give a concentration of 10 mg/ml of sodium lactate.[1]

6 Destruction of drug or contaminated articles

Incineration: 1000°C.

Chemical: Dexrazoxone may be inactivated by adding sodium hypochlorite solution (in the same strength as household bleach) until the dexrazoxone solution is decolorized.[4]

Contact with skin and eyes: Dexrazoxone is an irritant to mucous membranes, the affected areas should be washed with copious amounts of water, and a medical opinion sought.[4]

References

1 *US Data Sheet* (1995) Pharmacia Upjohn.
2 Anon. (1995) New drug counters doxorubicin cardio-toxicity not for use at start of chemotherapy. *Am. Health-Syst. Pharm.* **52**, 2076.
3 *Zinecard – Cardio-protective agent product monograph*, Pharmacia Upjohn.
4 Pharmacia Upjohn. Personal communications.

Prepared by Andrew Stanley

FILGRASTIM

1 General details

Approved name: Filgrastim.

Proprietary name: Neupogen.

Manufacturer: Amgen Ltd.

Supplier: Roche Products Ltd.

Presentation and formulation details: Filgrastim is a sterile, clear, colourless liquid, formulated in an aqueous sodium acetate buffer, pH 4, containing 4% mannitol and 0.004% polysorbate 80.

It is known chemically as non-glycosylated recombinant methionyl human granulocyte colony-stimulating factor (r-metHuG-CSF), and is produced by recombinant DNA technology using an *Escherichia coli* strain.

Filgrastim contains 30×10^6 IU (300 µg/ml). Neupogen 30 contains 300 µg of filgrastim in a 1 ml vial. Neupogen 48 contains 480 µg of filgrastim in a 1.6 ml vial.

Storage and shelf-life of unopened container: Filgrastim should be stored at 2–8°C. It should not be frozen. The pack is provided with an indicator to detect possible freezing. Vials that have been frozen (the indicator shows red) should not be used. A single brief period (up to seven days) of exposure to elevated temperatures (up to 37°C) does not affect stability. Unopened vials of filgrastim expire two years from the date of manufacture.[1]

2 Chemistry

Molecular structure: The amino acid composition of the mature r-metHuG-CSF sequence is:

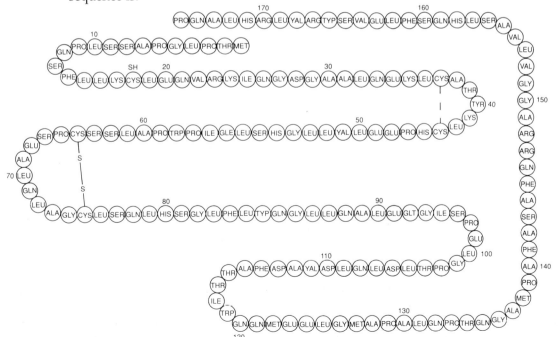

The solution contains filgrastim (r-metHuG-CSF) as a hydrophobic protein comprising 175 amino acids. The recombinant protein differs from natural human G-CSF by virtue of an additional amino terminal methionine residue and the absence of O-glycosylation. There are no potential sites of N-glycosylation on the natural human G-CSF or recombinant G-CSF molecules.

Molecular weight: Approximately 18–22 000.

Solubility: Filgrastim is soluble in aqueous solutions.

3 Stability profile

3.1 Physical and chemical stability

pH and physical stability: The pH of filgrastim is 4.0. Low pH and low salt concentration, together with additives, enhance filgrastim stability by preventing protein aggregation. The product should not be vigorously shaken when diluting, in order to avoid the formation of protein aggregates which might induce undesirable effects in the patient (i.e. formation of antibodies).

Stability on dilution: Diluted filgrastim solutions should not be prepared more than 24 hours before administration and should be stored at between 2 and 8°C. Solutions of filgrastim at concentrations of 15 µg/ml or higher, are stable at room temperature for up to one week.[2]

Container compatibility: Filgrastim diluted in 5% glucose or in 5% glucose plus human albumin is compatible with a variety of plastics. These include: PVC, polyolefin (co-polymer of polypropylene and polyethylene) and polypropylene.[2] If filgrastim is to be used as an infusion with the administration set composed of unknown material, human serum albumin (HSA) should always be added as a protective protein to the diluent to a concentration of at least 2 mg/ml. It is not necessary to protect filgrastim from light when the drug is being prepared for administration, but it is recommended that filgrastim is stored within the dispensing pack.[2]

Drug compatibility: The compatibility of filgrastim with other products and solutions has not been evaluated, therefore filgrastim should not be given together with any other drugs in the same infusion set and also should not be diluted in any other solution containing sodium chloride.

3.2 Stability in clinical practice

Undiluted filgrastim in tuberculin syringes (Becton-Dickinson)[2] is stable for up to 24 hours at controlled room temperature (25°C and not exceeding 37°C) or for up to seven days in the refrigerator 2–8°C. Filgrastim does not contain any preservatives. The manufacturer recommends that, in order to reduce the possibility of bacterial proliferation, filgrastim in syringes should be stored at 2–8°C and used within 24 hours of preparation.[1]

Filgrastim may be diluted in 5% glucose intravenous solution. Very dilute solutions of filgrastim may be adsorbed on to glass and plastic materials. Therefore, dilution to a final concentration of less than 0.2×10^6 IU (2 µg/ml) is not recommended.[2]

For solutions diluted to concentrations below 1.5×10^6 IU (15 µg/ml), HSA should be added to a final concentration of 2 mg/ml; i.e. in a final injection volume of 20 ml. Total doses of filgrastim less than 30×10^6 IU (300 µg) should be given with 0.2 ml of 20% HSA.[2]

4 Clinical use

Indications: Filgrastim is indicated for the reduction in both the duration of neutropenia and the incidence of febrile neutropenia in patients treated with established cytotoxic chemotherapy for non-myeloid malignancy. This allows the clinician to optimize cytotoxic chemotherapy and to reduce the incidence of febrile neutropenia and its clinical sequelae. The indication includes the reduction in duration of neutropenia and its clinical sequelae after myeloablative therapy which is followed by bone marrow transplantation.

In patients with severe congenital, cyclic, or idiopathic neutropenia (with an absolute neutrophil count (ANC) $\leqslant 0.5 \times 10^9/l$), or a history of severe or recurrent infections, long-term treatment with filgrastim is indicated to increase the ANC and reduce incidence and duration of infection-related events.

Filgrastim mobilizes peripheral blood progenitor cells (PBPCs) (as a single mobilizing agent, or following myelosuppressive chemotherapy) for autologous PBPC transplant. The infusion of filgrastim-mobilized PBPCs accelerates haemato-poietic recovery, reducing the need for platelet transfusions after myelosuppressive chemotherapy.

Filgrastim is also indicated in patients with advanced HIV infection and neutropenia (ANC $<1 \times 10^9/l$), allowing scheduled dosing of myelosuppressive medication.

Dosage:

▼ established cytotoxic chemotherapy (adults): when filgrastim is administered as an adjunct to standard dose chemotherapy, the recommended dose is $5\,\mu g/kg/day$. Individual patients may require dose escalation if the time taken to respond, or if the magnitude of the neutrophil response, is unacceptable after five to seven days of filgrastim therapy. A maximum tolerated dose has not yet been identified. Patients have received doses as high as $115\,\mu g/kg/day$, with no toxic effects attributable to filgrastim

▼ myeloablative therapy followed by bone marrow transplantation: filgrastim administration should not commence during the initial 24 hours after bone marrow infusion. The initial dosage of $10\,\mu g/kg/day$ is reduced to $5\,\mu g/kg/day$ once the neutrophil nadir has passed and ANC has exceeded $1.0 \times 10^9/l$ for three consecutive days

▼ mobilization of PBPCs: as a single agent, $10\,\mu g/kg/day$ subcutaneously for six consecutive days is the recommended dose to achieve effective mobilization of PBPCs. Alternatively, in conjunction with myelosuppressive chemotherapy, $5\,\mu g/kg/day$ subcutaneously is given daily from the first day post-chemotherapy until the expected neutrophil nadir is passed and the neutrophil count has recovered to the normal range. For patients who have not had extensive chemotherapy, a single apheresis is often sufficient. In other circumstances, additional leukaphereses are recommended

▼ severe chronic neutropenia (children or adults): for the treatment of congenital neutropenia, the initial recommended dose is $12\,\mu g/kg/day$ subcutaneously, but a lower dosage of $5\,\mu g/kg/day$ subcutaneously is used for idiopathic, or cyclic neutropenia. Treatment is continued until an ANC $>1.5 \times 10^9/l$ can be maintained; then minimum doses required to maintain this level are ascertained and administered

▼ advanced HIV infection: for the treatment of neutropenia, an initial dose of 1–$4\,\mu g/kg/day$ subcutaneously is recommended until a normal neutrophil count (ANC $\geqslant 2.0 \times 10^9/l$) is reached, and can be maintained. Subsequent maintenance doses of 300 µg/day subcutaneously are recommended. Further dose adjustment (and possibly long-term administration) may be necessary to maintain the ANC $\geq 2.0 \times 10^9$/l.

Filgrastim can be administered either as a bolus subcutaneous injection or as a short (30 minute) or continuous IV or subcutaneous infusion.[1]

Timing of administration: Filgrastim administration should be initiated at least 24 hours after the last dose of chemotherapy and should be discontinued at least 24 hours before the next chemotherapy dose. This is because filgrastim stimulates neutrophil precursor cell proliferation and, since many antineoplastic agents target rapidly proliferating cells, co-administration of filgrastim and antineoplastic therapy may theoretically lead to abolition of neutrophil precursors. Filgrastim administration should be continued throughout the expected chemotherapy-induced nadir until the patient achieves an ANC more than or equal to 10 000 cells/ml.[1]

Patients receiving dose-intensified chemotherapy should be continued on filgrastim until two consecutive ANCs register more than 10 000 cells/ml. The time to achieve this ANC level will vary, based on the chemotherapy regimen, the patient's underlying disease, prior treatment history and dose of filgrastim.[1]

5 Preparation of injection

Reconstitution: Not applicable.

Extravasation: Not irritant; no recommendations available (*see* Chapter 6).

6 Destruction of drug or contaminated articles

Disposal: Excess filgrastim solution may be disposed of into a drain with copious amounts of water. All other waste, including contaminated packaging or cleaning materials and used protective clothing must be placed with clinical waste for incineration. When dealing with broken vials, disposable gloves, eye protection and a face mask should be worn.

Contact with skin: This is thought not to be a serious problem; a general procedure should be adopted of removing contaminated clothing and washing skin thoroughly with soap and water. If the eyes are contaminated, irrigate with water and obtain medical advice.

References

1 *ABPI Data Sheet Compendium 1995–96* (1995) DataPharm Publications Ltd, London, pp. 1455–8.
2 Amgen (UK) Ltd. Personal communication.

Prepared by Andrew Stanley

GRANISETRON

1 General details

Approved names: Granisetron hydrochloride.

Proprietary name: Kytril.

Manufacturer or supplier: SmithKline Beecham Ltd.

Presentation and formulation details: Kytril injection is a clear, colourless, slightly straw-coloured liquid in clear glass ampoules.[1] Each 3 ml of isotonic saline contains 3 mg granisetron as the hydrochloride.

Storage and shelf-life of unopened container: Three years when protected from light. Do not freeze.

2 Chemistry

Chemical name: Endo-N-(9-methyl-9-azabicyclo [3.3.1] non-3-yl)-1-methyl-1H-idiazole-3-carboxamide hydrochloride.

Physical form: White to off-white solid.

Structural formula:

Molecular formula: $C_{18}H_{24}N_4O.HCl$.

Molecular weight: 348.9 (312.4 free base).

Solubility: Readily soluble in water and 0.9% sodium chloride.

3 Stability profile

3.1 Physical and chemical stability

Granisetron has been reported to be relatively stable after dilution in 5% glucose or 0.9% sodium chloride. Stability was maintained for at least three days at 20°C, or seven days at 4°C.[2,3]

Container compatibility: Granisetron solutions containing 0.056 or 0.15 mg/ml in 50 ml 5% glucose or 0.9% sodium chloride infusions were stable and compatible when stored in PVC bags or plastic syringes.[2,3]

Compatibility with other drugs: Granisetron solutions containing 0.056 or 0.15 mg/ml in 50 ml 5% glucose or 0.9% sodium chloride infusions were compatible with dexamethasone (20 or 40 mg) or methylprednisolone (120 mg) for 72 hours at ambient temperature.[3] Granisetron was chemically stable under these conditions.[3]

3.2 Stability in clinical practice

Granisetron is reported to be stable for 24 hours after preparation of infusions as recommended by the manufacturer.[1] Granisetron solutions containing 0.15 mg/ml in 5% glucose, 0.9% sodium chloride and a range of other infusions were tested for stability and compatibility when stored at 5°C in the dark, ambient temperature in a mixture of daylight and fluorescent light, or under temperature cycling conditions between 5°C and ambient temperature. Results confirmed that granisetron was physically and chemically stable under all conditions tested for 48 hours.[2]

Granisetron solutions containing 0.056 mg/ml in 50 ml in 5% glucose or 0.9% sodium chloride stored in PVC bags or in 20 ml syringes, or 0.15 mg/ml in 20 ml plastic syringes, has been reported to be chemically and physically stable for three days at 20°C, seven days at 4°C followed by three days at 20°C, or 30 days at –20°C, followed by seven days at 4°C and three days at 20°C.[3]

3.3 Stability in specialized delivery systems

No information available.

4 Clinical use

Main indication: Granisetron injection is indicated for the prevention or treatment of nausea and vomiting induced by cytostatic therapy.[1,2]

Dosage:

▼ adults: 3 mg granisetron injection administered either in 15 ml infusion fluid as an intravenous bolus over not less than 30 minutes or diluted in 20–50 ml infusion fluid and administered over five minutes. Prevention: in clinical trials the majority of patients have required only a single dose of granisetron to control nausea and vomiting over 24 hours. Up to two additional doses of 3 mg granisetron may be administered within a 24 hour period. Prophylactic administration of granisetron should be completed prior to the start of cytostatic therapy. Treatment: the same dose of granisetron should be used for treatment as prevention. Additional doses should be administered at least ten minutes apart
▼ children: prevention (injection): a single dose of 40 µg/kg body weight (up to 3 mg) should be administered as an intravenous infusion, diluted in 10–30 ml infusion fluid and administered over five minutes. Administration should be completed prior to the start of cytostatic therapy. Treatment: the same dose of granisetron should be used for treatment as prevention. One additional dose of 40 µg/kg body weight (up to 3 mg) may be administered within a 24 hour period. This additional dose should be administered at least ten minutes apart from the initial infusion.

5 Preparation of injection

The required volume is withdrawn from the ampoule and diluted either to 15 ml with 0.9% sodium chloride (for bolus administration) or in infusion fluid, to a total volume of 20–50 ml in any of the following solutions: 0.9% sodium chloride; 0.18% w/v sodium chloride and 4% w/v glucose; 5% w/v glucose; Hartmann's solution; sodium lactate injection; or 10% mannitol injection.

References

1 *ABPI Data Sheet Compendium 1995–96* (1995) DataPharm Publications Ltd, London, pp. 1736–7.
2 SmithKline Beecham Ltd. Personal communication.
3 Pinquet F *et al.* (1995) Compatibility and stability of granisetron, dexamethasone and methylprednisolone in injectable solutions. *J. Pharm. Sci.* **84**, 267–8.

Prepared by Andrew Stanley

LENOGRASTIM

1 General details

Approved name: Lenograstim.

Proprietary name: Granocyte.

Manufacturer or supplier: Chugai Pharma UK Ltd, Rhone-Poulenc Rorer Ltd.

Presentation and formulation details: Lenograstim is presented as a single-use vial of lyophilized product with, or without, an ampoule of solvent containing water for injections. The reconstituted product is formulated in an aqueous phosphate buffer at pH 6.5 and contains 5% mannitol, 0.1% human albumin and 0.01% polysorbate-20.[1]

Lenograstim is glycosylated recombinant human G-CSF, produced by recombinant DNA technology, expressed and glycosylated in a mammalian host cell system, Chinese hamster ovary (CHO) cells. Lenograstim (rHuG-CSF) belongs to the cytokine group of biologically active proteins which regulate cell differentiation and growth. Lenograstim is a factor which stimulates the neutrophil precursor cells as demonstrated by the CFU-S and CFU-GM cell count increases in peripheral blood.

Composition of the lyophilizate:[1]

Lenograstim	33.6 MIU	13.4 MIU
	263 µg	105 µg
Human albumin	1 mg	1 mg
Mannitol	50 mg	50 mg
Polysorbate-20	0.1 mg	0.1 mg
Disodium phosphate		
Sodium dihydrogen phosphate	pH 6.5	pH 6.5

2 Chemistry

Type: Lenograstim, human G-CSF, is a recombinant glycoprotein identical to the naturally produced human granulocyte colony stimulating factor isolated from CHU-2, a human cell line.

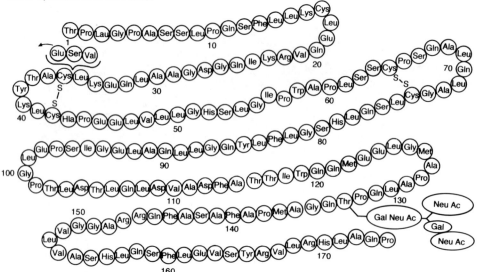

Molecular weight: Approximately 19 000.

Solubility: Soluble in aqueous solutions.

3 Stability profile

3.1 Physical and chemical stability

pH and physical stability: Lenograstim is formulated in a buffer and after reconstitution, the pH of the solution is 6.5. Protein aggregates may form when the solution is shaken vigorously, therefore, during reconstitution and when in solution lenograstim should not be shaken vigorously.[1,2]

Stability on reconstitution: Reconstituted lenograstim is stable in vials for up to seven days at room temperature.[2]

Stability on dilution: Lenograstim should not be reconstituted and diluted more than 24 hours before administration. Diluted solutions should be stored in a refrigerator at 2–8°C.[1,2]

Container compatibility: When diluted in a saline solution, lenograstim is compatible with the polyvinyl chloride giving sets.[1]

If the material of the giving set is not known the human albumin in the formulation acts as a protective protein to stabilize lenograstim against adsorption on to plastics.[1,2]

Compatibility with other drugs: The compatibility of lenograstim has been tested with intravenous fluids at room temperature for 24 hours. Lenograstim is compatible with 0.9% sodium chloride, 5% glucose and compound sodium lactate solutions for up to 24 hours.[1,2]

Compatibility with admixtures of other drugs has not been evaluated, therefore lenograstim should not be given together with any other drugs in the same infusion set.[1,2]

3.2 Stability in clinical practice

Lenograstim should be stored in a refrigerator between 2–8°C. However, the stability of lenograstim is unaffected by exposure to temperatures up to 30°C, for a period of 14 days. After a single exposure within these limits lenograstim may be returned to refrigeration and the original expiry date considered to apply.[2]

Lenograstim has been tested after storage for six months at 30°C. After this period the product was within the quality specification and therefore would be acceptable for use. The effect of this period of exposure on ultimate shelf-life is not defined. For periods of exposure longer than two weeks at room temperature, but less than six months, lenograstim should be returned to refrigeration and used within six months of the date of first exposure.[2]

Lenograstim reconstituted with 1 ml of water for injections is stable in polypropylene syringes for up to 14 days after storing at 30°C for 24 hours, then at 5°C.

Lenograstim should be diluted in 0.9% sodium chloride for intravenous infusion.[1] The maximum dilution which should be performed is one vial into 100 ml of fluid (0.32 MIU/ml; 2.5 µg/ml).

Since human albumin solution is included in the formulation, it does not need to be added when dilution is performed.

4 Clinical use

Main indications: Lenograstim is indicated for reduction in the duration of neutropenia and associated complications in patients with non-myeloid malignancy who have undergone bone marrow transplantation, or treatment with established cytotoxic chemotherapy regimens. By earlier recovery of neutrophil counts, the risk and severity of infection may be reduced and cytotoxic chemotherapy schedule may be maintained in a higher proportion of patients.[1]

Dosage: The recommended dose of lenograstim is 150 µg/m^2/day (19.2 MIU/m^2/day). The 33.6 MIU vial of lenograstim is sufficient to treat patients with a body surface area (BSA) of up to 1.8 m^2; the 13.4 MIU vial is sufficient to treat patients with a BSA of up to 0.7 m^2.

▼ Chemotherapy-induced neutropenia: lenograstim should be administered daily at the recommended dose as a subcutaneous injection starting on the day following completion of chemotherapy. Daily administration of lenograstim should continue until the expected nadir has passed and the neutrophil count returns to a stable level compatible with treatment discontinuation, with a maximum of 28 consecutive days of treatment. Treatment with lenograstim should be discontinued at least 24 hours before starting a course of cytotoxic chemotherapy, since lenograstim-induced proliferation of bone marrow precursor cells could theoretically enhance susceptibility to cytotoxic chemotherapy, increasing toxicity to the myeloid lineage.

If receiving dose-intensified chemotherapy, patients should continue lenograstim treatment until two consecutive ANC measurements $>1 \times 10^9/l$ are achieved.

▼ Bone marrow transplantation: lenograstim should be administered as a 30 minute intravenous infusion, diluted in isotonic saline solution, starting the day following transplantation. Dosing should continue until the expected nadir has passed and the neutrophil count returns to a stable level compatible with treatment discontinuation, with a maximum of 28 consecutive days of treatment, if necessary.

5 Preparation of injection

Reconstitution: Immediately prior to administration, lenograstim should be reconstituted by adding the extractable contents of one ampoule of solvent (water for injections) to the lenograstim vial and agitating gently. The contents should not be shaken vigorously. Dissolution should be complete in approximately five seconds and the final concentration of lenograstim in the solution is 263 µg/ml.[1]

Extravasation: Non-irritant. No recommendations available.

6 Destruction of drug or contaminated articles

Disposal: Excess lenograstim may be disposed of into a drain with water. All other waste, contaminated packaging, cleaning materials, protective clothing, should be incinerated as clinical waste.

Contact with skin: There have been no reports of problems following skin contact. General measures such as removal of contaminated clothing and washing thoroughly with soap and water should be taken.

Contact with eyes: Irrigate with an appropriate eyewash solution, and seek medical advice.

References

1 Granocyte Data Sheet. Rhone-Poulenc Rorer Ltd. October 1993.
2 Data on File: Chugai Pharma UK.

Prepared by Andrew Stanley

MESNA

1 General details

Approved name: Mesna.

Proprietary name: Uromitexan.

Manufacturer or supplier: ASTA Medica Ltd.

Presentation and formulation details: Clear glass ampoules containing an aqueous solution of mesna, 400 mg in 4 ml and 1000 mg in 10 ml.[1]

Each ampoule also contains disodium edetate 0.25 mg/ml and sodium hydroxide as buffer.

Storage and shelf-life of unopened container: When stored below 30°C and protected from light, mesna has a shelf-life of five years.[1]

2 Chemistry

Type: Sulphydryl compound (not cytotoxic).

Molecular structure: Sodium 2-mercapto-ethanesulphonate, HS-CH-CH-SO.Na.

Molecular weight: 164.2.

Solubility: Water soluble.

3 Stability profile

3.1 Physical and chemical stability

Mesna degrades by oxidation to form dimesna. Mesna should be protected from light, but it is stable under normal lighting conditions during administration.[2]

Container compatibility: Compatible with glass, PVC and polypropylene.

Compatibility with other drugs: Compatible with ifosfamide in 0.9% sodium chloride, 5% glucose and Ringer's lactate infusions.[2]

3.2 Stability in clinical practice

Mesna is stable for up to 24 hours in a solution of 0.9% sodium chloride or in a solution of ifosfamide in 0.9% sodium chloride.[1] Mesna (3.3 g and 5 g/l) and ifosfamide (also at concentrations of 3.3 g and 5 g/l, respectively) were admixed in 5% glucose solution and Ringer's lactate injection. Mesna exhibited approximately 5% decomposition over 24 hours, while ifosfamide showed no decomposition during this period.[2]

Admixtures of mesna (40 mg/ml) and ifosfamide (50 mg/ml) in water for injections (10 ml) were stable in polypropylene syringes at 4 and 20°C over 28 days, with less than 5% loss of each component present.[3] At 50 mg/ml the admixture was stable for 24 hours at 37°C,[4] thus enabling ambulatory continuous infusion of this regimen. The undiluted formulation of mesna was found to be stable when stored in polypropylene syringes at 5, 24 or 35°C for at least nine days.[5] (Mesna was also stable for at least one week when diluted 1:2 with various syrups for oral use and stored at 24°C.[5] Dilutions of mesna ranging from 1:2 to 1:100 in a variety of carbonated drinks, fruit juice and milk which were stored at 4°C, exhibited no clinically significant change in drug concentration.[5])

3.3 Stability in specialized delivery systems

Ifosfamide in combination with mesna (each 50 mg/ml) was stable for 24 hours at 37°C in Graseby 9000 Medication devices.[4]

4 Clinical use

Dosage: This is dependent on the dose and dosing schedule of ifosfamide or cyclophosphamide. The Data Sheet[1] should be consulted for detailed information to determine mesna dose and schedule in each case. Special schedules apply, for example, to children and patients receiving pelvic irradiation. Details of oral use of mesna injection are also described. Mesna is also available in oral form as tablets containing 400 or 600 mg mesna as the sodium salt.

5 Preparation of injection

Dilution: Use undiluted for bolus administration. Add to oxazaphosphorine infusion for 24 hour infusion regimens. For oral administration, mesna should be taken in a soft drink immediately after opening the ampoule.

Bolus administration: Mesna is given over 15 minutes as 20% of the oxazaphosphorine dose and is repeated after four and eight hours.

Intravenous infusion: Mesna is given as a concurrent infusion. Initially 20% of the oxazaphosphorine dose is given by intravenous bolus injection, followed by the oxazaphosphorine dose over 24 hours. A further infusion of 60% w/w of the oxazaphosphorine dose is then given over 12 hours.

Extravasation: Non-irritant.

6 Destruction of drug or contaminated articles

Mesna is not cytotoxic.

References

1 *ABPI Data Sheet Compendium 1995–96* (1995) DataPharm Publications Ltd, London, pp. 108–11.
2 Trissel LA *et al.* (1985) *Investigational drugs pharmaceutical data.* NCI, Bethesda, Maryland, USA.
3 Adams PS *et al.* (1987) Pharmaceutical aspects of home infusion therapy for cancer patients. *Pharm. J.* **238**, 476–8.
4 Sewell GJ *et al.* (1994) Stability of drug infusions in ambulatory infusion devices. *Aust. J. Hosp. Pharm.* **24**, 102–10.
5 Goren MP *et al.* (1991) The stability of mesna in beverages and syrup for oral administration. *Cancer Chemother. Pharmacol.* **28**, 298–301.

Prepared by Graham Sewell

ONDANSETRON

1 General details

Approved name: Ondansetron hydrochloride.

Proprietary name: Zofran.

Manufacturer or supplier: GlaxoWellcome.

Presentation and formulation details: Zofran injection is a clear, colourless, sterile solution. Each 1 ml of aqueous solution contains 2 mg ondansetron as the hydrochloride dihydrate. Ondansetron injection is available in glass or plastic ampoules and as a pre-filled syringe. Glass or plastic ampoules contain ondansetron 4 mg in 2 ml or 8 mg in 4 ml. Pre-filled syringe contains ondansetron 4 mg in 2 ml.[1]

Storage and shelf-life of unopened container: Ondansetron ampoules, either glass or plastic presentations, have a shelf-life of three years. Odansetron pre-filled syringe has a shelf-life of two years. Ondansetron injection should be protected from light and stored below 30°C.[2]

2 Chemistry

Chemical name: 1,2,3,9-tetrahydro-9-methyl 3-[(2-methylimidazole-1yl) methyl] carbazol-4-one, hydrochloride dihydrate.[3]

Physical form: White crystalline powder.

Molecular structure:

Molecular formula: $C_{18}H_{19}N_3O.HCl.2H_2O$.

Molecular weight: 365.8.

3 Stability profile

3.1 Stability in clinical practice

Ondansetron injection should not be administered in the same syringe or infusion as any other medication.

Compatibility with intravenous fluids: Ondansetron injection should only be admixed with those infusion solutions which are recommended.[2] Ondansetron injection has been shown to be stable for seven days at room temperature (below 25°C) under fluorescent lighting, or in a refrigerator, with the following intravenous infusion fluids:

▼ 0.9% sodium chloride

▼ 5% glucose
▼ 10% mannitol
▼ Ringer's
▼ 0.3% potassium chloride and 0.9% sodium chloride
▼ 0.3% potassium chloride and 5% glucose.

Compatibility studies have been undertaken in polyvinyl chloride infusion bags and polyvinyl chloride administration sets. It is considered that adequate stability would also be conferred by the use of polyethylene infusion bags or Type 1 glass bottles.[4]

Dilution of ondansetron in 0.9% sodium chloride or in 5% glucose has been demonstrated to be stable in polypropylene syringes. It is considered that ondansetron injection diluted with other compatible infusion fluids would be stable in polypropylene syringes.[4]

Compatibility with other drugs:[1-5] Ondansetron may be administered by intravenous infusion at 1 mg/hr, e.g. from an infusion bag or syringe pump. The following drugs may be administered via the Y-site of the ondansetron giving set for ondansetron concentrations of 16–160 µg/ml (e.g. 8 mg/500 ml and 8 mg/50 ml, respectively).

▼ *Cisplatin*: concentration up to 0.48 mg/ml (e.g. 240 mg/500 ml) administered over one to eight hours.
▼ *5-Fluorouracil*: concentrations up to 0.8 mg/ml (e.g. 2.4 g/3 l, or 400 mg/500 ml) administered at a rate of at least 20 ml per hour (500 ml per 24 hours). Higher concentrations of 5-fluorouracil may cause precipitation of ondansetron. The 5-fluorouracil infusion may contain up to 0.045% magnesium chloride, in addition to other excipients shown to be compatible.
▼ *Carboplatin*: concentrations in the range 0.18–9.9 mg/ml (e.g. 90 mg/500 ml to 990 mg/100 ml), administered over ten minutes, to one hour.
▼ *Etoposide*: concentrations in the range of 0.144–0.25 mg/ml (e.g. 72 mg/500 ml to 250 mg/1 l), administered over 30 minutes, to one hour.
▼ *Ceftazidime*: doses in the range 250–2000 mg, reconstituted with water for injections as recommended by the manufacturer (e.g. 2.5 ml for 250 mg and 10 ml for 2 g ceftazidime) and given as an intravenous bolus injection, over approximately five minutes.
▼ *Cyclophosphamide*: doses in the range 100 mg to 1 g, reconstituted with water for injections, 5 ml per 100 mg cyclophosphamide, as recommended by the manufacturer, and given as an intravenous bolus injection, over approximately five minutes.
▼ *Doxorubicin*: doses in the range 10–100 mg reconstituted with water for injections, 5 ml per 10 mg doxorubicin, as recommended by the manufacturer and given as an intravenous bolus injection, over approximately five minutes.
▼ *Dexamethasone*: dexamethasone sodium phosphate 20 mg may be administered as a sow intravenous injection over 2–5 minutes via the Y-site of an infusion set delivering 8 or 32 mg of ondansetron diluted in 50–100 ml of a compatible infusion fluid over approximately 15 minutes. Compatibility between dexamethasone sodium phosphate and ondansetron has been demonstrated, supporting administration of these drugs through the same giving set resulting in concentrations in line of 32 µg–2.5 mg/ml for dexamethasone sodium phosphate and 8 µg–1 mg/ml for ondansetron.

4 Clinical use

Main indications: Ondansetron tablets and injection are indicated for the management of nausea and vomiting induced by cytotoxic chemotherapy and radiotherapy. Ondansetron tablets and injection are also indicated for the prevention of post-operative nausea and vomiting.[1]

Dosage: For chemotherapy- and radiotherapy-induced nausea and vomiting.

▼ Adults: the emetogenic potential of cancer treatment varies according to the doses and combinations of chemotherapy and radiotherapy regimens used. Ondansetron is available for oral, parenteral and rectal use to allow the route of administration and dosing to be flexible.

▼ Emetogenic chemotherapy and radiotherapy:[6] for patients receiving emetogenic chemotherapy or radiotherapy, ondansetron can be given by rectal, oral (as tablets or syrup), or intravenous administration. The recommended oral dose is 8 mg one to two hours before treatment, followed by 8 mg orally, 12 hours later. The recommended intravenous dose of ondansetron is 8 mg administered as a slow intravenous injection immediately before treatment. To protect against delayed or prolonged emesis after the first 24 hours, oral or rectal treatment with ondansetron should be continued for up to five days after a course of treatment. The recommended oral dose is 8 mg to be taken twice daily.

▼ Highly emetogenic chemotherapy:[7] for patients receiving highly emetogenic chemotherapy, e.g. high dose cisplatin, ondansetron can be given either by intravenous or rectal administration.

When given intravenously, ondansetron may be administered as a single 8–32 mg intravenous dose immediately before chemotherapy. When administering doses of greater than 8 mg, ondansetron should be diluted in 50–100 ml of saline or other compatible infusion fluid and infused over not less than 15 minutes.

Alternatively a dose of 8 mg of ondansetron may be administered by slow intravenous injection immediately before chemotherapy, followed by two further intravenous doses of 8 mg two to four hours apart, or by a constant infusion of 1 mg/hr for up to 24 hours.

The selection of dose regimen should be determined by the severity of the emetogenic challenge.

The efficacy of ondansetron in highly emetogenic chemotherapy may be enhanced by the addition of a single intravenous dose of dexamethasone sodium phosphate, 20 mg administered prior to chemotherapy, or as 8 mg 15 minutes prior to chemotherapy, followed by 4 mg 6 hourly over the subsequent 24 hours.

To protect against delayed or prolonged emesis after the first 24 hours, oral or rectal treatment with ondansetron should be continued for up to five days after a course of treatment. The recommended oral dose is 8 mg to be taken twice daily.

▼ Children: in children ondansetron is administered as a single intravenous dose immediately before chemotherapy, followed by 4 mg orally twelve hours later. 4 mg orally twice daily should be continued for up to five days after a course of treatment.

▼ Patients with hepatic impairment: clearance of ondansetron is significantly reduced and serum half-life significantly prolonged in subjects with moderate or severe impairment of hepatic function. In such patients, a total daily dose of 8 mg should not be exceeded.

5 Preparation of injection

Ondansetron injection should not be administered in the same syringe or infusion as any other medication. Ondansetron should only be admixed with those infusion solutions which are recommended (*see* Stability profile).

Ondansetron injection can be used for intramuscular or intravenous administration; however doses in excess of 4 mg should not be administered intramuscularly.

When given intravenously, ondansetron may be administered as a single 8 mg intravenous dose. When administering greater than 8 mg ondansetron should be diluted in 50–100 ml of 0.9% sodium chloride or compatible infusion fluid (*see* Stability profile) and infused over not less than 15 minutes.

References

1 *ABPI Data Sheet Compendium 1995–96* (1996) DataPharm Publications Ltd, London, pp. 659–61.
2 GlaxoWellcome. Personal communication.
3 McKinnon JWM, Collin DT (1989) The chemistry of ondansetron. *Eur. J. Clin. Oncol.* **25** (Suppl. 1), 561.
4 Leak RF, Woodford JD (1989) Pharmaceutical development of ondansetron injection. *Eur. J. Cancer Clin. Oncol.* **25** (Suppl. 1) 576–69.
5 Trissel LA (1994) *Handbook on Injectable Drugs*, 8th edn. American Society of Hospital Pharmacists, Betheda, Maryland, USA, pp. 794–800.
6 Dicato MA *et al.* (1992) Efficacy of twice daily versus three times daily oral ondansetron in the prevention of chemotherapy induced emesis: a randomised single blind multicentre study. *Clin. Oncol.* **4**, 275–9.
7 Seynaeve C *et al.* (1992) Comparison of the anti-emetic efficacy of different doses of ondansetron given as either a continuous infusion or a single intravenous dose, in acute cisplatin-induced emesis. A multicentre, double-blind randomised parallel group study. *Br. J. Cancer* **66**, 192–7.

Prepared by Andrew Stanley

This section provides and identifies suitable sources of essential basic information on unlicensed cytotoxic agents known to be of current clinical interest. The interferons, interleukins and related biologically-derived compounds, now all known generically as cytokines, have been intentionally excluded since they do not present to pharmacy staff the same problems of handling as do more conventional cytotoxic agents.

Much of the content draws heavily on information provided by the National Cancer Institute (NCI) of the National Institute of Health of the US. Copies of two books, *NCI investigational drugs: pharmaceutical data* and *Investigational drugs: chemical data*, which are updated annually, may be obtained by post, free of charge from:

Pharmaceutical Resources Branch
National Cancer Institute
Executive Plaza North
Suite 818
Bethesda, Maryland 20892
USA.

More comprehensive information may also be available from the NCI in clinical brochures for individual drugs, or via the Internet NCI pharmaceutical database, or from investigators currently working with the compounds concerned.

Other useful sources of information regarding drugs in trials are:

EORTC
New Drug Development Office
Free University Hospital
PO Box 7057
1007 MB Amsterdam
The Netherlands

Telephone: + 31 (20) 444 2795
Fax: + 31 (20) 444 2767

CRC Phase I/II Clinical Trials Committee Formulations Unit
Department of Pharmaceutical Science
University of Strathclyde
204 George Street
Glasgow
G1 1XW

Telephone: 0141 552 4400 Ext. 2454
Fax: 0141 552 6443

DOXORUBICIN LIPOSOMAL

1 General details

Approved names: Liposomal doxorubicin hydrochloride, Doxil.

Proprietary name: Dox-SL.

Manufacturer or supplier: Sequus Pharmaceuticals Inc. (formerly Liposome Technology Inc.).

Presentation and formulation details: Liposomal doxorubicin is provided as a sterile translucent, red suspension in 10 ml glass vials.[1,2] Each vial contains 20 mg doxorubicin hydrochloride at a concentration of 2 mg/ml.[2] The lipid carrier is fully hydrogenated soy-phosphatidyl-choline (HSPC) cholesterol and methoxy-polyethylene glycol carbamate of distearoyl phosphatidylethanolamine (MPEG-DSPE).[1,2] Other ingredients are sucrose, ammonium sulphate and histidine.[2] The main particle size is approximately 100 nm, with more than 90% of the drug encapsulated in liposomes. Dox-SL is buffered to pH 6.5.

Storage and shelf-life of unopened container: Stored at between 2–8°C. Stability studies are in progress.

2 Chemistry

Type: Cytotoxic anthracycline antibiotic.

Molecular structure: As for doxorubicin, but encapsulated in liposomes coated with biocompatible polyethylene glycol polymer. The entrapment of doxorubicin in the liposome bilayer is significantly enhanced by the presence of negatively charged phospholipids, such as egg-derived phosphatidylglycerol (PG). Initial studies were carried out with a 'first generation' liposome carrier of short circulation time (L-DOX). The currently-used liposome carrier is a 'second generation' liposome of longer circulation time.[3]

Molecular formula: See doxorubicin monograph, page 241.

Molecular weight: 580.0.

3 Stability profile

3.1 Physical and chemical stability

DOX-SL is supplied as a 'liquid'. The dose required is normally diluted before use in 5% glucose infusion. 0.9% sodium chloride is also permissible.

4 Clinical use

Rationale: Liposomes are microscopic vesicles made of phospholipids, identical to those found in cell membranes. Liposomes are non-toxic and can safely transport their load through the vascular compartments without dilution or degradation. When the liposomes reach diseased tissues, they deliver concentrated doses of medication. Doxorubicin encapsulated in liposomes coated with biocompatible polymers has been shown in animal models to be less toxic and to distribute more selectively to tumours, when compared with the same dose of conventional doxorubicin. These liposomes are also claimed to evade rapid detection and uptake by cells of the reticuloendothelial system, unlike conventional liposomes that are rapidly cleared from the bloodstream. The treatment rationale for the use of liposome-encapsulated doxorubicin is to improve tumour deposition of the drug, thereby improving the disease response rate in solid cancers.[3,4]

5 Preparation of injection

Intravenous infusion: Dilute the required dose with 250 ml 5% glucose and infuse over 30 minutes. Do not administer as a bolus injection. Do not mix with other drugs.

Extravasation: Reported to be less serious than with conventional doxorubicin in animal models.

6 Destruction of drug or contaminated articles

If the raw material is spilled, contain the spill with an absorbent and deactivate with 1% w/v sodium hypochlorite solution, until colourless. Dispose of waste in accordance with local regulations.[2]

Contact with skin: If doxorubicin liposomal comes into contact with skin or mucosa wash immediately and thoroughly with soap and water.

References

1 Alpar O (1989) Liposomes as drug carriers. *Pharm. J.* **243**, 254–355.
2 Liposome Technology Inc. (1991) Personal communication.
3 Stealth liposomal doxorubicin hydrochloride injection (S-Dox). Liposome Technology Inc. *Clinical Study Protocol*, April 1991.
4 Gabison A *et al.* (1994) Clinical studies of liposome-encapsulated anthracyclines. *Acta Oncol.* **7**, 779–86.

Prepared by Yaacov Cass

FLOXURIDINE

1 General details

Approved name: Floxuridine.

Proprietary names: FUDR, fluorodeoxyuridine, 2-deoxy-5-fluorouridine.

Manufacturer or supplier: Hoffman La Roche.

Presentation and formulation details: White powder in vials containing 500 mg floxuridine.

Storage and shelf-life of unopened containers: Three years stored at 15–30°C.

2 Chemistry

Type: Nucleoside consisting of the pyrimidine base fluorouracil and the sugar deoxyribose.

Molecular structure: 5-fluoro 2'-deoxyuridine 5'-phosphate (FUDR monophosphate).

Molecular weight: 246.2.

3 Stability profile

3.1 Physical and chemical stability

The manufacturer indicates that floxuridine is soluble in water and that it is relatively stable in aqueous solutions. After reconstitution the solution has a pH of 4.0–5.5. The pH for optimum stability is pH 4 and 7.[1]

Floxuridine, diluted in 0.9% sodium chloride or 5% glucose, to a concentration of 0.5 mg/ml, and stored in glass or PVC containers, is stable for seven days at 20°C. Diluted solutions containing 5 or 10 mg/ml floxuridine in 0.9% sodium chloride, 5% glucose or water of injections are stable (<10% loss) for 14 days at 20°C. Storage at 2–8°C is likely to exhibit similar stability.[1,2]

Floxuridine at concentrations of 2.5–12.5 mg/ml in sodium chloride was shown to be stable for up to 12 days stored in the reservoir of the Infusoid Model 400 pump.[3]

Compatibility with other drugs: Floxuridine has been shown to be compatible with cisplatin, etoposide, fluorouracil, fludarabine, heparin, leucovorin, calcium, ondansetron, paclitaxel, vinorelbine and sargomostin.[2]

4 Clinical use

Type: Anti-metabolite, metabolized to fluorouracil after administration.

Main indications: It is primarily used intro-arterially to treat hepatic metastases from colorectal or gastrointestinal carcinoma.[1]

Dosage: The usual dosage of floxuridine by continuous infusion is 0.1–0.6 mg/kg daily. Higher dosages (0.4–0.6 mg/kg daily) are usually used for hepatic artery infusion, since the liver metabolizes the drugs and thus reduces the risk of systemic toxicity.[1]

Floxuridine has been administered intravenously in the treatment of solid tumours. A dose of 0.5–1 mg/kg for 6–15 days, or until toxicity occurs, has been used. By single intravenous injection the usual dosage is 30 mg/kg daily for five days, followed by 15 mg/kg every other day for up to 11 days, or until toxicity occurs.[1]

5 Preparation of injection

Reconstitution: Floxuridine should be reconstituted with 5 ml of water for injections to provide a solution containing 100 mg/ml, reconstituted vials are stable for two weeks at 2–8°C.[1,2]

The desired dose is diluted in 0.9% sodium chloride or 5% glucose in the required volume.

Extravasation: Non-irritant.

6 Destruction of drug or contaminated articles

Incineration: No specific information available.

Chemical: No specific information available.

Contact with skin: No specific information available.

References

1 *Drug Information* (1995) American Hospital Formulary Service, American Society of Hospital Pharmacists, Bethesda, USA.
2 Trissel LA (1994) *Handbok of Injectable Drugs*, 8th edn. American Society of Hospital Pharmacists, Bethesda, Maryland, USA.
3 Keller JH and Ensminger WD (1982) Stability of cancer chemotherapeutic agents in a totally implanted drug delivery system. *Am. J. Hosp. Pharm.* **39**, 1321–3.

Prepared by Yaacov Cass

IRINOTECAN

1 General details

Approved names: Irinotecan, camptothecin 11.

Proprietary name: Campto.

Manufacturer or supplier: Rhône-Poulenc Rorer (France).

Presentation and formulation details: Irinotecan is supplied as a powder in 2 ml and 5 ml vials, containing 80 mg and 200 mg, respectively.[1]

Storage and shelf-life of unopened container: The unopened vials should be stored at room temperature (15–25°C) and are stable for 18 months.

2 Chemistry

Type: Synthetic derivative of camptothecin, a plant alkaloid obtained from the Chinese tree *Camptotheca acuminata*.[2]

Molecular structure: 7-ethyl-10 [4-(1-piperidino)-1-piperidino] carbonyloxycamptothecin.

Molecular formula: $C_{31}H_{36}O_6N_4$.

Molecular weight: 677.2.

3 Stability profile

3.1 Physical and chemical stability

A pale yellow, crystalline powder, freely soluble in glacial acetic acid, but only slightly soluble in water (3 g per 100 ml). The pH of an aqueous solution (2% w/v) is 3.5–4.5.[1]

Irinotecan reconstituted and diluted in 0.9% sodium chloride or 5% glucose is stable (less than 10% loss) for two hours at room temperature (15–25°C) for four days at 2–8°C. Infusions containing irinotecan are compatible with PVC infusion containers, with no evidence of extraction of plasticizers during four days storage at 4–8°C.[1,3]

4 Clinical use

Type: DNA topoisomerase-1-inhibitor.

Main indications: Irinotecan is indicated in second-line treatment of metastatic colorectal cancer, following the failure of primary chemotherapy. The recommended initial dose is 350 mg/m^2 administered as an intravenous infusion over not less than 30 minutes. This dose should be administered at three week intervals.[1]

If the patient experiences severe asymptomatic neutropenia (neutrophil count <500/mm^3), or febrile neutropenia (temperature 38°C and neutrophil count 1000/mm^3) the dose to be administered during later courses should be reduced to 300 mg/m^2.[1,3]

5 Preparation of injection

Reconstitution: Irinotecan should be reconstituted in water for injections. Add the appropriate volume (2 ml or 5 ml, respectively) to the vial and shake to dissolve, to give a solution containing 40 mg irinotecan per ml.[1]

Dilution: The reconstituted dilution should be added to 250 ml 0.9% sodium chloride or 5% glucose.

Administration: Infuse into a peripheral or central vein over not less than 30 minutes.[1]

Extravasation: Non-irritant.

6 Destruction of drug or contaminated articles

Incineration: No specific information available.

Chemical: No specific information available.

Contact with skin: Wash immediately with soap and water. If undiluted solution should come into contact with mucous membrane, rinse immediately with copious water.

References

1 *Campto. Brochure for Hospital Pharmacists* (1995) Rhone-Poulenc Rorer, France.
2 *Campto. Colorectal Cancer at the eve of the 21st century and the first specific topoisomerase inhibitor* (1995) Rhone-Poulenc Rorer, France.
3 Irinotecan. *Drug Evaluation Monographs 1994–95* (1995) Micromedex Inc., 84.

Prepared by Yaacov Cass

STREPTOZOCIN

1 General details

Approved name: Streptozocin.

Proprietary name: Zanosar.

Manufacturer or supplier: In the UK, supplied on a 'named patient' basis through IDIS Ltd.

Presentation and formulation details: Pale yellow, freeze-dried powder containing 1 g streptozocin. Contains sodium hydroxide to adjust pH. Each vial also contains 220 mg citric acid. Contains no preservatives.

Storage and shelf-life of unopened container: Store at 2–8°C, protected from light.

2 Chemistry

Type: Nitrosourea.

Molecular structure: 2-deoxy-2-(methyl-nitrosoamino)carbonylamino-β-D-gluco-pyranose.

Molecular weight: 265.2.

Solubility: Soluble in water, 0.9% sodium chloride and ethanol.

3 Stability profile

3.1 Physical and chemical stability

Effect of temperature: Streptozocin was reconstituted in 1 l of 20% glucose. The final concentration of the solution was 1 mg/ml. The study indicated less than 10% degradation after 72 hours at both 5°C and 22–24°C.[1]

The injection was stable for more than 60 hours at 4 and 25°C when reconstituted with water for injection or 0.9% sodium chloride.[1]

1 g vials were reconstituted with 9.5 ml of 0.9% sodium chloride irrigation, 20% glucose, and deionized water. The vials were stored at 3 and 24°C. pH fell slightly after 48 hours at 24°C, consistent with initial degradation of streptozocin. All solutions were clear, pale yellow at reconstitution and no colour changes were discernible over 48 hours. No particulates or cloudiness was observed in the vials.[1]

Effect of light: A significant loss of potency was observed after 340 days and 740 days of exposure to light.[1]

The freeze-dried product, when stored under conditions of minimal light exposure, did not show significant potency reduction.[1]

Compatibility: Streptozocin may be reconstituted in water for injections, 0.9% sodium chloride or 5% glucose.[2]

Container compatibility: Vials containing 1 g of streptozocin were reconstituted with 9.5 ml of 5% glucose or 0.9% sodium chloride. Aliquots of 10 ml were transferred to 1 l plastic IV bags (Abbott). Samples were assayed for DEHP over a 48 hour period. No leeching of DEHP from the plastic into the streptozocin solution was observed.[1]

4 Clinical use

Main indications: Metastatic islet cell tumours of the pancreas.

5 Preparation of injection

Reconstitution: Reconstitute each 1 g vial with 9.5 ml of diluent, to yield a solution containing 100 mg/ml streptozocin.[2]

Intravenous infusion: In 250–500 ml 0.9% sodium chloride or 5% glucose; over 30–60 minutes. Bolus not recommended because it is extremely uncomfortable for the patient.[2]

Extravasation: The drug solution is vesicant. No specific recommendations for management (*see* Chapter 6).

6 Destruction of drug or contaminated articles

Incineration: No specific information.

Chemical: No specific information.

Contact with the skin: No specific information.

7 Centres with a known interest in this drug

▼ The Royal Marsden Hospital, London.
▼ Hammersmith Hospital, London.

References

1 Upjohn (UK) Ltd (1990) Personal communication.
2 Zanosar Data Sheet.

Prepared by Tim Root

TENIPOSIDE

1 General details

Approved names: Teniposide, VM26, PTG, thenylidene-ligan-P.

Proprietary name: Vumon.

Manufacturer or supplier: Bristol-Myers Squibb, Clinical Cancer Research Department, Bristol-Myers Squibb, UK.

Presentation and formulation details: 5 ml ampoules containing a solution of teniposide 10 mg/ml. Each 5 ml also contains benzyl alcohol 150 mg, N,N-dimethylacetamide 300 mg, polyoxyetholated castor oil 2.5 g, absolute alcohol 4.7 g and maleic acid to adjust pH.[1,2]

Storage and shelf-life of unopened containers: Store at room temperature, protected from light. The stability of the contents of the ampoules appears unaffected by exposure to light or by freezing.[3]

2 Chemistry

Type: Podophyllotoxin derivative.

Molecular structure: Epipodophyllotoxin, 4-demethyl-9-(4,6-o-2-thenylidene-β-D-glucopyranoside).

Molecular weight: 656.

3 Stability profile

Teniposide exhibits physical instability in aqueous solutions in varying periods of time depending on concentration, solution, and container type. The manufacturer recommends the following utility times for dilutions of the drug stored at either 4 or 25°C.

Infusion solution	Container type	Teniposide concentration (µg/ml)	Use within (hr)
0.9% sodium chloride	Glass	100	24
	Glass	400	24
	Plastic	100	8
5% glucose	Glass	100	24
	Glass	200	24
Water for injections	Glass	100	24
	Glass	200	24
	Plastic	100	8

More recent work from Amsterdam suggests that at a concentration of 0.4 mg/ml in 5% glucose or 0.9% sodium chloride in both glass and PVC infusion containers, teniposide is physically and chemically stable for at least four days at room temperature. Even at the lowest recommended concentrations of 0.1 and 0.2 mg/ml precipitation of teniposide from aqueous solution may occur unpredictably. Precipitation may be initiated by several factors including excessive agitation and contact with incompatible substances or surfaces.[3]

3.1 Stability in clinical practice

Once diluted for infusion, solutions should be stored at room temperature. Because of the unpredictability of the risk of precipitation, solutions should be used as soon as possible and certainly within 24 hours of preparation. Solutions of 1 mg/ml should be used within four hours.[3] Solutions showing visible evidence of precipitation should be discarded.

As with some other surfactant-containing preparations, contact between the concentrate and plastic disposables has been observed to result in softening, cracking and leakage. Variable degrees of leaching of plasticizers from PVC infusion containers of both 5% glucose and 0.9% sodium chloride solutions have been observed and appear to be dependent on several factors including time, concentration and size of container.[3–5] From this point of view the use of non-PVC infusion containers may be preferable.

4 Clinical use

Main indications: Treatment of acute leukaemia.

5 Preparation of injection

Reconstitution: Dilute with the desired volume of 5% glucose or 0.9% sodium chloride solution to a concentration between 0.1 and 1 mg/ml. Avoid violent agitation during mixing.

Administration: By slow intravenous infusion over at least 30–60 minutes.

Extravasation: Vesicant. Avoid extravasation. No specific management recommended (*see* Chapter 6).

6 Destruction of drug or contaminated articles

Incineration: No specific information available.

Chemical: No specific information available.

Contact with skin: No specific information available.

References

1 *NCI Investigational Drugs* (1990) Pharmaceutical Data, National Cancer Institute, Bethesda, Maryland, USA.
2 Beijnen JH *et al.* (1991) Chemical and physical stability of etoposide and teniposide in commonly used infusion fluids. *J. Parenter. Sci. Technol.* **45**, 108–12.
3 Trissel LA (1994) *Handbook of Injectable Drugs*, 8th edn. American Society of Hospital Pharmacists, Bethesda, Maryland, USA.
4 Pearson SD, Trissel LA (1993) Leaching of diethylhexyl phthalate from polyvinyl chloride containers by selected drugs and formulation components. *Am. J. Hosp. Pharm.* **50**, 1405–9.
5 Faouzi MA *et al.* (1994) Leaching of diethylhexyl phthalate from PVC bags into intravenous teniposide solution. *Int. J. Pharmac.* **105**, 89–93.

Prepared by Tim Root

TOPOTECAN

1 General details

Approved names: Topotecan, hycamptamine, SKF 104864-A, NSC-609699.

Proprietary name: Hycamptin.

Manufacturer or supplier: SmithKline Beecham.

Presentation and formulation details: Vials of pale yellow, lyophilized powder containing topotecan as hydrochloride 5 mg, manitol 65 mg, tartaric acid 75 mg.

Storage: Store at room temperature.

2 Chemistry

Type: Topoisomerase I inhibitor, water soluble derivative of the alkaloid, camptothecin.

Molecular structure: (S)-10-[(dimethylamino)methyl]-4-ethyl-4,9-dihydroxy-1H-pyrano[3′,4′:6,7]indolizino[1,2-b]-quinoline-3,14-(4H,12H)-dione.

Molecular formula: $C_{23}H_{23}N_3O_5$.

Molecular weight: 421.45.

3 Stability profile

3.1 Physical and chemical stability

Data on stability and compatibility of topotecan with diluents and other drugs are limited. Solutions containing 10, 20 and 500 μg/ml in 0.9% sodium chloride and 10 and 500 μg/ml in 5% glucose exhibit less than 3% loss when stored for up to four days (10 and 500 μg/ml solutions) or three days (longest period tested), in the case of 20 μg/ml solutions, at room temperature in Viaflex (Baxter Healthcare) PVC infusion bags.[1] Similar data have been presented in a report stating that dilutions of topotecan containing 20 and 100 μg/ml in 5% glucose or 0.9% sodium chloride in PVC exhibit no loss of activity during 48 hours of storage at room temperature.[2]

Topotecan is compatible with 0.9% benzyl alcohol. This has been used as a preservative in CADD-1 infusion pump reservoirs containing a dose of 4.2 mg/m² topotecan in 40 ml water, for delivery over a seven day period.[1]

4 Clinical use

Type: Inhibitor of the enzyme topoisomerase I which facilitates DNA replication by making reversible breaks in DNA permitting torsional relaxation of the molecule during transcription.[3]

Main indications: Topotecan is under investigation in a variety of malignant conditions including cancers of the lung,[4-6] bowel,[7] ovary[8] and breast.[9] It seems most likely that the first product licences for topotecan granted during the life of this edition will be for ovarian and/or lung cancers.

Dose: A range of intravenous dosage schedules are under investigation. Because the activity of topotecan appears to be schedule dependent, these generally utilize repeated daily dosing (1.25–2 mg/m²/day for five days in every 21[4-6,8,9]) or prolonged intravenous infusion (0.6 mg/m²/day for 21 days in 28[7]).

5 Preparation of injection

Reconstitution: Each 5 mg vial of powder should be dissolved in 5 ml water.

Dilution: The appropriate quantity of reconstituted injection solution should be further diluted in an appropriate volume of 5% glucose or 0.9% sodium chloride prior to infusion.

Bolus administration: Not recommended.

Extravasation: No specific information.

6 Destruction of drug or contaminated articles

No special instructions.

References

1 Data on File, SmithKline Beecham.
2 Anon. (1988, 1990) *NCI investigational drugs pharmaceutical data.* National Cancer Institute, Bethesda, Maryland.
3 Anon. (1995) Topoisomerase I inhibitors: a novel class of antineoplastic drugs. *Drugs Ther. Perspect.* **5**, 7–9.
4 Perez-Soler R *et al.* (1995) Phase II study of topotecan in patients with squamous cell carcinoma of the lung previously untreated with chemotherapy. *Eur. J. Cancer* **31A** (Suppl. 5), S224.
5 Perez-Soler R *et al.* (1995) Phase II study of topotecan in patients with small cell lung cancer (SCLC) refractory to etoposide. *Proc. Am. Soc. Clin. Oncol.* **14**, 355.
6 Hutson PR *et al.* (1995) Pharmacodynamic evaluation of the response of extensive stage small cell lung cancer to topotecan. *Proc. Am. Soc. Clin. Oncol.* **14**, 460.
7 Creemer GJ *et al.* (1995) Phase II study with topotecan (T) administered as a 21-day continuous infusion to patients with colorectal cancer. *Eur. J. Cancer* **31A** (Suppl. 5), S146.

8 Armstrong D *et al.* (1995) A phase II trial of topotecan as salvage therapy in epithelial ovarian cancer. *Proc. Am. Soc. Clin. Oncol.* **14**, 275.

9 Chang AY *et al.* (1995) Clinical and laboratory studies of topotecan in breast cancer. *Proc. Am. Soc. Clin. Oncol.* **14**, 105.

Prepared by Max Summerhayes

TRIMETREXATE

1 General details

Approved name: Trimetrexate.

Proprietary names: TMTX, NSC-352122.

Manufacturer or supplier: Warner-Lambert.

Presentation and formulation details: Trimetrexate is supplied as a pale greenish yellow-to-tan coloured, lyophilized powder for injection. The powder is freeze-dried with glucuronic acid to form the glucuronate salt. The powder plug is presented in a 6 ml flint glass vial, each vial containing 25 mg of trimetrexate.

Storage and shelf-life of unopened containers: The unopened vials should be stored at room temperature (15–25°C). Unopened vials are stable for two years.

2 Chemistry

Type: Anti-metabolite, a folate antagonist, related to methotrexate.

Molecular structure: 6-([[(3,4,5-trimethoxyphenyl)amino]methyl)-5-methyl-2,4-quinazolinediamine-D-glucuronic acid.

Molecular formula: $C_{19}H_{23}N_5O_3(C_6H_{10}O_7)$.
Molecular weight: 564.0.

3 Stability profile

3.1 Physical and chemical stability

The pH of the reconstituted solution is 3.5–5.5. Trimetrexate may develop a precipitate in solutions above pH 5. Trimetrexate is incompatible with 0.9% sodium chloride injection and other chloride-containing solutions.[1]

4 Clinical use

Main indications: Trimetrexate has been tried in phase II studies in a wide variety of tumours. However, principal interest remains in colorectal, lung and breast cancers.[1]

5 Preparation of injection

Reconstitution: Trimetrexate should only be reconstituted with water for injections. 2 ml are added to each vial to give a final solution containing 12.5 mg/ml trimetrexate.[1]

Dilution: Trimetrexate can be further diluted in 5% glucose. It should never be added to chloride-containing solutions.[1]

Administration: Intravenous bolus or by slow intravenous infusion.

Extravasation: Irritant and vesicant.

6 Destruction of drug or contaminated articles

Incineration: No specific information available.

Chemical: No specific information available. However, the addition of alkali or chloride-containing solution should inactivate the trimetrexate.

Contact with skin: No specific instructions available, wash area with copious amounts of water and/or 0.9% sodium chloride.

Reference

1 NCI Investigational Drugs – Pharmaceutical Data (1994).

Prepared by Andrew Stanley